Anatomy of the Living Human

Atlas of Medical Imaging

ANDRÁS CSILLAG

Anatomy of the Living Human

Atlas of Medical Imaging

KÖNEMANN

András Csillag

Department of Anatomy, Histology and Embryology,
Semmelweis University of Medicine, Budapest, Hungary

Contributors

Kinga Karlinger and Erika Márton

Department of Radiology and Oncotherapy,
Semmelweis University of Medicine, Budapest, Hungary

With the advice and expertise of

Adrian K. Dixon

Professor and Head, Department of Radiology, University of Cambridge,
Addenbrooke's Hospital, Cambridge, UK

and

Miklós Réthelyi

Professor and Head, Department of Anatomy, Histology and Embryology,
Semmelweis University of Medicine, Budapest, Hungary

© 1999 Könemann Verlagsgesellschaft mbH
Bonner Str. 126, D-50968 Köln

Project editor: Vince Books, Budapest
Editor: Péter Teravagimov
Drawings: Csaba Piller
Water paintings: János Kálmánfi
Design: Almagro Bt., Budapest
Desktop publishing: Gabriella Haász, Róbert Balázs Piri

Printing and binding: Amilcare Pizzi, Milan
Printed in Italy

ISBN 3-8290-4264-7
10 9 8 7 6 5 4 3 2 1

To the unfading memory of the eminent Hungarian neuroscientist and devoted teacher of anatomy, János Szentágothai.

Contents

Authors' Preface

With the advent and development of modern diagnostic imaging techniques, there is an increasing need for students to have a sound anatomical background in keeping with the level of definition these imaging techniques provide. The last few years have seen continual progress in medical imaging, both in terms of technology and in imaging expertise. The amount of detail and the degree of structural definition that can be obtained using the latest equipment allow the interior of the human body to be visualized with remarkable anatomical precision. Studies no more than a few years old may have already been rendered obsolete.

Previous anatomical imaging manuals have aimed to facilitate evaluation of clinically relevant structures and pathological alterations. In a sense, anatomy served clinical radiology. Now, it is increasingly feasible to use imaging techniques to obtain a better understanding of anatomical relationships themselves. The study of cross-sectional anatomy has long been an integral part of anatomical education. However, its impact may be greatly enhanced when it is linked to a study of real clinical cases.

The majority of the material in this book covers conventional X-ray imaging and more advanced techniques such as computed X-ray tomography (CT), magnetic resonance imaging (MR) and ultrasonography. CT is the method of choice for a large number of diagnostic examinations, particularly in body cavities (thorax, abdomen, pelvis). It is now in routine use in diagnostic departments worldwide. Advances in CT technology mean that CT units have improved almost beyond

recognition. Not only does this mean improved quality of X-ray images but also an impressive range of off-line image processing and archiving facilities. MR is particularly recommended for examination of the cranial cavity and the brain and has numerous other applications. Images have a high degree of anatomical precision – like those of CT. MR is still rather costly and less widely used than CT; but its use is rapidly spreading worldwide. Ultrasonography is the least expensive and most readily accessible imaging technology. In most cases, however, ultrasound images do not have quite the same level of anatomical precision as can be achieved with other modalities. Even so, the frequent application of the method and rapid advances in image quality justify inclusion of representative samples here.

The use of both conventional X-ray studies and more advanced techniques such as CT or MR can be complemented by injection of contrast material, e.g. for demonstration of blood vessels (angiography), bile ducts (cholangiography) or kidney structures (urography). Contrast-enhanced images are highly informative, showing anatomical relationships and branching patterns that would be difficult to identify otherwise, even on careful cadaver dissection. Frequently, pathological alterations can highlight morphological details that normally blend into the surrounding tissue. For example, the presence of a pathological exsudate in the abdominal cavity (ascites) allows the borders of the notoriously complex peritoneal pockets and folds, which are hardly visible under normal circumstances, to be seen with remarkable clarity.

In addition to material from conventional X-ray, CT, MR and ultrasonography, the book also contains images obtained using the most up-to-date methods in nuclear medicine such as single photon emission tomography (SPECT) and positron emission tomography (PET). These techniques enable the visualization of events occurring at the molecular level with an imaging window in the nanosecond range. PET, for example, is now capable of localizing the brain centres that are active at the time an image is taken, allowing us almost to 'read a person's thoughts' in a way.

This Atlas of Medical Imaging has a dual purpose. First, it is intended to help graduate students of medicine understand the three-dimensional position of structures within the human body, thus complementing their studies of systematic (descriptive) and topographical anatomy. Anatomical details can be seen as they are to be found in living patients. Second, it is intended as an aid to medical students, young medical graduates and medical practitioners in evaluating diagnostic images obtained using the latest in imaging techniques.

Although the book covers the entire human body, including the extremities and body cavities, a fully-comprehensive description of the body was not our aim. By no means should the Atlas be used as a substitute for descriptive or systematic anatomy books. On the contrary, we should note there are certain limitations to those parts of the anatomy that can be identified in diagnostic images. For example, some very large nerves (spinal nerves, sciatic nerve) and cranial nerves can be seen with some of the methods discussed here, but most peripheral nerves are either invisible or poorly discernible using the methods in this book.

To assist the reader, the original diagnostic images have been paired with matching colour drawings showing exactly what can be seen. The various diagnostic modalities are distinguished by the background colour.

We should like to thank the reviewers of the book, Adrian K. Dixon, Professor and Head of Radiology, University of Cambridge, UK, and Miklós Réthelyi, Professor and Head of the Department of Anatomy, Histology and Embryology, Semmelweis University of Medicine, Budapest, Hungary, for their painstaking and conscientious work.

The bulk of the conventional X-ray, CT and SPECT material was obtained from the diagnostic units in the Department of Radiology and Oncotherapy, Semmelweis University of Medicine, Budapest. We should like to thank our colleagues in the Department for their invaluable help, in particular Ernő Makó, Professor and Head, Ádám Mester, Senior Lecturer, Anikó Tőkés and Andrea Maléta, radiographers. We should also like to express our gratitude to the following colleagues in other departments and institutions: The International Medical Centre, Budapest, in particular Péter Bazsó, Director, Richárd Asbóth, Senior Consultant, and Viktor Rohonczy, radiographer, for kindly providing MR images and echocardiograms; Senior Consultant Ferenc Molnár, Angiology Laboratory, Haynal Imre University of Health Sciences, Budapest, for angiocardiograms and valuable discussions concerning this part of the work; Senior Consultant László Szentpéteri, Central Hospital of the Ministry of the Interior, Budapest, for kindly donating angiograms of the limbs, abdomen and pelvis and László Bodrogi, Senior Lecturer, Department of Neurology, Semmelweis University of Medicine, Budapest, for cerebral angiograms; Senior Consultant György Székely, Szent János Hospital, Budapest, and György Harmat, Director-in-Chief, Madarász Children's Hospital, Budapest, for ultrasonograms; Kornélia L. Szluha, Department of Radiology, University Medical School, Debrecen, for lymphangiograms; Senior Lecturer Levente Pataky, Department of Oral Surgery and Dentistry, Semmelweis University of Medicine, Budapest, for dental tomograms; Senior Consultant László Bohár, Kerepestarcsa Hospital, Hungary, for MR images of the shoulder region; Professor Balázs Gulyás, Department of Neuroscience, Karolinska Insitute, Stockholm, Sweden, for MR based brain maps in relation to PET activation. Special thanks must go to our departmental photographer, Róbert Nagy, for his skilled assistance and to János Kálmánfi and Csaba Piller, whose artistic skills have made a great contribution to the impact of this work. The professional, editorial and technical assistance of Vince Books, Budapest, is also acknowledged.

Budapest, 19th April, 1999

The Authors

Introduction

The images shown in this atlas were obtained using various diagnostic methods that are characteristic for specific organs or regions of the human body. The following introductory chapter provides a concise summary of the physical basis, diagnostic application and technical background of these methods.

DIAGNOSTIC X-RAY

When on a dim November evening in 1895 Wilhelm Conrad Röntgen discovered X-rays, in fact he merely realized and named the physical basis of an existing phenomenon. Understanding X-ray radiation requires a knowledge of Bohr's atomic model (1913), and the electromagnetic spectrum. According to Bohr's mechanistic atomic model, each atom consists of a central nucleus with electrons orbiting around it. The nucleus is composed of positively charged protons and uncharged neutrons. The mass of the atom is virtually all within its nucleus due to electrons having virtually no mass. The number of negatively charged electrons orbiting the nucleus is equal to the number of protons in the nucleus; therefore, their charges cancel each other out. The electrons occupy distinct orbits or shells, representing different energy levels, which increase from the inner to the outer shells, named K-L-M-N. Every physical system prefers lower energy states; if an electron is pushed to an orbit that is higher than its own level, it will endeavour to get back to the original (i.e.

lower) energy state in order to stabilize the system. Each electron orbit accommodates a finite number of electrons. However, this does not imply that it is actually occupied by just so many electrons. In a stable condition, the atom shows no external charge because those of its electrons and protons cancel each other out and, provided all its electrons occupy their normal orbits, there is no energy surplus either. These defined electron orbits represent specified levels of energy, determined by the motional energy and the potential energy of the electromagnetic field. Accordingly, the total energy of electrons in the outer shells, i.e. orbits of greater diameter, is greater than the total energy of electrons occupying more proximal (inner) shells. Following transmission of energy to an atom, some of its electrons are pushed to outer orbits of higher energy, a process called excitation. The energy required for excitation always equals the difference between the energy levels of the two orbits. Therefore, an atom can only be excited by a given quantum of energy. As already mentioned, unstable physical systems tend toward the lowest possible level of energy. Thus, in the excited atom, an electron temporarily occupying an outer orbit of higher energy will soon fall back to a proximal (inner) orbit of lower energy, whilst its surplus energy (the difference between the values of the two orbits) will be discharged in the form of radiation. Such radiation belongs to the spectrum of electromagnetic waves. When electrons leave an outer orbit, the radiation is given off as thermal waves (microwaves) or visible light. With electron movement nearer the nucleus, the wavelength of radiation emitted decreases and the energy level increases, thus giving off X-rays. Atomic excitation is a well-known phenomenon in everyday life – we only have to think of fluorescent lights or television screens. When an atom is excited by a very high energy source, the electron will escape its atom altogether rather than merely being displaced from its orbit; this electron is released as a free photoelectron whereas the remaining particle becomes a positive ion: a phenomenon called ionization. Rays that are powerful enough to give rise to such a process are termed ionizing radiation. X-rays belong in this category; but, under certain conditions, ultraviolet (UV) or visible light, ultrasound waves of great intensity, or even massive electric discharges (lightning) may bring about similar, e.g. atmospheric, ionization phenomena. In the electromagnetic spectrum, the shortest wavelength (i.e. highest energy) domain is occupied by the so-called cosmic rays, which are of extremely high penetrating capacity. These are followed by gamma rays, originating from isotopes, and then by X-rays. These are spread across a fairly broad range, starting from the so-called hard X-rays of high energy, used for irradiation therapy, through the region of diagnostic X-rays to those soft X-rays used in surface therapy. Next in the sequence are UV and visible light rays, followed by thermal waves and microwaves (used in domestic microwave ovens). With some overlap, these are followed by ultrashort radio waves and then short and medium radio waves. The lowest energy and shortest wavelength domain in the electromagnetic spectrum is occupied by the radiation due to alternating current.

X-rays are generated in large quantity when electrons of high kinetic energy collide with a particular material (target) and deceleration of the electrons causes a discharge of energy (*Figs. 1–2*).

The greater the speed of the colliding electrons, i.e. the greater the voltage of the X-ray tube, the shorter the wavelength of the resulting radiation. The discharge from any X-ray tube is a compound one, meaning that it contains both soft and hard X-rays (i.e. rays of longer and shorter wavelength, respectively). Just as white light can be separated into colours representing components of different wavelength in the spectrum using a glass prism, compound X-rays can also be separated with the help of a special 'prism' (containing arrays of crystalline minerals) to yield X-ray diagrams. Apart from the deceleration (braking) process described above, X-rays can be generated by other means, too. When the electron

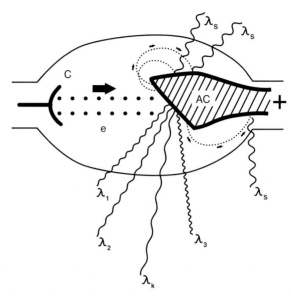

Figure 1. The principle of the X-ray tube. C – cathode, AC – anti-cathode (anode), e – electrons, λ_1-λ_3 – X-ray photons of variable energy (wavelength), λ_k – characteristic radiation, λ_s – X-ray photons due to secondary radiation.

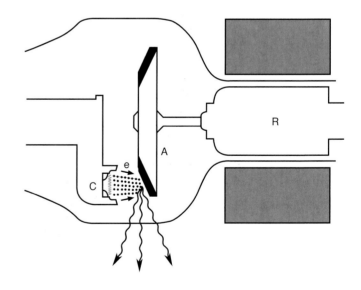

Figure 2. X-ray tube with rotating anode. C – cathode, e – electron beam, A – anodal disc, R – rotor.

beam (cathode ray) collides with the target it destabilizes its electron structure. An electron displaced from the innermost K orbit will be replaced by another electron falling back from the neighbouring L orbit. Thus, the entire intrinsic energy of the atom is reduced, and this energy deficit appears as electromagnetic waves (i.e. X-rays) emitted by the atom. The wavelength of such radiation is specific to the material of the target. It is therefore termed characteristic (characteristic rays are represented by sharp bands in the X-ray spectra or diagrams mentioned above). In conventional X-ray, the image is formed as a shadow cast by objects which attenuate the beam. Unlike the shadows caused by visible light, however, the X-ray shadow is invisible to the human eye. Since the time of Röntgen's discovery, X-ray images have either been viewed on a fluorescent screen or made permanent using photographic procedures.

Highly radiopaque structures, when placed in the path of X-rays, give full shadows, whereas those objects which are partially radiopaque and partially radiolucent cast intermediate shadows (penumbra). The images obtained in human diagnostics largely belong to the latter category, since the organs of the body are of heterogeneous composition. When evaluating X-rays it should be noted that, because of the linear path of the beam and the finite size of the source, the image is generated by central projection, i.e. the closer the object is to the source and the farther from the screen the greater the distortion and enlargement will be (*Fig. 3*).

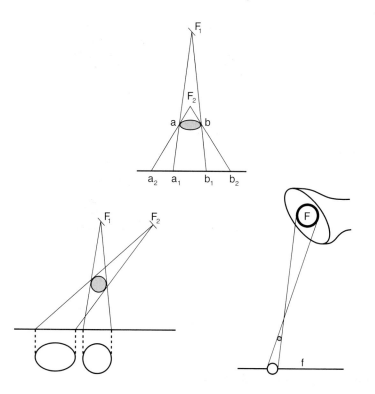

Figure 3. Axial projection (above), lateral distortion (left) and virtual enlargement (right) in X-ray studies. F – focal plate, f – plane of film.

Therefore, the recording film should be placed close to the patient's skin, while the focus of the source should be as far away as possible (even as much as 150–200 cm). Furthermore,

those structures near to the centre of the object are less likely to undergo distortion than those lying near to the periphery.

1. Owing to their calcium content, bones show the highest opacity and are therefore most conspicuous in X-ray images.
2. Attenuation of the soft tissues is approximately equal to that of water.
3. Attenuation of the fatty tissue is less than that of soft tissues.
4. Air and gases are completely translucent.

The final X-ray image is based upon differential attenuation, according to the density, specific weight and thickness of the various tissues. Attenuation is also dependent on the physical properties of the X-rays used; the absorption is greater with long wavelength (soft rays) than with short wavelength (hard rays). The attenuation scale of different human tissues is shown below (*Fig. 4*).

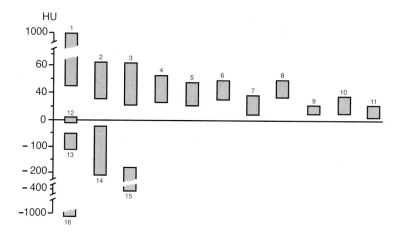

Figure 4. Radiopacity ranges of different human tissues in computed tomography. HU – Hounsfield unit. 1 – bone; 2 – blood; 3 – liver; 4 – tumour; 5 – heart; 6 – spleen; 7 – pancreas; 8 – kidney; 9 – adrenal gland; 10 – bowel; 11 – bladder; 12 – water; 13 – breast; 14 – fat; 15 – lung; 16 – air.

It should be noted that the overall opacification (blackening of the X-ray film) reflects the additive value of all tissues lying in the beam path (summation image).

For elimination of secondary radiation from interaction with tissues in the human body, focussing tubes and/or Bucky-grids are applied, which filter out X-rays of inappropriate direction and intensity that might cause interference. X-ray examinations can be performed using various beam directions: anteroposterior, posteroanterior or lateral. It is also possible to take specially targeted X-rays, by positioning the part of the body under the fluorescent screen. Fluoroscopy is used for the examination of moving structures, for monitoring the passage of contrast material within the organs, or for three-dimensional imaging (by turning the patient with respect to the screen). The value of fluoroscopy is now greatly enhanced by the use of image amplification and improved recording systems. It is widely used in traumatology and angiography, as well as functional examinations such as swallowing tests. Apart from traditional X-ray films (radiographs), permanent records are now also obtained by multiplication, digitization and other post-processing methods.

Contrast studies are essential in conventional radiography, mainly for imaging of hollow organs such as the gastrointestinal tract. A non-toxic salt of very high radiopacity (finely dispersed barium sulphate) is used either as a fluid cast to fill the organ, or as a thin film covering the inner surface of the organ (mucosal relief study). In some cases, air is introduced after barium for better visualization of surface disorders (double contrast study). The upper (stomach, duodenum) or lower (colon) abdominal organs can be studied using barium meal or barium enema, respectively. Barium can also be injected through a special nasojejunal tube e.g. for study of the small intestine (enteroclysis).

COMPUTED TOMOGRAPHY (CT)

Essentially, in X-ray based imaging, the rays attenuated by the human body through which they pass are visualized using analogue techniques as a summation picture. The chest X-ray can be readily understood. Though also based on X-ray, CT offers a fundamentally novel approach.

Joint application of new technical advances in space technology (signal detection, amplification, noise elimination, linear scanning) and computer science enabled Hounsfield and Cormack (Nobel laureates, 1979) to realise the first CT apparatus. In traditional radiology, the entire region to be examined is exposed to radiation, so that most of the rays fogging the X-ray film derive from scattered rather than modulated radiation. Analogue roentgenograms (radiograms) represent summational images, whereby the layers through which the beam passes are added up or subtracted from each other. This is the case even with classical X-ray tomography, except that those layers irrelevant to the investigation are blurred. Conversely, CT is capable of forming images that are free

from summation. The basic principle of CT is that a very thin (collimated) beam emitted by a constant output X-ray tube (gun) is detected and measured by a constantly coupled detector. The latter responds only to the attenuation of the primary beam, without picking up the background noise due to secondary radiation. As the patient is being examined in the required planes, a point-to-point absorption profile is generated by the detector according to the linear attenuation of the beam. In passing through matter (the human body) X-rays undergo attenuation due to absorption and scattering. This factor is an exponential function, termed the attenuation coefficient. In materials of constant thickness, the number of X-ray photons passing through is determined by the linear attenuation coefficient. This depends on the density of the material (tissue), the atomic number of its components and the energy of X-ray photons. Given the constant energy output of CT equipment, the value of the linear attenuation coefficient is influenced only by the atomic number of the tissue components and the density of the tissue.

While passing through the body, the X-ray beam passes through organs of varying attenuating capacity. Such heterogeneous organs yield different absorption profiles when scanned in differerent planes. In accordance with various mathematical algorithms, the attenuation profiles corresponding to various scanning directions determine the number of picture elements (pixels) or, more precisely, volume elements (voxels) – remember that the beam always has a certain width, too – i.e. the spatial resolution. Voxels represent slabs of 0.5–10 mm side length, whose depth depends on the width of the beam and whose absorption can be computed and numerically expressed by measuring the absorption values for different directions of the beam. The image of the investigated tissue profile is constituted by such voxels, in modern CT equipment in the form of a 512 by 512 matrix. Thanks to the algorithms used in the most up-to-date CT units, image processing is remarkably fast, virtually real-time. In order to visualize the computed data as real images, the data are displayed on a screen as grades of a grayscale with the help of a digital/analogue converter. Rather than showing absolute values of attenuation, the CT image represents, for practical reasons, a relative value of attenuation, as compared to a reference (baseline) level (water, air). This scale of relative attenuation is named after Hounsfield. The value for water is zero, for air -1000, and for the hardest compact bone 2000. The CT image results from transverse X-ray tomograms in which the absorption values of a given body profile are visualized as a matrix image in accordance with their spatial arrangement and resolution. Such cross-sectional images are composed solely of the absorption values of the measured layer and are not confounded by the shadow of other layers. In brief, the CT image represents computed, rather than directly measured values.

Even minute differences of absorption can be discerned in a CT image. These differences can be numerically expressed, as described above, but it proves more informative for the human eye to visualize grades of tones as an analogous grayscale picture. Since the human eye can distinguish only about 15–20 grades of the grayscale, one step of tone would cover approximately 100 Hounsfield units using the entire practical range (-1000 for air, 0 for water and +1000 for hard tissue). However, the examiner may use the 15–20 grades at his disposal over a limited range of the scale. Thus, for example, by assigning one step of tone to 2–3 HU, the absorption resolution (i.e. the contrast) within the relevant range can be considerably improved and fine differences of contrast can be detected with a higher sensitivity (the absorption resolution is limited by the signal/noise ratio). It is also possible to select the level around which the absorption resolution is enhanced (window level). The range of tones viewed above or below this level is called the window width. Should a higher anatomical precision be required, the window has to be 'opened wider'. Accordingly, when small differences of density are to be visualized, a 'narrow window' at a level close to the attenuation value of the organ itself should be selected. Attenuation values above the upper or below the lower limits of the window width will appear on the screen as white or black spots, respectively. The visualized range, determined by the window width, is distributed over the 15–20 grades of grayscale.

For reliable measurement of attenuation values, the X-ray generator must be working at a constant tube voltage of 30–150 kV, the intensity of current ranging between 200 and 500 (700) mA, in continuous or pulse mode. The anode may be of the fixed or revolving type but in both cases high stability of voltage is of paramount importance. The X-ray detectors are situated opposite the gun and revolve simultaneously with the X-ray tube (*Fig. 5*).

The detectors contain scintillating crystals (NaI or CaF_2), organic crystals or high pressure gas chambers (xenon). The

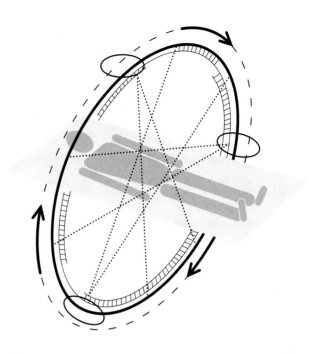

Figure 5. Schematic drawing demonstrating the principle of CT.

X-ray gun and the detectors are mounted on a ring-shaped device called a gantry, affording both high precision of movement and mechanical stability. The gantry has to ensure perfectly coordinated movements of the gun and the detectors, whilst maintaining vibration-free operation, despite the massive centrifugal force generated by the rapidly revolving X-ray tube. In modern CT systems, the detectors can be arranged in parallel rows (rather than in a single row), enabling several body sections to be visualized in a single revolution of the gantry. The measured values are then fed into a high performance computer for processing of the composite grayscale (sometimes colour-coded) images. The computer can add several mathematical algorithms, e.g. edge and contrast enhancement, and it can eliminate artifacts.

As long as raw data are available, several post-processing manipulations can be performed in order to improve image quality or for analysis of the images. However, due to a lack of sufficient capacity, the raw data are not normally stored for long, except for a limited amount of data required for filming (several photographic procedures are used in the different CT systems). Only the most informative frames are saved and used to select the window levels and widths required for diagnosis. Measurements can be made and documented on the selected pictures: length (distance), angle, density, area; the region of interest (ROI) can be enlarged; individual pictures can be subtracted from each other or superimposed. The factors of greatest importance in determining the quality and informative value of CT pictures are the absorption resolution, scanning time and layer thickness. However, the radiation burden must also be kept in mind, since we are working with X-rays.

The following post-processing methods are used. Measurement of distance: CT gives real data for body parameters without linear or depth distortion. The data measured in the pictures correspond to realistic values. The same holds for measurement of angles around the X and Y axes. These are particularly important in the examination of bones or in the planning of orthopedic and reconstruction surgery. A region of interest (ROI) can be drawn around either manually or using a built-in program, and the area of the delineated region can be calculated from the number of pixels it contains. By performing the same measurement in serial slices, the volume of the organ or mass in question can be calculated from the slice thickness and the area values. Histogram analysis: the distribution of attenuation values within a ROI or along a line drawn on the screen is shown by histograms. Normal histograms are bell-shaped (Gaussian curve), e.g. the distribution of attenuation values for a water phantom, where the standard value is modified only by statistic fluctuations of photon emission (quantum noise). In heterogeneous masses, i.e. organs of the body, the histograms are usually asymmetric, not following a Gaussian distribution. In mixed tissues, histograms have additional peaks. Subtraction of images is possible in the case of native and intravenous (IV) contrast-enhanced images taken in parallel at identical levels. A change of attenuation can be better judged this way than by the naked eye or by separate measurements. Addition of images is used to increase the thickness of adjacent slices, making the attenuation more discernible. Another valuable method, the density profile, gives the distribution of density values (y axis) along a line (x axis).

Clearly, CT has several advantages over conventional X-ray methods (including traditional tomography). The CT image is free from dimensional reduction or distortion: two-dimensional images are actually visualized in two dimensions, whereas in conventional X-ray the originally three-dimensional structures are seen as two-dimensional and distorted projected images. CT images do not suffer from the distorting effects of central projection, overlap due to superposition, summation or subtraction of densities. Both the size, proportions and angles shown in CT are true representations of the original. Minute differences in contrast enable visualization of the interior of the body and differentiation of the structures lying inside the skull as well as other bones. Thus, normal and abnormal structures can be distinguished by their shape, density or perhaps the accumulation of contrast material. CT images are obtained in the transverse (axial) plane. Whether this is an advantage over conventional radiography depends on the diagnostic problem. In any case, even if it is a disadvantage, it is more than compensated for by a better visual impression. However, it should be noted that the geometric resolution of conventional analogue X-ray pictures exceeds that of CT images (the refinement of analogue images can only be approximated, depending on the matrix size). Furthermore, the burden of radiation is several times greater in the case of CT than with the traditional X-ray method. Nevertheless, with the highly collimated 'hard' beam of CT, the amount of scattered radiation is reduced. Therefore, the patient's total burden of radiation is moderate, unless particularly sensitive parts, such as the lens of the eye or gonads (ovary, testis) fall in the path of the beam.

Nowadays, CT has encroached upon virtually all the territory of traditional X-ray diagnostics. Particularly important benefits of CT are spatial orientation and tissue differentiation (though not at the level of histology). A major application of CT is in neuroradiology, where it plays a crucial role in the diagnosis of stroke, in particular the early differentiation of haemorrhage and infarction. In addition to soft tissues, bones can also be successfully visualized with CT. The method requires no specific preparation in the investigation of the central nervous system, bones, soft tissues, musculoskeletal system or thorax. However, for examinations of the gastrointestinal system or pelvis, oral administration of contrast material is necessary. Such contrast materials are either dilute water-soluble diagnostics or finely dispersed barium sulfate in high dilution. For a typical gastrointestinal test, the patient is given 1000–1500 ml of contrast material to be consumed within 1 hour in instalments and a further 300 ml of contrast material to fill the stomach immediately before the CT examination. By filling the stomach and the small intestine, this amount of contrast material makes it possible to separate these structures from neighbouring, non-gastrointestinal parts and to distinguish coarse thickening of the wall from larger intraluminal lesions. For investigation of the colon, contrast material is administered in the form of an enema. Improved delineation of the organs of the female pelvis is assisted by the use of intravaginal tampons. A further improvement in the anatomical differentiation of vascular structures is achieved with the help of water-soluble contrast materials administered intravenously (IV) before or during the CT examination. Another option is IV administration in bolus form, followed by a further rapid infusion of iodinated contrast material during the course of the CT examination. Modern, fast CT systems (helical or spiral CT) enable dynamic investigation of organs in the arterial, tissue perfusion and venous phases. This is achieved using a timed delay, depending on the estimated velocity of circulation and the distance of the organ to be investigated from the site of administration of contrast material. Apart from demonstrating parenchymal disorders, the path of contrast material can also be indicative of functional states, e.g. renal excretion. Sequential (repeated) CT of the same body slice (seriography) is used to judge the accumulating capability of given organs, tissues, deformations or masses. With modern fast CT equipment, the course of contrast material in the blood vessels can almost be 'chased' by rapidly advancing the table. Computed reconstructions of such sequences are termed CT angiography, which may replace traditional (invasive, hence hazardous) angiographic methods.

CT examination is performed as follows. The patient is laid on a scanning table, the longitudinal axis of which lies perpendicular to the gantry. Prior to examination, a lengthwise overview image (topogram or scout radiograph) is taken with the help of a fixed X-ray tube and detectors, in anteroposterior or lateral beam direction. This topogram (though based on a digital matrix) resembles traditional X-ray images, and is used to mark the region to be investigated. If required, the gantry can be tilted up to 25–30 degrees (depending on the equipment) for better visualization of structures, e.g. the intervertebral discs. Similarly, the head and neck can be examined in the frontal (coronal) plane with the patient lying prone, head up (reflected) or supine, head hanging down, and the gantry tilted appropriately. For thoracic or abdominal CT, it is necessary for the patient to hold his breath to avoid artifacts due to respiratory movements. Even so, distortions owing to the contractions

of the heart or the pulsation of major blood vessels cannot be eliminated since the data acquisition time is longer than the cardiac cycle. When absolutely necessary (examination of the heart), the problem can be overcome by ECG triggered CT. Marking of the required region is followed by selection of the slice thickness (i.e. the degree of collimation of the beam). The serial sections can be contiguous, overlapping (when the table step is less than the slice thickness) or non-contiguous (when the table step is greater than the slice thickness). The collimation of the beam can be reduced, which improves spatial resolution, but in this case the signal/noise ratio is also decreased and, therefore, longer data acquisition times are needed. To create reconstruction images, contiguous slices of adequate thickness are combined using special software which recognizes and merges adjacent pixels to generate sections in the sagittal, coronal or other required planes. This procedure is called multiplanar reconstruction (MPR).

In helical (spiral) CT equipment, the X-ray tube and the line of detectors opposite it revolve continuously, the attenuation values being collected non-stop while the table moves forward. The density of data in what is called continuous volume recording depends on the collimation (width) of the beam and the speed of table advance. In fact, in this procedure, rather than simple slices being taken, the data are collected along a helical line, still enabling true reconstruction of slices in the transverse (or any other required) plane. With volume recording, three-dimensional imaging of the organs (e.g. surface shaded display – SSD) is feasible. The undistorted character of CT makes it the method of choice in radiotherapy, since both the density data and the size proportions shown in the transverse sections are realistic.

High resolution CT (HRCT) is a procedure in which a very narrow beam is used with a specified computer reconstruction. This leads to a reduction in pixel diameter in the central region of the image, with a considerable improvement in local resolution. Currently, the smallest attainable pixel diameter is ca. 0.3 mm. Clearly, a reduction in pixel (i.e. voxel) size makes the signal/noise ratio worse because the image noise increases. This must be compensated for by longer data acquisition times. HRCT is particularly useful in the imaging of bones or the lung parenchyma.

Invasive methods of diagnostic imaging

Angiography

Following injection of contrast material, the blood vessels of the body can be visualized by X-ray based imaging techniques. The method of injecting of the contrast material is either direct puncturing of the artery or vein, or catheterization, the latter enabling selective or superselective filling of the individual branches.

Catheterization is performed using one of two techniques: (1) preparation of the blood vessel selected for introduction of the catheter; (2) percutaneous puncture followed by catheterization. The catheter can be inserted through a vein (downstream injection) or through an artery (upstream injection). The objective of catheter examinations is visualization of the peripheral circulation of the limbs, brain and visceral organs or of the central circulation such as the heart and the large (principal) vessels.

In summation type investigations, the contrast material is introduced at a site from which a complete filling of the required vascular circuit or organ can be ensured. An example of this is summational abdominal aortography, in which the contrast material injected into the aorta simultaneously fills the right and left renal arteries, or the aortic arch. In selective arteriography, the renal arteries are cannulated individually, so that the circulation and perfusion of a kidney can be examined at a greater density and using much less contrast material. In the case of the lung, summational pulmonary angiography is performed with contrast material injected into the main pulmonary artery, completely filling the vessels of both lungs. Single lobes or segments can be visualized by pushing the catheter further into one of the pulmonary arteries and then on to the lobar and segmental branches.

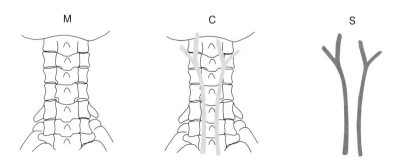

Figure 6. Digital subtraction angiography. M – matrix image, C – compound image, S – subtracted image.

Angiographic manipulations require sterile surgical conditions and purpose-built equipment. More recent angiographic machines are equipped for digital subtraction angiography (DSA); here summational imaging is no longer used. The principle of DSA is that an X-ray image taken from the body region in question serves as the background for a subsequent image taken after injection of vascular contrast material (*Fig. 6*).

The images are converted by an analogue/digital converter into a digital image matrix. Following inversion, the first image is then subtracted from the second, contrast-enhanced image by the computer. Thus, the contrast material that fills the vessels shows up without any interfering background, since the subtracted image contains only the information which was not present before the injection of contrast material, i.e. the vascular system. Following digital/analogue reconversion, the processed digital data can be seen as real images on the visual display unit. Not only does the method provide good quality peripheral angiograms with low amounts of contrast material but it is also adequate for arteriography following intravenous injection. The storage and processing capacity of modern computers allows viewing not only in the form of sequential 'frozen' images but also as a continuous, quasi-cinematographic replay of the images, subtracted on-line.

The catheter is introduced by the method of Seldinger. The Seldinger hypodermic needle (cannula) consists of three parts: an outer blunt cannula, the puncturing needle and a stylet. For temporary closure the device is equipped with an obturator (tap). The plastic cannula with the needle inside is inserted in an oblique position into the required blood vessel, after which the needle is removed and replaced by a flexible guide wire in order to find the vascular segment to be catheterized. Having reached this, a flexible, antithrombotic catheter of appropriate diameter is passed along the guide wire. Near the end the catheters have side openings to ensure an easy flow of the contrast material. Using an approach from the femoral artery, abdominal investigations require catheters of 60–80 cm length, whereas for a selective examination of the aortic arch and the cervical branches 100–110 cm catheters are necessary. The technique for inserting the cannula is as follows. Under local anaesthesia, a tiny cutaneous incision is made three to four fingers' breadth distal to the inguinal ligament (of Poupart). The femoral artery can be easily palpated, fixed and compressed at this site, and it has no major branches. For the femoral vein, the point of insertion lies 1 cm medial to the artery (it is good practice to make the patient perform the Valsalva manoeuvre for better filling of the vein). Should one fail to puncture the femoral artery (local tumour, infection, atherosclerosis, recent traumatic injury etc.) the axillary artery is recommended as an insertion site, although this may be more risky due to the proximity of the brachial plexus and may cause haematomas. If the right femoral vein cannot be used for reasons similar to those mentioned above, a cubital or axillary vein can be used. Importantly, the punctured vessel should lie on a bony floor because it can be compressed more successfully after catheterization.

Direct puncture of arteries for arteriography (e.g. the common carotid artery for investigation of the cerebral circulation) is no longer in use, except in an emergency. However, translumbar aortography is still occasionally performed in the following way: with the patient lying prone, a strong and long needle is inserted under the twelfth rib, left of the midline ca. one palm's width in the direction of the contralateral shoulder. Having reached the vertebra, the needle is retracted slightly and then pushed in again, directed slightly more forward to puncture the aorta. This investigation is performed under local or general anaesthesia in those patients whose femoral arteries are not palpable and who suffer from 'high' claudication. The contrast material is administered under high pressure with the help of a motorised injector, allowing simultaneous examination of the iliac and femoral systems on both sides.

Demonstration of the inferior vena cava is necessary in cases of suspected neoplasmic invasion or thrombotic occlusion. The purpose of the examination is to establish the precise height and extent of the occlusion and the position of collaterals. In such cases, the contrast material is usually injected directly into the femoral vein but catheterization of the jugular vein is also feasible. Opacification of the superior vena cava is required in cases of superior vena cava syndrome for demonstration of the site of the occlusion and the presence of collateral circulation. Here the contrast material is injected simultaneously into both basilic veins. Angiographic investigation of portal hypertension is a complex task. The site of occlusion, in particular whether it is intra- or extrahepatic, has to be established, and the hepatofugal and hepatopetal collateral systems visualized. Further methods worthy of mention are (on the arterial side) celiacography, angiography of the superior mesenteric artery, hepatic artery and splenic artery

(indirect portography) and (on the venous side) measuring the pressure in the hepatic vein. Superselective angiography of the left gastric artery is used for the demonstration of oesophageal varicosities. Using the Seldinger method for the catheterization of arteries (puncturing the femoral, occasionally the axillary arteries), selective and superselective filling of very small arteries, such as the suprarenal, bronchial, spinal, intercostal arteries can be attained. Direct portography with the help of percutaneous transhepatic puncture or by transjugular invasion is also feasible.

The investigation of the heart comprises the following procedures.

Atriography: injecting the right atrium to establish the thickness of the atrial wall and the full size of this heart chamber.

Dextrocardiography: aimed at dynamic testing of the central circulation. The contrast material is injected into the region of the superior vena cava – atrium transition. Selective or superselective variants of this investigation involve angiography of the right ventricle or the pulmonary arteries.

Coronary angiography: This method provides essential information for coronary surgery. Several selective methods are known which are used for separate catheterization of the right and left coronary arteries. The main arteries, even tertiary and quaternary branches, anomalous anastomoses, collaterals, constrictions or occlusions, deformations of the vascular wall, anomalies and variations of the vascular supply can all be well demonstrated.

Lymphangiography (LAG)

This technique is rather rarely used nowadays. Strictly speaking, lymphangiography means only the imaging of the lymphatic vessels, whereas the imaging of lymph nodes is termed lymphadenography. The method has been all but superseded by more advanced ones (US, CT, MR). Nevertheless, due to its exceptional ability to highlight individual lymphatic vessels, it still has a place in an anatomically oriented book. One difficulty with LAG is that lymph vessels are invisible to the naked eye, let alone through the skin. Therefore, a lymphotropic dye marker has to be injected first, usually in the dorsum of the foot or, occasionally, in the hand. This dye is now considered hazardous, since it may cause sensitization and subsequent anaphylaxis in some patients.

Another problem is that LAG requires very good dexterity. After the dye marker has sufficiently labelled the lymph vessels, these can be prepared under local anaesthesia and punctured with a special needle, using surgical binoculars. Through the inserted and fixed needle the lymphatic system is filled very slowly with an oily contrast material, using a special hypodermic syringe and a thermostated container to keep the contrast material at the right viscosity (body temperature). The total time required for a complete filling of the lymphatic system from the lower limb is 1.5–2 hours. The first images are taken immediately after injection to check if the dye is indeed in the lymph vessels. Then further X-rays are taken of the leg and the thigh to monitor the filling of the vessels. After completion of the injection, the pelvis and abdomen are investigated. Images are taken in both the anteroposterior and oblique positions to detect filling deficits. After 24 hours, the lymph vessels are no longer visible, only the lymph nodes themselves where medullary sinuses and filling deficits due to cellular deposits (metastases) can be clearly discerned. The contrast material is present in the nodal reticulum cells. The lymph nodes remain labelled for as long as 4–12 months, enabling long term follow-up of structural changes.

Retrograde pyelography and ureterography

With recent, more effective, methods at hand, these techniques are less frequently used, except in combination with therapeutic interventions. Their aim is opacification of the urinary passages of the kidney and ureter. The contrast material is introduced via a cystoscope and ureteral catheter (this intervention must never be done bilaterally at the same time or even at short intervals). Either an iodinated contrast material, heated to body temperature, is used to fill the renal pelvis and calyces or it is also possible to use air, oxygen or CO_2 for the imaging of negative calculi (pneumopyelography). By combining these positive and negative contrast techniques, double contrast effects can even be achieved. The examination is performed with a fluoroscopic control followed by selective radiograms. The main fields of application of retrograde pyelography and ureterography are deformations, destructive scars or tumours of the urinary passages in cases when the excretory capacity of the kidney is too low for urography. It is also possible to demonstrate calculi, tumours and obstruction of the urinary tract. Nowadays, the method is confined to those cases where unilateral disorders of the kidney or ureter cannot be clarified with US, CT, infusion urography or X-ray tomography and, particularly, where the examination has immediate therapeutic consequences.

Cystography

This procedure is used for the imaging of the urinary bladder. Briefly, a water-soluble iodinated contrast material (sometimes treated with a viscosity enhancer) is injected through a catheter, or an appropriate volume of carbon dioxide is introduced (pneumocystography). Diluted barium should never be used for cystography. Double contrast methods are also used for demonstration of the contours of the urinary bladder. Retrograde cystography with positive contrast is useful for the demonstration of the position, contours and internal disorders of the bladder. With gradual filling, the compliance and occasional rigidity of the bladder can be investigated. However, the method does not show the thickness of the wall. Pictures taken sequentially in the different phases of filling can be combined in a single image. Retrograde cystography can also be supplemented with micturition cystography, particularly for a better demonstration of the neck of the bladder together with the internal orifice of urethra. Advantages of cystography over IV urography are better opacification and a more informative image. The disadvantage is that the highly dense contrast material may mask the faint or negative shadows of some calculi. Pneumocystography is useful in the demonstration of stones but not for disorders affecting the wall of the organ.

Urethrography

Two methods are known for the imaging of the urethra, micturition cystography (see above) and direct retrograde filling. In the latter method, the terminal part of the urethra is filled with iodinated urographic contrast material (with or without viscosity enhancer). Images can be taken during filling (strictures are shown best at this time) or, following a complete filling of the bladder, during micturition. The latter method is suitable for demonstration of the dislocations of the posterior urethra and for inspection of the neck of the bladder and its surroundings. The images are taken in anteroposterior and oblique planes. Typical disorders that can be well demonstrated by cystography comprise malformations, fistulae, diverticula, scars, neoplasmic obstruction of the urethra, or a narrowing due to compression from abscesses or prostatic hypertrophy, for example.

Hysterosalpingography (HSG)

This examination is used for opacification of the uterus and the Fallopian tubes and requires collaboration of the radiologist and gynaecologist. An aqueous contrast material is introduced transvaginally into the uterine cavity and the uterine tubes under the guidance of fluoroscopy. The method is particularly important in cases of infertility, for example, disorders of the internal cervical os and cervical canal, occasionally even genital tuberculosis. Patency of the Fallopian tube and its communication with the peritoneal cavity can also be verified.

Myelography

This method is still used to visualize the structures of the spinal cord and the spinal nerve roots in the thecal sac. Under fluoroscopic control an iodinated contrast material is given percutaneously into the thecal sac through a long needle placed caudal to the lower end of the cord (conus). A good distinction can be made between the intra- and extradural masses. However, MRI has superseded this technique.

Bronchography

Opacification of the bronchial system with an iodinated aqueous and isotonic contrast material is recommended in cases of disorders that are potentially associated with the bronchi (tumour, abscess, bronchiectasis) and cannot be clarified either by conventional X-ray or CT. Since this examination has a lasting and adverse effect on respiratory function, it is never done bilaterally except with a few days' interval. Full opacification of the lung parenchyma is not required; the examination is acceptable when bronchi of the fifth to sixth order are filled. Contrast material is introduced through a flexible catheter, usually following (and guided by) bronchoscopy. This is done under anaesthesia to prevent cough and subsequent dissipation and fading of contrast material. Rather than using pressure injection, the examiner allows the

contrast material to trickle down one of the main bronchi with the help of gravity and the respiratory activity of the patient, who is kept in an appropriate body position. X-rays are taken during and after contrast filling from at least two directions.

Endoscopic methods

Modern flexible fibre-optic systems enable investigation of the interior of organs. Apart from their diagnostic use, other manipulations (e.g. taking histological samples, biopsy) are also feasible. Contrast material can also be introduced with the help of endoscopes, for example for imaging the bile passages or pancreatic ducts (endoscopic retrograde cholangiopancreatography, ERCP).

ULTRASONOGRAPHY (US)

As an imaging method, ultrasonography is fundamentally different from all the other techniques mentioned so far. Whilst the latter exploit some part of the electromagnetic spectrum as an energy source, this is not the case with ultrasonography. Ultrasound waves do not belong to the electromagnetic spectrum, instead they represent mechanical oscillations travelling in air or other conducting media. Such mechanical oscillations also generate audible sound. The human ear can detect oscillations between the frequency limits of 20 Hz and 20 kHz. Those below 20 Hz are termed infrasounds, whereas those above 20 kHz are called ultrasounds.

The waves generated by propagating mechanical oscillations make the molecules of the conducting medium oscillate around their resting position, maintained by inertia. In a given medium whose particles are in close contact, sound waves travel at a characteristic speed of propagation, influenced by the density and compliance (elasticity, resilience) of the medium. Sound travels slowest in air: at a speed of 340 m/s. It is considerably faster in water (1500 m/s) and in compact bone (around the biological average) it travels at an impressive 4000 m/s. The speed of propagation also depends on frequency and wavelength. Travelling sound waves are also characterized by their intensity: the amount of energy passing through a unit surface within a unit of time. A widely used relative measure of sound intensity is the decibel (dB), determined by the amplitude of sound.

For diagnostic purposes, ultrasound is generated with the help of a device called a transducer by transforming one form of energy into another. This is achieved by means of a piezo-electric crystal, which changes its shape under an electric potential to yield mechanical oscillations (*Fig. 7*).

Thus, electric energy is turned into mechanical energy, which travels through the conducting medium in the form of sound (ultrasound) waves. A similar transformation of energy, albeit in the opposite direction, can also occur in the trans-ducer: mechanical oscillations travelling in the piezoelectric crystal induce an electric potential field. Hence the same transducer can act as both transmitter and receiver, i.e. it is capable of both generating and detecting ultrasound waves. Therefore, in practice, ultrasound waves are emitted as pulses by exposing the piezoelectric crystal to short bursts of electric impulses (current, potential) at regular intervals (ca. 1000/s).

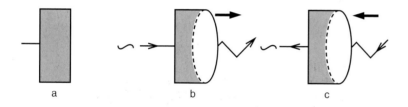

a   b   c

Figure 7. The principle of ultrasonography. a – piezoelectric crystal (transducer), b – transformation of electrical energy into high frequency mechanical oscillations (ultrasound waves), c – transformation of reflected ultrasound waves into electrical signals.

During the time windows elapsing between pulses (approx. 1 ms) the reflected ultrasound waves are detected by the trans-ducer. If sound/ultrasound waves arrive at an interface (the bor-der between two conducting media), one part of their energy passes through that interface, while the other part is reflected. As with optical phenomena, both reflection and absorption vary according to the properties of the interface. If the direc-tion of sound is perpendicular to the surface then it will not be deflected at all, only the speed of travel will be altered according to the properties of the new medium. Should an ultrasound wave hit the surface at an angle, however, its course will be altered, too, as in the refraction of light. Soft tissue/soft tissue interfaces hard-ly modify the speed of travel of ultrasound waves. The propaga-tion of ultrasound is virtually the same in all soft tissues. Conversely, the speed of propagation is considerably greater in bones and, as a result, a significant deflection (refraction) of ultra-sound waves can be observed at bone/soft tissue interfaces.

A further characteristic of sound propagation is termed the acoustic impedance of the medium, which depends on the density of the medium and the speed of travel therein. In a given conducting medium, the intensity and amplitude of an ultrasound beam exponentially decrease with the travelling distance. Such a decrease in intensity/amplitude is termed attenuation. When the frequency of sound is increased, the degree of attenuation is usually enhanced. In other words, the depth of penetration of ultrasound is reduced. Attenuation is due to the following factors: absorption, by which mechan-ical oscillation is turned into heat, reflection, refraction and scattering. The measure of attenuation is expressed as the thickness of the layer (in cm) capable of reducing the intensi-ty of a passing ultrasound beam by half. Attenuation values are one thousandth in water and one tenth in blood. In the soft tissues, the attenuation value reaches almost 1 in the liver, is higher than 1 in the cardiac muscle, over 10 in air and around 20 in the bone of the skull.

Ultrasound can be used in three different ways for imaging (i.e. the characterization of the media through which it passes).

1. *A-mode (amplitude mode)*. Here the reflected signals (echoes) appear as vertical bands (deflections, spikes) on the oscilloscope curve. The distance of bands measured on the base-line indicates the distance of the reflecting surface from the transducer, whilst the amplitude of deflections represents the magnitude of reflection at the given standard amplification. Based on the constant spreading velocity of ultrasound waves in soft tissues, the distance of peaks enables measurement of the true distance of reflective borders (tissue limits) inside the human body. This method is still in use, for example in ophthalmologic ultrasonography.

2. *M-mode (motional mode)*. In this method, the echoes appear as shining (glimmering) spots. The echo signals reflected from a moving surface constitute a curve on the oscilloscope screen. This technique is used in echocardiogra-phy, where the movements of the walls of heart chambers can be observed with high precision.

3. *B-mode (brightness mode)*. The echo signals appear on the screen as glimmering spots. The organ or part of an organ to be examined is scanned by the ultrasonic beam in an arbitrarily chosen plane. By summation of the echo signals, a true two-dimensional topographic image of the planar sections of the reflective surfaces is obtained. The follow-ing scanning methods are used (*Fig. 8*).

a. The beam is transmitted to the tissues by angular tilting of the transducer (sector scan)

b. The beam is passed along parallel lines (linear or parallel scan)

c. A combination of the two methods described above yields the convex scan. For all scanning, the transducer is operated manually or by a mechanical device.

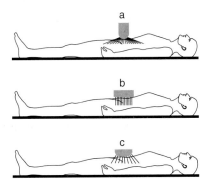

Figure 8. Scanning methods used in ultrasonography. a – sector scan, b – linear/parallel scan, c – convex scan.

The echographic signals (spots of light) are visualized on the screen according to their depth of origin, after which the ultrasound beam passes on. The echoes obtained in different transducer positions are stored by the apparatus and, after completion of scanning, the entire scanned section is displayed as a black and white (bistable) two-dimensional image. This image can now be printed on polaroid paper or film. More effective still, the light spots, whose intensity is proportional to the amplitude of echoes, can be visualized as grades of a grayscale, producing near-realistic images. A more modern version employs several motor-driven transducers with an electronic focussing of the beam. With this method, the time required for imaging can be reduced and the number of images obtained per second is sufficient for a dynamic visualization of organs, enabling real-time monitoring of movements.

Each organ or diagnostic problem has its optimal method of investigation. The diagnostic value of ultrasonographic examinations depends, more than anywhere else, on the correct scanning plane and the dexterity of the examiner. Rather than examining in all potentially available planes, we use standard planes and sections for a precise anatomical and pathological orientation. For example, the abdominal organs are examined with the patient in a supine position, in inspiration or expiration. The kidneys are examined with patients lying on their side with the transducer in the lumbar position. For an examination of the heart, the transducer is directed up from below through the acoustic window under the xiphoid process. Some organs are better visualized through specially designed acoustic windows: for example, the right suprarenal gland is scanned through the liver, or the pelvic organs through a full and distended bladder (the latter being highly permeable to ultrasound waves).

Ultrasound frequency shifts generated along the surfaces of organs in motion or currents of liquid (blood) can be examined by an apparatus utilizing the Doppler principle. As we know from everyday experience, the sound of an ambulance siren is perceived at a higher frequency (pitch) when the vehicle is moving towards us than when it is moving away. A similar principle is applied for the imaging of the blood flow inside the vessels. Two piezo crystals are used, one serving as a constant transmitter and the other receiving the modified signal (*Fig. 9*).

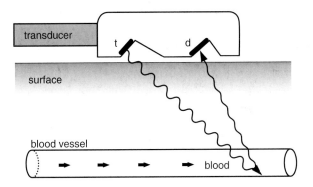

Figure 9. The principle of the Doppler technique in ultrasonography. t – transmitter, d – detector.

This way, the velocity of blood flow in the vascular system or the chambers of the heart can be measured. An acceleration due to constriction in the vessels or between heart chambers may signify meaningful pathological alterations. Doppler sonographic instruments can be used for the investigation of foetal heart beat, except in the earliest phases of embryonic life (before 4 months), when their use should be limited because of the continuous (twice normal) sonic energy discharge. In computer-linked Doppler sonographic equipment, not only can the velocity of the blood be measured but the direction of blood flow can be shown by colour-coding. By using this method, even pressure gradients or the amount of regurgitating blood (backflow, leak) can be measured in echocardiography. Moreover, the volume (capacity) of shunts (bypasses) can be determined, rendering invasive catheter tests unnecessary.

Contrary to expectation, tissue differentiation enabling direct histological evaluation is not considered to be a feasible approach in ultrasonography. However, the method is capable of distinguishing certain properties of tissues, mainly according to the number, extent and position of reflecting surfaces (interfaces). For example, in a cystic structure the interior is free of echo whilst the posterior (far side) wall gives intense echo signals, greatly improving the imaging quality of underlying structures (see the imaging of pelvic organs through the full bladder). Even with increased amplification, the interior of the structure remains free of echo, and translucency is only slightly reduced with increased frequency, i.e. the attenuation of fluid-containing structures is weak. The ultrasonic image of fluid substances is not influenced by their viscosity. Conversely, solid structures that are frequently of an irregular shape and whose contours are less smooth than in cystic structures tend to give some internal echo signal, while the posterior wall echo is either absent or weak. The imaging of regions beneath these structures is poor due to scattering of the beam. At an increased amplification, the internal echo signals become more frequent and the pattern may also change. Necrotic or homogeneous tumours may also have cystic components; in these cases amplification or enhancement of frequency may yield more echo signals from the interior of the structure. Some structures show the features of both cystic and solid formations. These are of mixed character and irregular shape with internal echoes: for example, cysts with inner partitions, fibrotic compartments, perhaps debris or scattered solid parts. Abscesses or necrotic metastases also belong to this category.

More than in any other imaging method, the success of ultrasonography greatly depends on the proficiency and skill of the examiner. Evaluation of sonographic images requires a good knowledge of physics, technology and pathology. One has to keep in mind that each and every image is a composite of a series of images.

Using Doppler ultrasonography, we can also assess the vascularization and circulation of organs. Avascular structures (with no vessels inside) yield no Doppler echo signal. Hypovascular structures are poor in Doppler echoes whereas hypervascular structures generate many such signals. The properties of blood flow also differ according to the type of vessels. Such differences can be well characterized in arteries and veins. In Doppler sonography, the echo signals reflected from moving red blood cells are visualized, rather than the blood vessels themselves. In two-dimensional images, blood vessels larger than 3–4 mm can be discerned, and even the vascular wall is visible. Two types of arteries can be distinguished: low resistance arteries, in which the diastolic flux is rather high as in the internal carotid or renal arteries, and high resistance arteries where the flux in the diastolic phase (after the systolic peak) is zero or even negative (retrograde) as in the external carotid or femoral arteries. Venous flow is continuous and of low speed as demonstrated, for example, in the femoral or portal veins. Ultrasonic perfusion tests, in which the blood flow in a given vessel is determined in a non-invasive fashion by computation, enjoy increasing popularity.

The examiner has to be aware of the physical properties that may lead to the formation of artifacts. Such artifacts comprise shadowing effects, distortion due to curvature of slanting reflective surfaces, and reverberation ('backtalk'). Backtalk is observed between two interfaces, when an already reflected ultrasonic beam gets re-reflected ping-pong fashion until its intensity drops below the level of detectability. In such cases, the delayed reverberating echoes give the false impression of multiple interfaces rather than a single, deep-lying one.

MAGNETIC RESONANCE IMAGING (MRI OR MR)

Of the routinely used imaging methods, MRI belongs to the group (together with US) which is not associated with ionizing radiation.

The imaging properties of X-ray based techniques depend on atomic number and attenuation capacity, and those of ultrasonography on the reflection of sound waves by tissue interfaces. MRI is a method based on a complex physical phenomenon, in which the image is formed under a constant magnetic field using the energy of radiofrequency impulses. Nuclear magnetic resonance was discovered in 1946 by Bloch and Purcell, and for decades the phenomenon has been used for the biophysical or biochemical analysis of materials. It was not until the 1970s that, thanks to space technology, the progress of computerization made the method available for diagnostic imaging.

The rather complicated physics behind MRI can be explained in a simplified fashion using a geometric model of the atom.

Nuclear magnetism

The atom is the smallest chemically derived particle of matter, consisting of a nucleus surrounded by shells of negatively charged electrons. The nucleus consists of protons and neutrons, collectively termed nucleons. Protons are positively charged, whereas neutrons possess no charge. The nucleons also have a spin, i.e. they behave as elementary magnets (dipoles) generating a magnetic field while rotating around their own axis. Therefore, each spinning atomic nucleus is associated with a minute external magnetic field.

Magnetic field is measured in a unit known as Tesla. 1 Tesla equals 10 000 Gauss. The value of the Earth's magnetic field is 0.3–0.7 Gauss. Elementary magnets have two poles called north and south. Identical poles repel while opposite poles attract each other. Those materials with magnetic properties tend to be aligned according to the magnetic lines of force. If an electric conductor is placed in a magnetic field, current is generated. Conversely, electric current (a stream of charged particles such as ions or protons in motion) can generate a magnetic force field.

In atoms with an even number of nucleons, the magnetic dipoles are neutralized, i.e. such atoms exhibit no magnetic dipole momentum. However, those atoms with an odd number of nucleons are unbalanced and show a manifest magnetic momentum, enabling the phenomenon of magnetic resonance. The nucleus of the hydrogen atom consists of a single proton. Of all the elements, this shows the highest magnetic momentum. Other elements are also capable of nuclear magnetic resonance. This was exploited in MR spectroscopy long before MRI and is still used in some cases (carbon, C_{13} 6 protons + 7 neutrons; fluorine, F_{19} 9 protons +10 neutrons; sodium Na_{23} 11 protons + 12 neutrons; phosphorus P_{31} 15 protons + 16 neutons). Even so, none of these elements can match the intensity of the nuclear magnetism of hydrogen, in which the single proton has no 'counterbalance'. Fortunately, this element happens to be the largest constituent (two thirds) of living tissues, and the intensity of its signal exceeds that of any other element by a factor of 1000. In practice, MRI investigates the distribution, behaviour and binding state of protons present in water and fat in relation to their environment.

Magnetic resonance

When dipoles of hydrogen, oscillating irregularly, are placed in an extrinsic magnetic field, the elementary magnets align in a parallel or antiparallel direction (north-south, south-north) (*Fig. 10*).

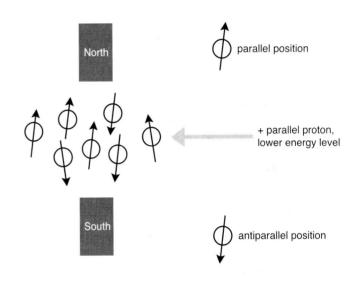

Figure 10. Orientation of protons in longitudinal magnetization.

Their signals cancel each other out. However, slightly more protons (one thousandth of a percent, with a 0.5 Tesla field and at 37 °C a mere 4 out of 2 million!) tend to align in a parallel direction, i.e. lower energy state, than in an antiparallel direction. This minute but constant shift in the number of aligned protons, known as longitudinal magnetization, enables the imaging with MR.

The rotation of protons is not perfectly axial but rather like that of a spinning top (or, for that matter, the Earth itself) whose axis rotates about the vertical direction, thereby sweeping out a cone (*Fig. 11*).

This is called precessional motion. The precessional frequency of protons equals the speed of such motion, i.e. the number of revolutions per second. The precessional frequency is directly proportional to the force of the external magnetic field and also depends on chemical structure and temperature.

Owing to the precessional motion, the protons, when placed in a magnetic field, possess a magnetic vector whose axis lies at an angle to the pivotal axis. The precessional motion is irregular because the protons are out of phase, i.e. the transverse components of movement are cancelled out.

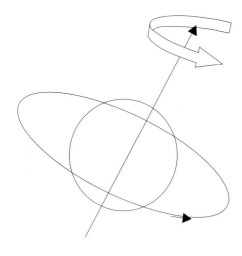

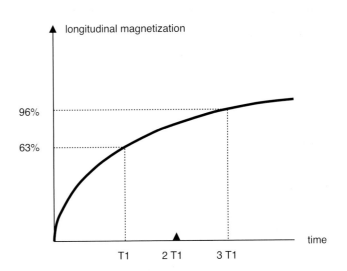

Figure 11. Precessional movement of the proton.

Figure 12. Time course of T1 relaxation.

Relaxation

Transverse magnetization is attained by an extrinsic impulse of radiofrequency (RF) waves. The frequency of such waves must be in the range of resonance (see above) and perpendicular to the pivotal axis. The axial shift (deflection) caused by this wave in a given proton depends on the intensity and duration of the RF wave: at 90 degrees the protons are deflected as far as the transverse plane. The high-energy state generated by the RF impulse is unstable. As soon as the impulse is gone, the protons begin to revert to their original state by precessional motion. This means they both approach the direction determined by the lattice and lose their previously acquired phase synchrony. Such longitudinal reordering of protons with a restoration of the original magnetic state is termed spin-lattice or T1 relaxation.

At the same time, independently of spin-lattice relaxation, a much faster process is observed: relaxation of transverse magnetism. This means that the protons lose the (transverse) phase synchrony imposed upon them by the RF impulse. Such desynchronization is called spin-spin or T2 relaxation.

T1 relaxation in living tissue follows an exponential curve, the time constant (T1 time) being characteristic of the given tissue (*Fig. 12*).

The T1 constant (the time required for the restoration of 63% of longitudinal magnetization) depends on histological conditions, phase state and also on the intensity of the magnetic field (the stronger the field the longer the T1 relaxation time). Energy discharge from fatty tissue is fast with a steep relaxation curve, i.e. short T1 value, whereas in water the discharge of energy is slower with a shallow curve and longer T1 value. In solid phase, the T1 value is reduced because the protons can easily pass their surplus energy on to the nearby lattice. This property of tissues, based on differences in relaxation times, enables a good separation of tissues and organs when using T1 weighted images.

T2 relaxation in the tissues follows an exponentially decreasing curve, corresponding to a gradual loss of transverse phase synchrony (*Fig. 13*).

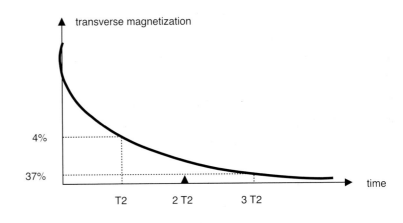

Figure 13. Time course of T2 relaxation.

The T2 time constant gives the time required for the disappearance of 63% of the transverse magnetization. Independent of T1 relaxation and orders of magnitude faster, T2 relaxation is due to an inhomogeneity of the magnetic field (generated locally or by the equipment), enabling further separation of tissues using T2 weighted images.

During the course of the exponential decrease, the transverse vector rotates. Since rotation of the elementary magnets is known to generate electromagnetic (RF) waves, a measurable current is induced in the coil surrounding the patient's body. Such a decreasing curve, denoted *FID* (free induction decay, i.e. free attenuation from excited state), is labeled *T2**.

Signal localization, image contrast, spatial resolution

Signal localization is achieved by a fine and even 'mistuning' of the homogeneous magnetic field. The magnet surrounding the patient ensures a homogeneous field intensity in the given volume of space. For the excitation of protons, an RF impulse of definite wavelength is required. During relaxation, the protons also discharge impulses of a similar wavelength. Due to this uniformity of RF waves, in cases of homogeneous magnetic fields, single protons cannot be identified. In order to locate the individual transmitters (i.e. to distinguish the protons of adjacent slices from those of other slices), the external magnetic field must be slightly altered by 'mistuning'. To this end, a consistent gradient ('slope') is introduced with the help of an electromagnetic coil (called a gradient coil). Thus, there is a detectable difference in the resonating frequency discharge of each proton according to the slope of the gradient. Any impulse of a given frequency meets with resonance only in a single plane that is perpendicular to the direction of the gradient, i.e. only those protons which lie in that particular plane are excited (the latter can also be an oblique one). Such gradients are introduced in each of the three dimensions of space: axial – transverse Z, sagittal X, frontal – coronal Y. This enables identification of individual image dots defined by adjacent slices, and, within slices, by rows and columns. Processing is performed by computer using Fourier transformation.

The thickness of the measured slice depends on the band width of the RF impulse and the slope of the gradient. The following gradients are used: slice selecting, phase coding, and readout or frequency gradients. Thus, all voxels in the space registered by the three gradients are true measured values (as opposed to the computed data in the quadratic matrix of the CT image). For a better understanding, let us consider a piano. Standing with one's back to the piano it is quite possible to tell the position of the key from the pitch of the sounding tone. Those with absolute pitch can even name the very tone. This is precisely what computerized MRI units do, except in a little more complex and precise fashion in all three dimensions of space (think of a 'three-dimensional piano'), when they locate a given proton by its precessional frequency. The direction of the slice selecting gradient decides the plane in which the image is obtained, whether the sections are anatomically in the sagittal, transverse (axial) or coronal (frontal) plane.

Factors influencing signal intensity, TR, TE

TR (repetition time). The time required for the re-establishment of the longitudinal magnetic vector (i.e. the time interval between the 90-degree RF impulses). The shorter the TR value the better emphasized the difference between T1 relaxation curves will be, those tissues with short T1 values giving an intense signal (bright spot) while those with long T1 values give a weak signal (dark spot). By increasing the TR, the difference in signal intensity gradually decreases and eventually disappears. Thus, short TR values correspond to T1 weighted images (with TR less than 700 ms).

TE (echo time). Indicates the time point of signal measurement in T2 relaxation. With long TE values the differences in transverse magnetism are emphasized, those tissues with long T2 values appearing more intense (bright) while those with short T2 values give weaker signals (dark). Thus, increasing TE values correspond to (proportionally enhanced) T2 weighted images.

Spin echo sequence. This commonly used imaging sequence is associated with both T1 and T2 relaxation, the density of protons, and is also sensitive to convectional phenomena. Following the instantaneous loss of phase synchrony due to the 90-degree impulse, the transverse magnetic vector of protons decays rapidly with very small differences remaining. If another, 180-degree, impulse is given at half TE, the protons of greater precessional velocity will be temporarily 'lagging behind' at the time of reversal but, by the end of TE, will catch up with the slower spinning protons. Therefore, the effect of relaxation is doubled during the same time period (TE).

Remember the story of the hare and the tortoise racing. They start together and, naturally, the hare is way off when the signal comes to turn back. Then, suddenly, the tortoise finds itself in a better position, since it has barely left the start line, now called finish. Eventually, they finish the race at the same time.

Careful selection of the parameters of examination is of great importance.

Magnetic signals of different tissues

Factors influencing tissue contrast
– density of protons
– longitudinal relaxation time (T1)
– transverse relaxation time (T2)
– resonating frequency
– chemical shift
– magnetic susceptibility
– convection, perfusion, molecular movements

Signal intensity is enhanced by
– increase of proton density
– longer T2 value
– shorter T1 value

Phenomena and disorders causing intense signals in T1 weighted images
– fat (droplets of lipid containing contrast material in the CNS)
– high protein content (cysts)
– haemorrhage, subacute or chronic forms (intra- and extra-cellular methaemoglobin)
– melanin (deposited in tumours)
– slow, marginal flow of liquid
– paramagnetic metals (iron, copper, e.g. Wilson's disease), dystrophic calcification, necrosis
– paramagnetic contrast material

Those materials attenuating the effect of the external magnetic field are called diamagnetic (99 % of human tissue falls into this category). Those that enhance the external magnetic field are termed paramagnetic (e.g. ferrous oxides). Those which possess magnetic properties without an external magnetic field and whose magnetic properties can be further enhanced by an external magnetic field are called ferromagnetic. Finally, those materials which are capable of inducing strong magnetic fields but lose their magnetism as soon as the external magnetic field is off are termed superparamagnetic.

Imaging technology

The magnets used for MR imaging are either permanent magnets (like a huge horseshoe magnet) or electromagnets. The former are made of solid metal, so they are very heavy and of limited force field (a maximum of 0.25 T). However, magnets have an advantage in that they can be 'open', allowing better access to the patient. Electromagnets are capable of generating stronger magnetic fields but the bulk of the energy fed into the coil is converted to heat. The magnetic force attainable by such systems does not exceed 0.35 T unless superconducting systems are used. In the systems, the wire of the coil is made of a special alloy and the system is kept at near zero-Kelvin temperature (-269 °C) with the help of liquid helium. In superconducting electromagnets, once fed into the system the electric current keeps circulating with virtually no resistance as long as cooling persists. Using superconducting magnets, a very high field strength can be achieved. Currently, the maximum used in clinical examinations is 2.0 T. Systems may be categorized as follows: low-field systems (up to 0.2 T), intermediate-field systems (0.35–0.5 T) and high-field systems (1–2.0 T). Experimental systems of 3.0 T are also available.

In the given range, the magnetic fields used in MR represent little biological hazard. However, patients with metallic implants of paramagnetic character (e.g. aneurysm clips) or electro-inductive devices (e.g. cochlear implants) should not be examined with MR. Examination of patients with electronic pacemakers is also forbidden, the more so because the electrode of the pacemaker unit may serve as a RF antenna and be unduly activated by the magnetic field. On the other hand, other non-magnetic metals (titanium, gold etc) cause only local signal deficit.

Convection phenomena, MR angiography

When examining human patients, a continuous or pulsating flow of liquids (blood, CSF) is often encountered. Such flow can be slow or fast, and its direction perpendicular or parallel to the plane of section. If the flow of liquid is fast enough, then the protons excited by the RF impulse will have left the slice by the time their discharged energy is to be detected, their place being taken by protons not yet excited. Accordingly, a signal void phenomenon will be observed in the relevant vessel or organ. This phenomenon is exploited by the TOF (time of flight) technique used for MR angiography in which the signal void makes the vessels clearly separable from background tissues of variable signal intensity. With very rapid sampling, the opposite effect can also be achieved, the vessels showing up more intense than the signals from the surrounding tissues.

Another phenomenon used for MR angiography is termed phase contrast (PC). Protons of rapidly flowing liquids undergo faster desynchronization than those of stationary tissues. This technique can even be used to measure the velocity of flow.

Several techniques are known for the elimination of artifacts arising from physiological movements: ECG gating, respiration gating, temporary suspension of peristalsis by drugs.

For better tissue differentiation, special contrast materials are used. These can modify the T1, T2 or both in certain tissues or organs in which they are accumulated. A member of the family of lantanides, gadolinium, is the most widely used MR contrast material. It accumulates preferentially in some tissues (mostly pathological, such as tumours) and shortens the T1 relaxation time with a subsequent increase in signal intensity.

NUCLEAR MEDICINE AND IMAGING METHODS

Employing radioactive isotopes as an open source of radiation, nuclear medicine is concerned with diagnostic, therapeutic and research tasks. Isotopes are forms of atoms which occupy the same position in the periodic system but differ in mass number. Due to an instability of the nucleus, certain isotopes undergo spontaneous transformation (decay), leading to corpuscular and electromagnetic radiations. Such isotopes are termed radioactive. Those isotopes used in diagnostics can be categorized by their source.

1. Nuclear reactor: e.g. iodine 131, chromium 51, iron 59, gold 198
2. Cyclotron: e.g. indium 111, gallium 67, iodine 123, thallium 201
3. Isotope generator: e.g. molybdenum 99, technetium 99 m (metastable)

Electromagnetic radiation originates from the following reactions:

1. Gamma radiation accompanying beta decay of the nucleus.
2. Characteristic X-ray from the electron shell of radionuclides whose decay is associated with K electron trapping.
3. Annihilation radiation (511 keV) arising from fusion of the positrons emitted by radionuclides with electrons.

Alpha-emitting radionuclides are not used in human diagnostics. Some radionuclides discharge beta particles, or the energy surplus remaining after the trapping of electrons, in a protracted fashion in the form of gamma radiation with a measurable half life. Such nuclei are called metastable (indicated by 'm' written after the mass number). Metastable isotopes are pure gamma emitters (with no corpuscular radiation) – a definite advantage for the patient because, unlike beta rays that are absorbed by the human body, gamma rays can be well detected externally and sufficient activities can be used without increasing the radiation burden.

Medical application of isotopes is based upon the fact that biological systems, such as the human organism, cannot distinguish isotopes of a given atom. Isotope-labelled compounds are processed in the body exactly as their natural counterparts, hence these can be monitored by radiation detectors. Owing to the high sensitivity of detectors, the amount of radioactivity introduced can be kept small enough to avoid interference with the organic system. Radioactive materials are therefore used as tracers. The tracer principle is attributed to the Hungarian-born physicist György Hevesy. The story has it that the eminent scientist had long suspected his landlady of serving leftovers from the previous day's meal in a 'reprocessed' form. Hevesy was desperate to find a way of pinpointing any traces from the previous meal without being noticed by the landlady. So he hit upon the idea of isotope tracing – according to the anecdote.

Radiopharmacons are used to monitor functional and morphological changes in the human organism by highly sensitive and non-invasive methods. The isotopes are administered orally, intravenously or by inhalation. Enrichment of the isotopes can be attained by active transport (^{131}I-NaI in the acini of the thyroid or ^{99}Tc-DNSA in the tubules of the kidney), phagocytosis (RES elements of the liver, spleen and lymph nodes); microembolization (lung scintigraphy); antigen-antibody reaction (marker antibodies for tumours and metastases); direct accumulation in blood-brain barrier lesions.

The electromagnetic radiation of radionuclides is detected by scintillation detectors, containing NaI crystals contaminated (activated) with thallium. The measurement is selective for photons of defined energy, enabling simultaneous detection of several radionuclides.

SPECT (Single Photon Emission CT). Emission CT studies the distribution of radiopharmacons in two-dimensional summation images. Similar to X-ray based CT, the image results from a computerized reconstruction of multiple data. Radiation is detected by a pair of revolving scintillation cameras moving along the longitudinal axis of the patient's body. Apart from tomograms, the method is also suitable for generating whole body images. Using special electronics for the detection of high energy (511 keV) annihilation photons, even positron emitting radionuclides can be studied.

PET (Positron Emission Tomography). The principle of the method has been known since 1978. The specific metabolites to be examined are labelled (in a nearby cyclotron) with very short half-life positron-emitting isotopes. The labelled metabolites are then injected intravenously or inhaled by the patient. When a positron collides with an electron, the ensuing annihilation yields a pair of high-energy (511 keV) gamma photons, which leave the body in opposite directions (180 degrees) *(Fig. 14)*. These photons are then detected by the numerous detectors surrounding the body of the patient and arranged at 180 degrees. For successful measurement of the coincidence of quantum pairs, the time window of data acquisition must be less then 10 nanoseconds. This requires

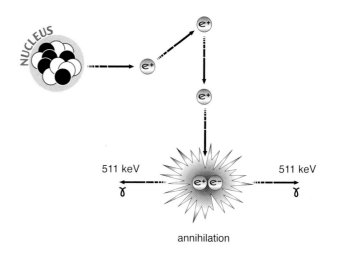

Figure 14. Scheme of positron annihilation. e⁺ – positron, e⁻ – electron.

high performance electronic equipment and powerful computers. Nowadays, PET units are the most costly of all imaging facilities used in nuclear medicine, the more so because they need a special cyclotron unit (or must be operated in collaboration with an existing cyclotron nearby). The method is suitable for quantitative assessment of metabolic activity in various organs with good spatial resolution. Currently, PET is used mainly for metabolic studies of the brain and the heart, allowing investigation of the viability, exposure and diseases of the organs. The method is particularly informative in revealing tumours, monitoring therapy and in early detection of disease recurrence.

HEAD

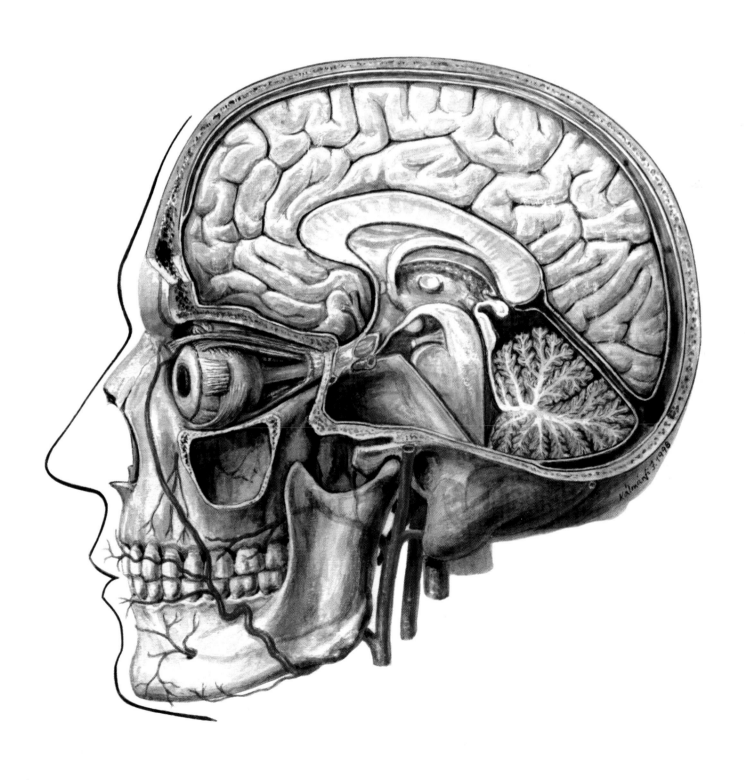

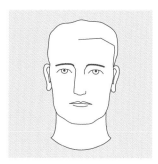

3D CT SSD reconstruction of skull, frontal view

1 - Temporal fossa
2 - Frontal bone (squamous frontal bone)
3 - Supraorbital notch
4 - Nasion
5 - Fossa for lacrimal sac
6 - Orbit
7 - Infraorbital foramen
8 - Nasal bone
9 - Zygomatic bone
10 - Nasal septum
11 - Nasal cavity (piriform aperture)
12 - Superior dental arch of maxilla
13 - Ramus of mandible
14 - Mental foramen
15 - Body of mandible

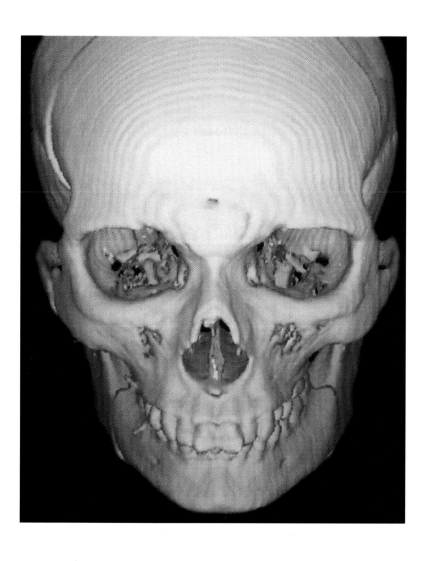

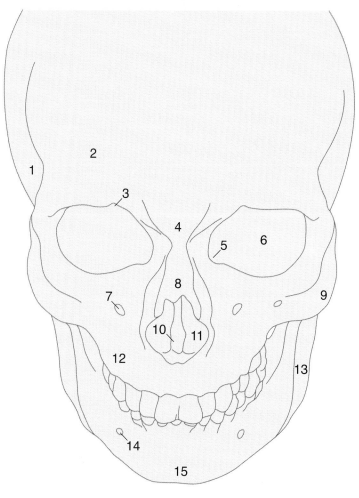

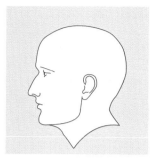

Internal cranial base, 3D CT SSD reconstruction, superior view

1 - Frontal sinus
2 - Crista galli
3 - Cribriform plate
4 - Orbital part of frontal bone and anterior cranial fossa
5 - Zygomatic arch
6 - Ala minor (lesser wing) of sphenoid
7 - Optic canal
8 - Anterior clinoid process
9 - Sella turcica, hypophyseal fossa
10 - Dorsum sellae
11 - Posterior clinoid process
12 - Foramen ovale
13 - Ala major (greater wing) of sphenoid, middle cranial fossa
14 - Carotid sulcus and foramen lacerum
15 - Foramen spinosum
16 - Petrous temporal
17 - Clivus
18 - Jugular foramen
19 - Foramen magnum
20 - Jugular tubercle
21 - Cerebellar fossa, posterior cranial fossa
22 - Internal occipital crest

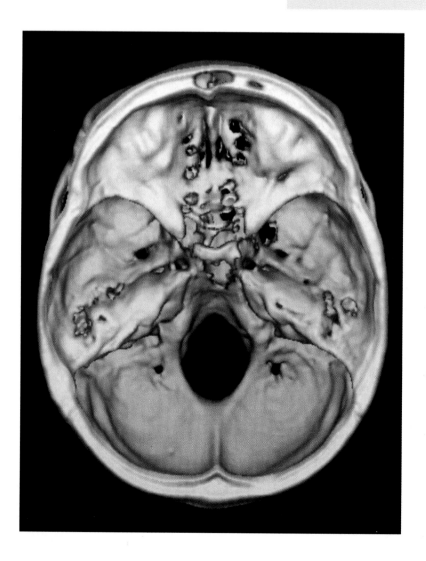

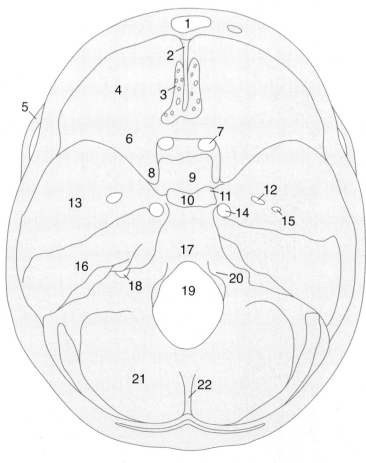

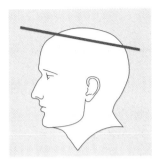

T2 weighted axial MR of the brain

1 - Scalp (galea aponeurotica and skin)
2 - Skull bone, dura mater and subdural space
3 - Subarachnoid space
4 - Superior frontal gyrus
5 - Falx cerebri and longitudinal cerebral fissure
6 - Superior frontal sulcus
7 - Middle frontal gyrus
8 - Precentral gyrus
9 - Central sulcus
10 - Postcentral gyrus
11 - Superior sagittal sinus

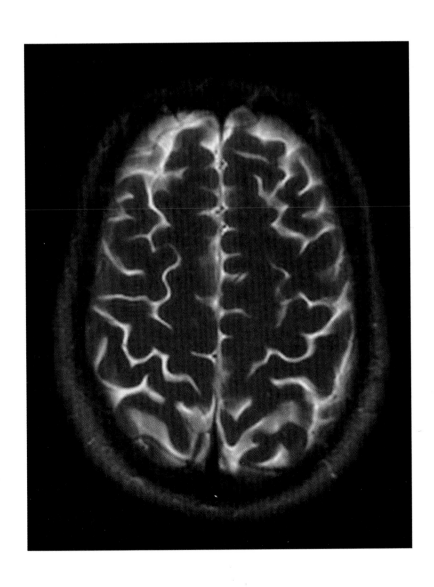

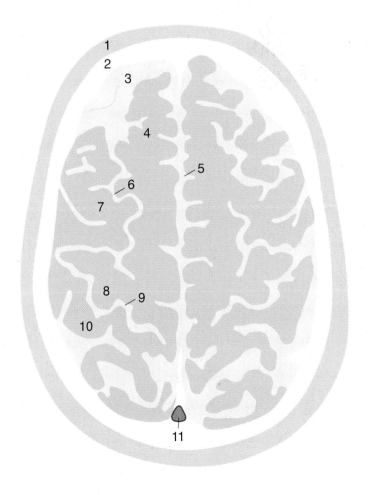

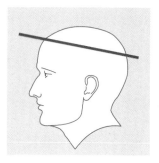

T2 weighted axial MR of the brain

1 - Scalp
2 - Centrum semiovale
3 - Longitudinal cerebral
    fissure
4 - Outer table of skull bone

5 - Diploë
6 - Inner table and dura
    mater
7 - Superior sagittal sinus

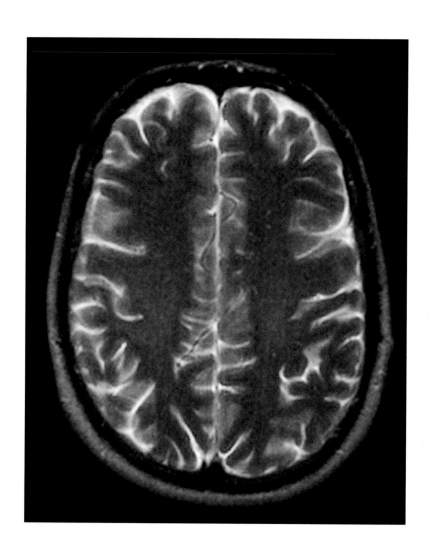

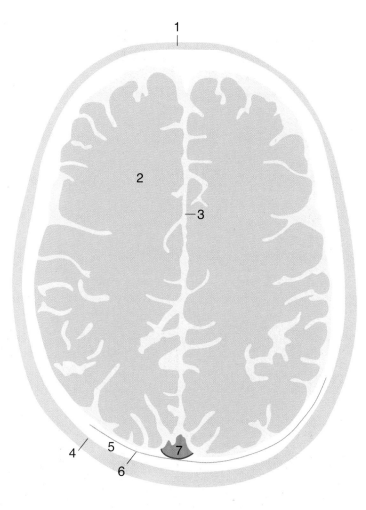

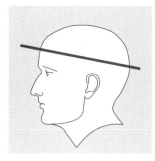

T2 weighted axial MR of the brain

1 - Frontal lobe
2 - Longitudinal cerebral fissure
3 - Anterior cerebral artery
4 - Genu of corpus callosum
5 - Lateral ventricle (central part)

6 - Corona radiata
7 - Lateral sulcus (posterior ramus)
8 - Occipital lobe
9 - Superior sagittal sinus

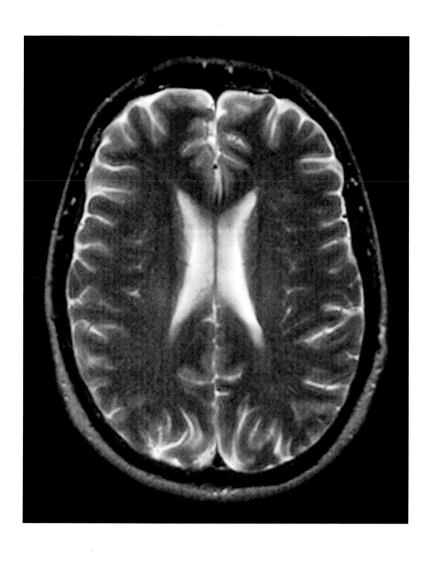

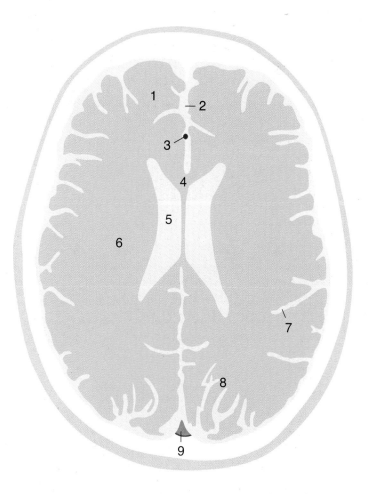

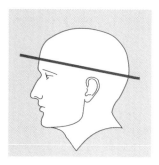

T2 weighted axial MR of the brain

1 - Frontal lobe
2 - Longitudinal cerebral fissure
3 - Genu of corpus callosum
4 - Frontal horn of lateral ventricle
5 - Septa pellucida

6 - Head of caudate nucleus
7 - Temporal operculum
8 - Insula
9 - Body of lateral ventricle
10 - Choroid vessels
11 - Falx cerebri
12 - Superior sagittal sinus

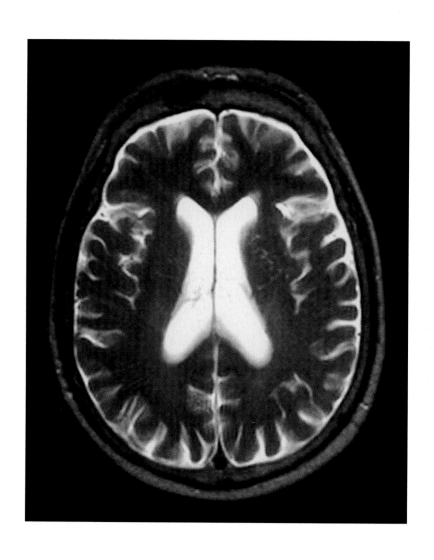

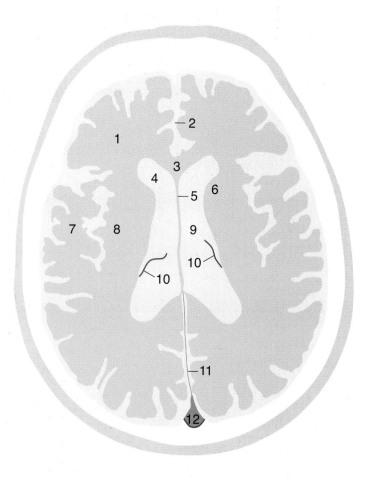

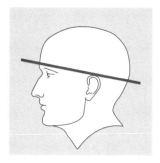

T2 weighted axial MR of the brain

1 - Orbital gyri
2 - Longitudinal cerebral fissure and falx cerebri
3 - Forceps minor
4 - Anterior cerebral artery
5 - Frontal horn of lateral ventricle
6 - Frontal operculum
7 - Lateral fossa
8 - Head of caudate nucleus
9 - Septa pellucida
10 - Insular gyri

11 - Fornix
12 - Interventricular foramen (of Monro)
13 - Thalamus
14 - Branch of middle cerebral artery in lateral sulcus (Sylvian fissure)
15 - Internal cerebral vein
16 - Lateral ventricle
17 - Forceps major
18 - Occipital lobe
19 - Superior sagittal sinus

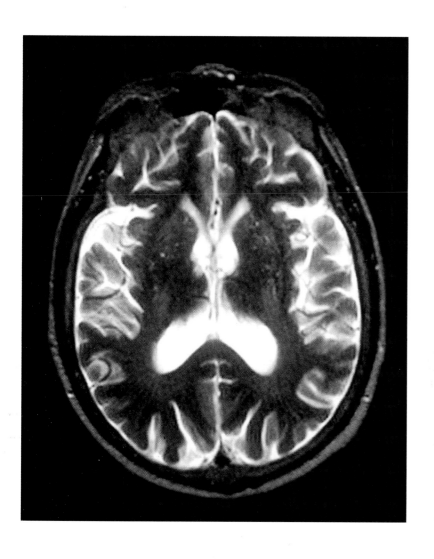

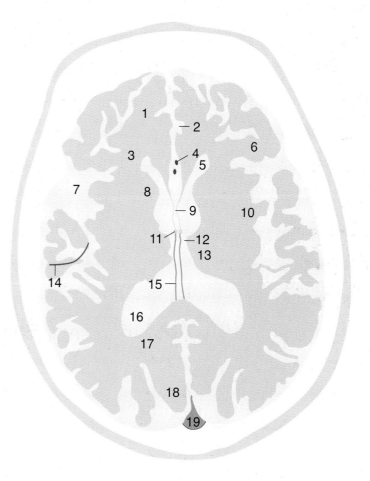

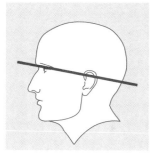

T2 weighted axial MR of the brain

1 - Nasal cavity
2 - Eyeball
3 - Optic nerve
4 - Gyrus rectus
5 - Anterior cerebral artery
6 - Temporal operculum
7 - Lateral sulcus
    (Sylvian fissure)
8 - Thalamus

9 - Third ventricle
10 - Insular gyri
11 - Internal cerebral vein
12 - Forceps major
13 - Trigone of lateral ventricle
    (collateral trigone)
14 - Straight sinus
15 - Superior sagittal sinus

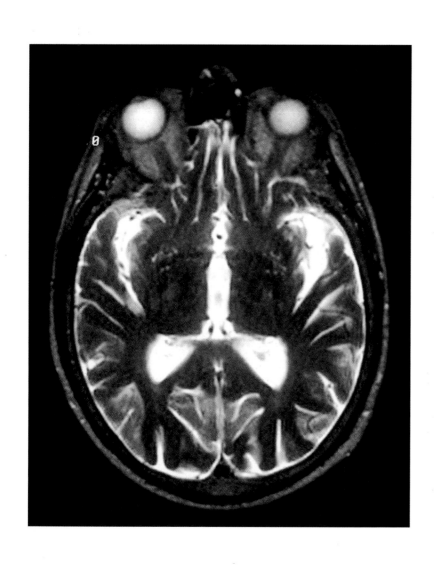

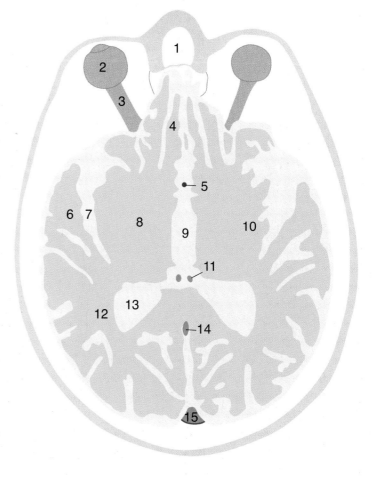

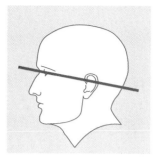

T2 weighted axial MR of the brain

1 - Nasal septum
2 - Eyeball
3 - Orbit
4 - Ethmoidal air cells
5 - Optic nerve
6 - Gyrus rectus
7 - Temporal lobe
8 - Middle cerebral artery
9 - Interpeduncular fossa and cisterna
10 - Anterior cerebral artery
11 - Optic tract
12 - Mesencephalon
13 - Posterior cerebral artery
14 - Cisterna ambiens
15 - Cisterna of great cerebral vein
16 - Trigone of lateral ventricle (collateral trigone)
17 - Great cerebral vein (of Galen)
18 - Straight sinus
19 - Calcarine fissure
20 - Calcar avis
21 - Occipital horn of lateral ventricle
22 - Superior sagittal sinus

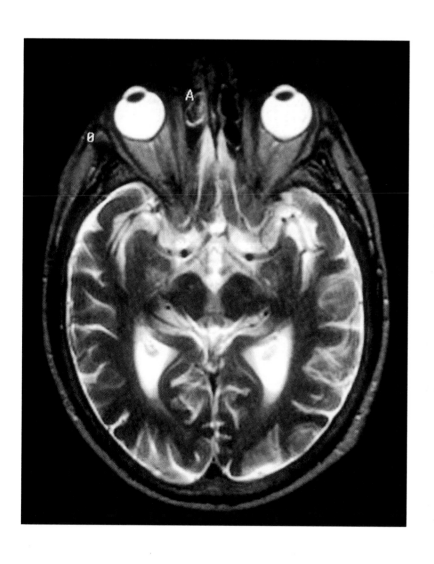

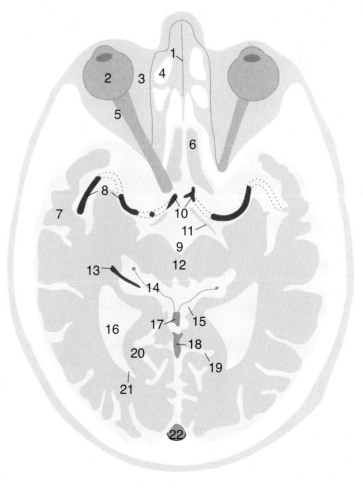

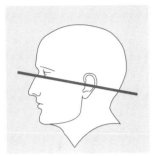

T2 weighted axial MR of the brain

1 - Nasal septum
2 - Ethmoidal air cells
3 - Eyeball
4 - Orbit
5 - Sphenoidal sinus
6 - Internal carotid artery
7 - Suprasellar cisterna and infundibulum
8 - Dorsum sellae
9 - Interpeduncular fossa and cisterna
10 - Crus cerebri
11 - Temporal horn of lateral ventricle
12 - Cisterna ambiens
13 - Tectum of mesencephalon
14 - Cisterna of great cerebral vein
15 - Great cerebral vein (of Galen)
16 - Optic radiation
17 - Superior sagittal sinus

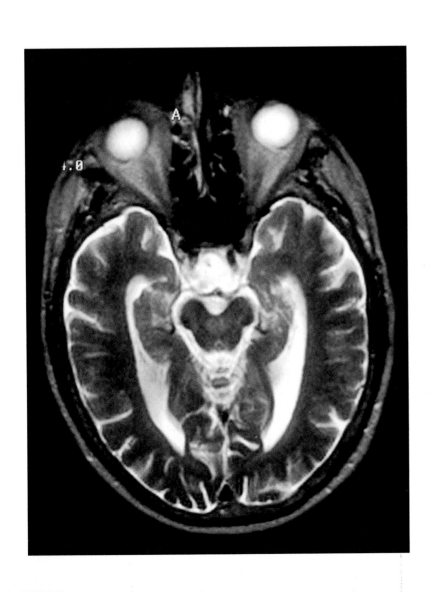

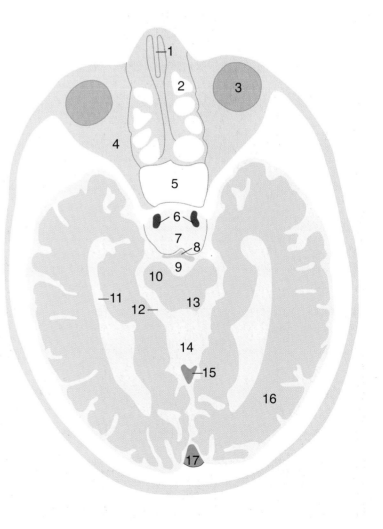

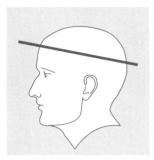

T1 weighted axial MR of the brain

1 - Scalp
2 - Outer table of skull bone
3 - Diploë
4 - Frontal lobe
5 - Temporalis muscle
6 - Lateral sulcus
 (Sylvian fissure)
7 - Frontal operculum
8 - Temporal operculum
9 - Insula
10 - Third ventricle

11 - Interthalamic adhesion
12 - Temporal lobe
13 - Trigone of lateral ventricle
 (collateral trigone)
14 - Splenium of corpus
 callosum
15 - Inferior sagittal sinus and
 straight sinus
16 - Occipital lobe
17 - Superior sagittal sinus

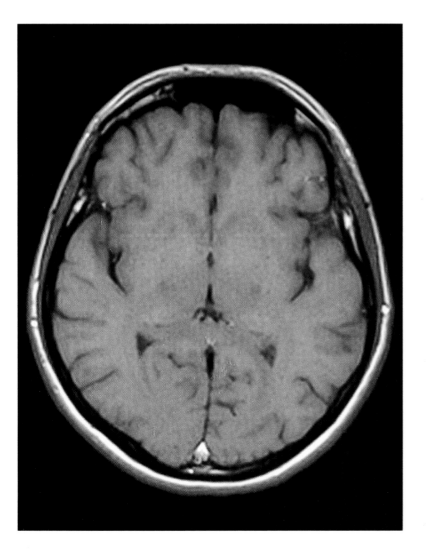

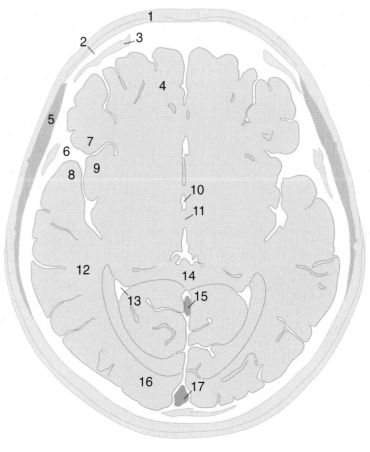

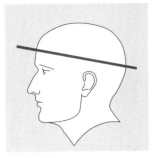

T1 weighted axial MR of the brain

1 - Orbit
2 - Frontal lobe
3 - Temporalis muscle
4 - Anterior cerebral artery
5 - Temporal operculum
6 - Lateral sulcus
　　(Sylvian fissure)
7 - Third ventricle
8 - Hypothalamus
9 - Posterior commissure

10 - Optic radiation
　　(geniculo-cortical
　　tract of Gratiolet)
11 - Calcar avis
12 - Calcarine fissure
13 - Internal cerebral vein
14 - Straight sinus
15 - Trigone of lateral ventricle
　　(collateral trigone)
16 - Superior sagittal sinus

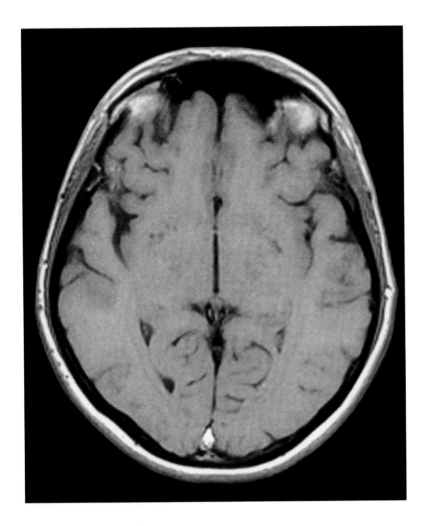

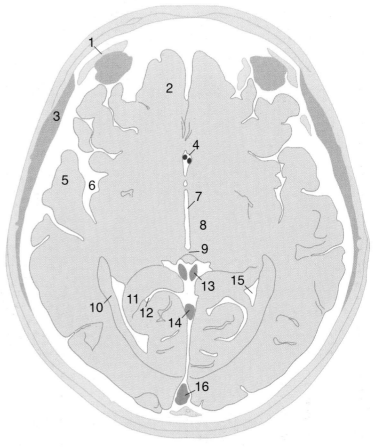

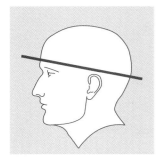

T1 weighted axial MR of the brain

1 - Orbit
2 - Gyrus rectus
3 - Temporalis muscle
4 - Optic tract
5 - Hypothalamus
6 - Crus cerebri
7 - Cerebral aqueduct

8 - Superior colliculus
    (midbrain)
9 - Internal cerebral vein
10 - Occipital lobe
11 - Straight sinus
12 - Superior sagittal sinus

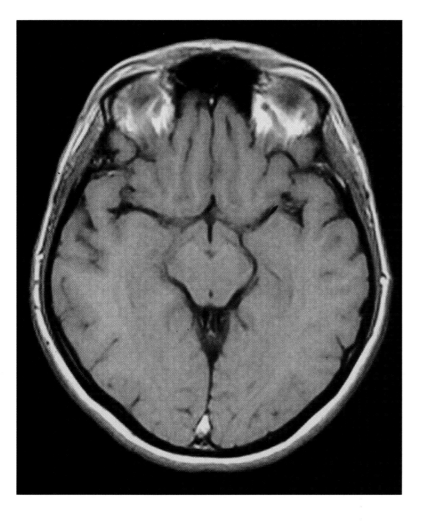

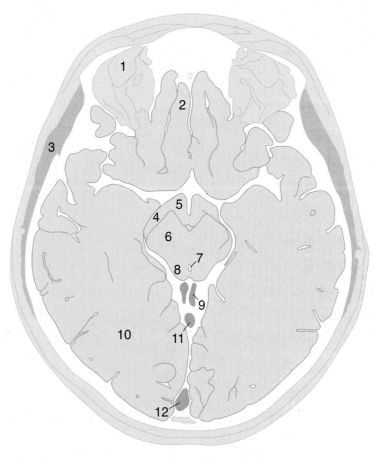

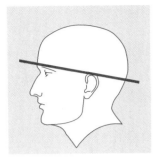

T1 weighted axial MR of the brain

1 - Eyeball
2 - Nasal cavity
3 - Orbit
4 - Gyrus rectus
5 - Superior ophthalmic vein
6 - Optic chiasma
7 - Infundibulum

8 - Temporal lobe
9 - Interpeduncular fossa
10 - Crus cerebri
11 - Cerebral aqueduct
12 - Cerebellum
13 - Occipital lobe
14 - Superior sagittal sinus

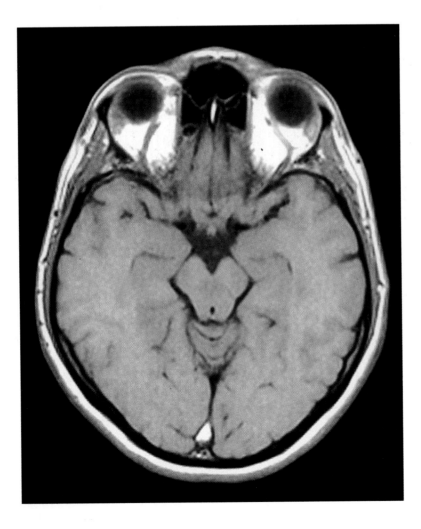

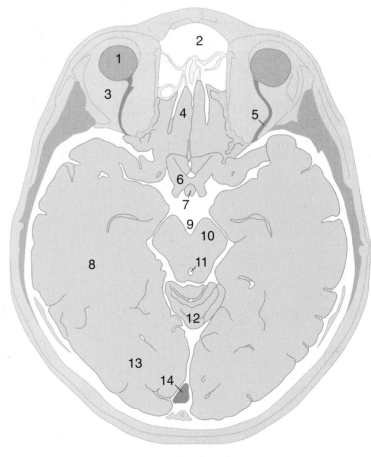

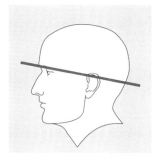

T1 weighted axial MR of the brain

1 - Eyeball
2 - Nasal cavity
3 - Optic nerve
4 - Sphenoidal sinus
5 - Extraocular muscle
6 - Temporal lobe

7 - Ophthalmic artery
8 - Sella turcica
9 - Pons
10 - Fourth ventricle
11 - Vermis of cerebellum
12 - Occipital lobe

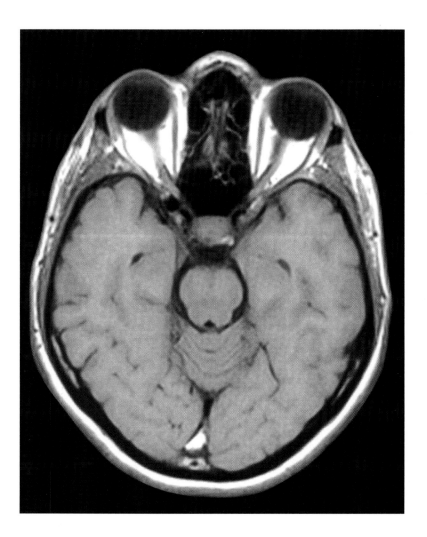

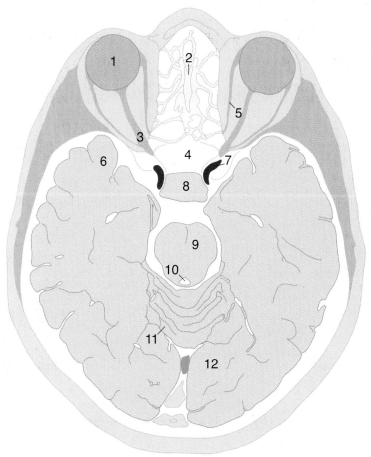

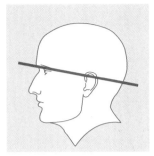

T1 weighted axial MR of the brain

1 - Lens of the eye
2 - Nasal septum
3 - Rectus lateralis muscle
4 - Rectus medialis muscle
5 - Spheno-ethmoidal recess
6 - Sphenoidal sinus
7 - Temporal pole
8 - Sella turcica and
pituitary gland

9 - Internal carotid artery
10 - Dorsum sellae
11 - Pons
12 - Cisterna ambiens
13 - Pinna of the ear
14 - Fourth ventricle
15 - Vermis of cerebellum
16 - Superior sagittal sinus
17 - Occipital lobe

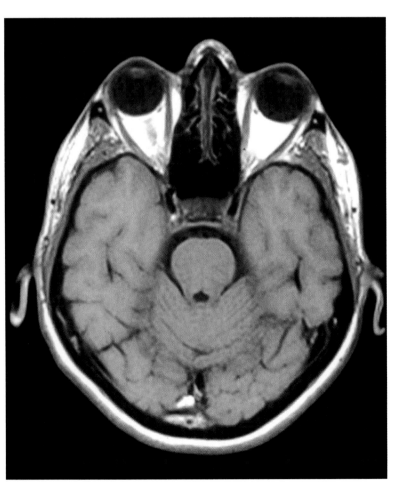

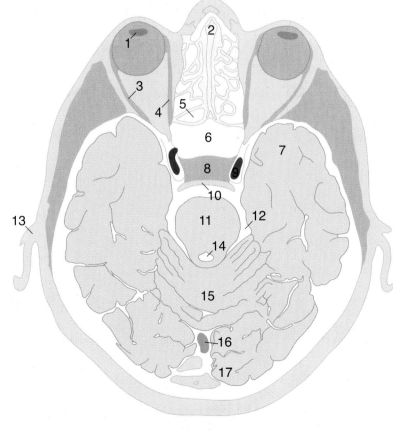

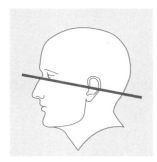

T1 weighted axial MR of the brain

1 - Eyeball
2 - Orbit
3 - Ethmoidal air cells
4 - Temporal pole
5 - Sphenoidal sinus
6 - Internal carotid artery
7 - Clivus
8 - Basilar artery
9 - Trigeminal nerve
10 - Pons

11 - Middle cerebellar peduncle (brachium pontis)
12 - Fourth ventricle
13 - Pinna of the ear
14 - Cerebellar hemisphere
15 - Vermis of cerebellum
16 - Confluence of venous sinuses (torcular Herophili)
17 - Internal occipital protuberance

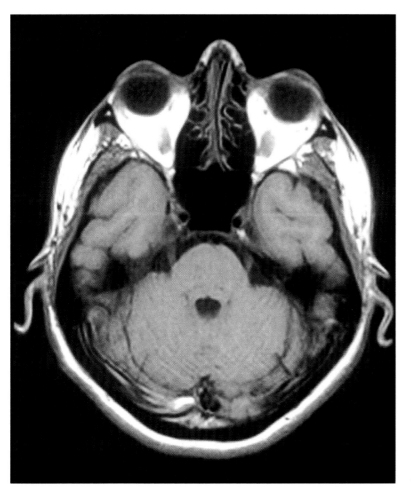

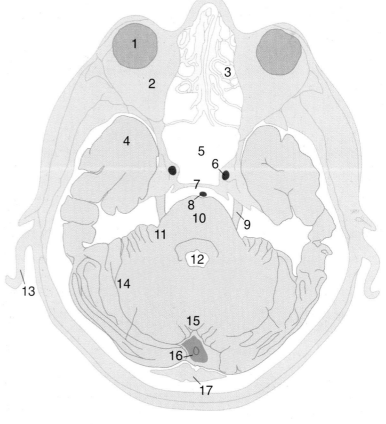

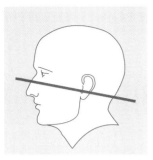

T1 weighted axial MR of the brain

1 - Nasal septum
2 - Nasolacrimal duct
3 - Zygomatic bone
4 - Maxillary sinus
    (of Highmore)
5 - Lateral pterygoid muscle
6 - Sphenoidal sinus
7 - Auditory tube
8 - Internal carotid artery

9 - Petrous temporal bone
10 - Prepontine cisterna
11 - Concha of ear
12 - Pons
13 - Fourth ventricle
14 - Cerebellar hemisphere
15 - Vermis of cerebellum
16 - Internal occipital crest

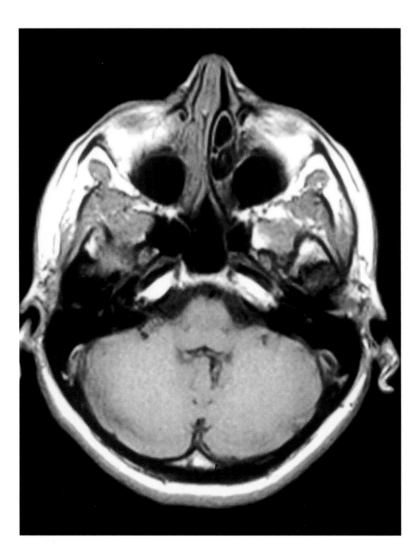

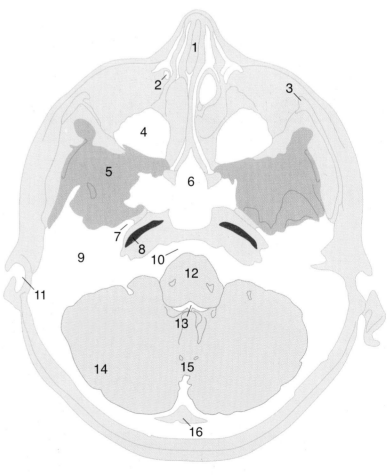

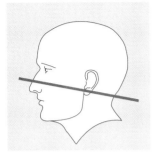

T1 weighted axial MR of the brain

1 - Nasal septum
2 - Inferior nasal concha
3 - Nasolacrimal duct
4 - Middle nasal concha
5 - Maxillary sinus
    (of Highmore)
6 - Masseter muscle
7 - Lateral pterygoid muscle
8 - Tensor veli palatini
    muscle
9 - Head of mandible
10 - Longus capitis muscle
11 - Auditory tube
12 - Internal carotid artery
13 - Occipital bone,
    basilar part
14 - Mastoid air cells
15 - External acoustic meatus
16 - Medulla oblongata
17 - Tonsilla of cerebellum
18 - Vermis of cerebellum

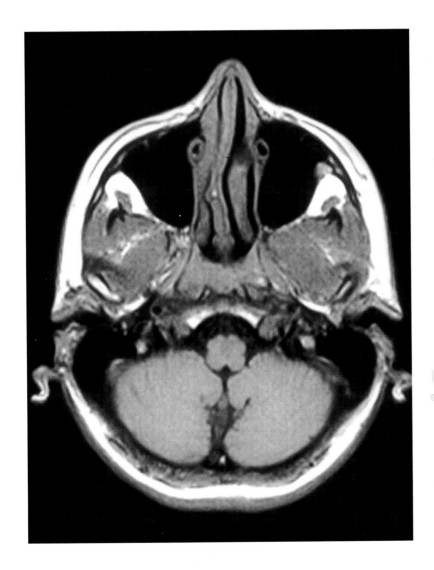

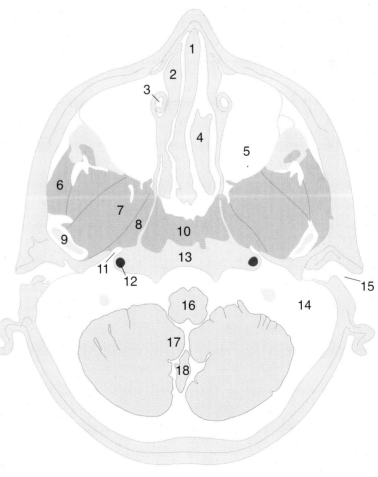

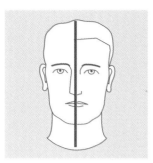

Sagittal MR of brain

1 - Skull bone
2 - Subdural and subarachnoid spaces
3 - Cortical vein
4 - Medial frontal gyrus
5 - Paracentral lobule
6 - Cingulate gyrus
7 - Cingulate sulcus
8 - Precuneus
9 - Genu of corpus callosum
10 - Trunk of corpus callosum
11 - Frontal sinus
12 - Rostrum of corpus callosum
13 - Lateral ventricle
14 - Fornix
15 - Anterior cerebral artery
16 - Thalamus
17 - Splenium of corpus callosum
18 - Parieto-occipital sulcus
19 - Sphenoidal sinus
20 - Pituitary gland and sella turcica
21 - Optic chiasma in suprasellar cisterna
22 - Interpeduncular fossa
23 - Tectum of mesencephalon
24 - Tentorium cerebelli
25 - Calcarine fissure
26 - Basilar artery
27 - Pons
28 - Fourth ventricle
29 - Cuneus
30 - Medulla oblongata
31 - Vermis of cerebellum (arbor vitae)
32 - Confluence of venous sinuses
33 - Cerebellomedullary cistern
34 - Spinal cord

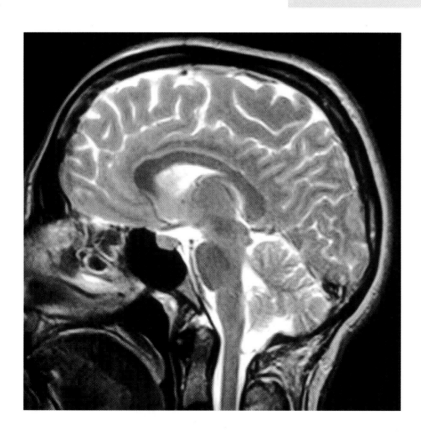

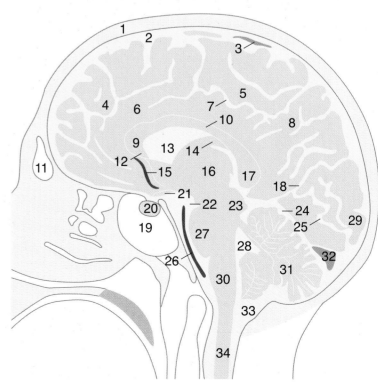

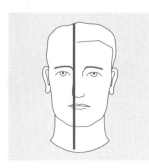

Sagittal MR of brain

1 - Skull bone
2 - Subdural and
    subarachnoid spaces
3 - Frontal lobe
4 - Frontal horn of
    lateral ventricle
5 - Corpus callosum
6 - Body of lateral ventricle
7 - Precuneus

8 - Frontal sinus
9 - Head of caudate nucleus
10 - Thalamus
11 - Parieto-occipital fissure
12 - Cuneus
13 - Internal carotid artery
     (intracavernous part)
14 - Tentorium cerebelli
15 - Cerebellum

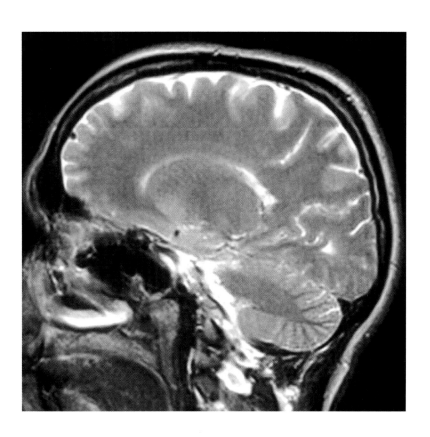

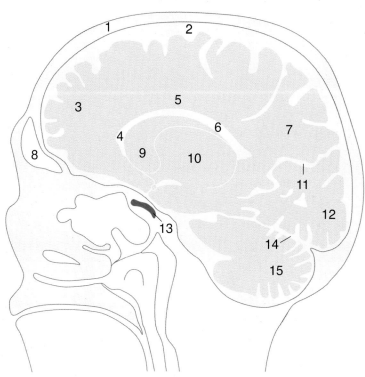

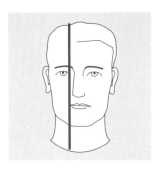

Sagittal MR of brain

1 - Skull bone
2 - Subdural and
    subarachnoid spaces
3 - Parietal lobe
4 - Frontal lobe
5 - Head of caudate nucleus
6 - Body of lateral ventricle
7 - Orbit
8 - Temporal horn of lateral
    ventricle

9 - Hippocampus
10 - Choroid plexus of lateral
     ventricle
11 - Occipital lobe
12 - White matter of
     cerebellum (medulla)
13 - Gray matter of cerebellum
     (cortex)

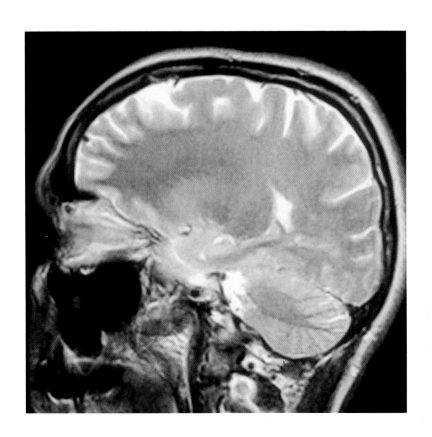

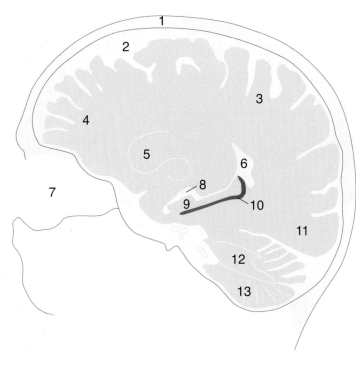

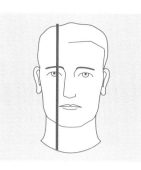

Sagittal MR of brain

1 - Skull bone
2 - Subdural and
    subarachnoid spaces
3 - Parietal lobe
4 - Frontal lobe
5 - Lentiform nucleus
6 - Tail of caudate nucleus
7 - Eyeball
8 - Rectus inferior muscle
9 - Optic nerve
10 - Temporal pole
11 - Temporal horn of lateral
     ventricle
12 - Hippocampus
13 - Occipital horn of lateral
     ventricle
14 - Tentorium cerebelli
15 - Cerebellum (cortex)
16 - Cerebellum (medulla)

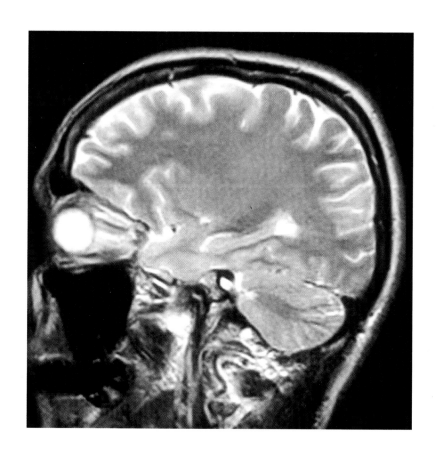

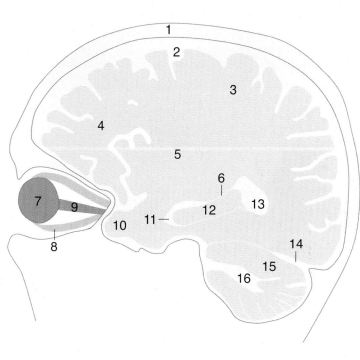

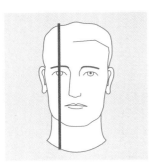

Sagittal MR of brain

1 - Skull bone
2 - Subdural and
   subarachnoid spaces
3 - Frontal lobe
4 - Frontal operculum
5 - Lateral (Sylvian) sulcus
6 - Insular gyri

7 - Parietal lobe
8 - Eyeball
9 - Orbit (maxilla)
10 - Temporal lobe
11 - Occipital lobe
12 - Tentorium cerebelli
13 - Cerebellum

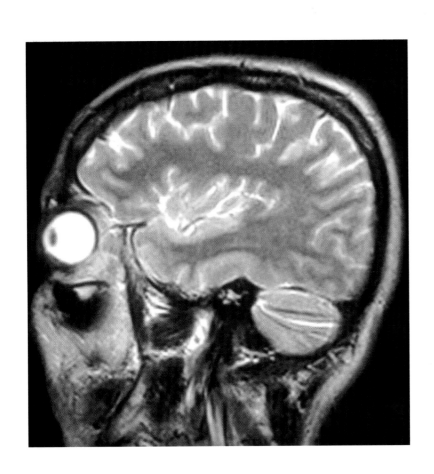

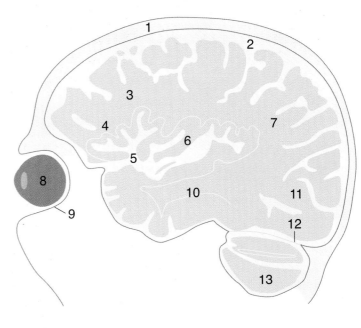

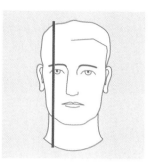

Sagittal MR of brain

1 - Skull bone
2 - Subdural and
    subarachnoid spaces
3 - Frontal lobe
4 - Parietal lobe

5 - Eyeball
6 - Lateral (Sylvian) sulcus
7 - Temporal lobe
8 - Occipital lobe
9 - Cerebellum

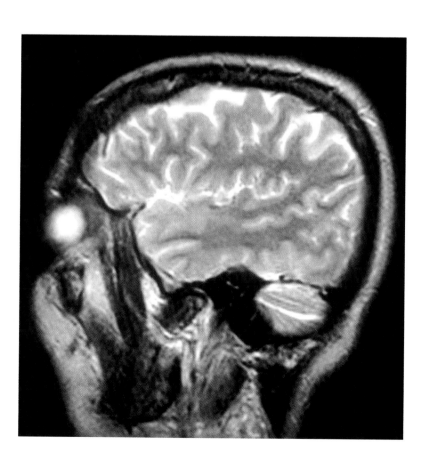

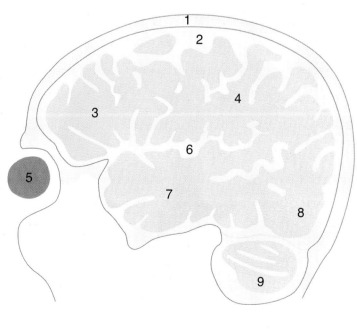

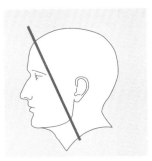

Coronal MR of brain

1 - Skull bone
2 - Subdural and
    subarachnoid spaces
3 - Longitudinal cerebral
    fissure and falx cerebri
4 - Frontal lobe

5 - Orbital gyri
6 - Ala minor (lesser wing)
    of sphenoid
7 - Temporal pole
8 - Sphenoidal sinus
9 - Gyrus rectus

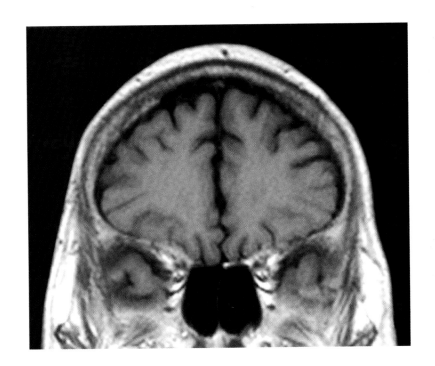

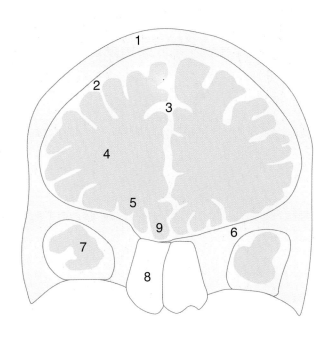

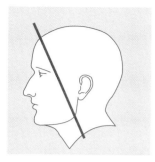

Coronal MR of brain

1 - Skull bone
2 - Subdural and
    subarachnoid spaces
3 - Frontal lobe
4 - Longitudinal cerebral
    fissure and falx cerebri

5 - Genu of corpus callosum
6 - Frontal horn of lateral
    ventricle
7 - Gyrus rectus
8 - Temporal lobe
9 - Sphenoidal sinus

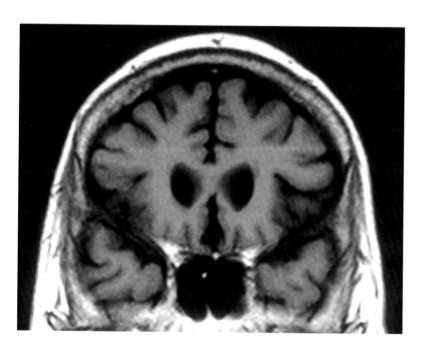

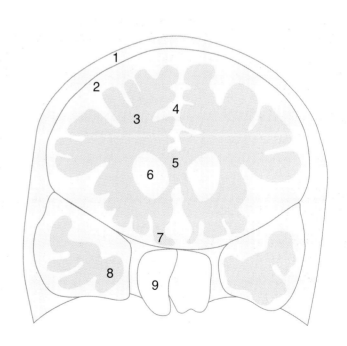

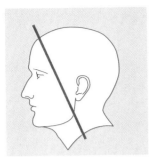

Coronal MR of brain

1 - Skull bone
2 - Subdural and subarachnoid spaces
3 - Frontal lobe
4 - Longitudinal cerebral fissure and falx cerebri
5 - Corpus callosum
6 - Frontal horn of lateral ventricle
7 - Septum pellucidum
8 - Frontal operculum
9 - Lateral (Sylvian) sulcus
10 - Insula
11 - Temporal operculum
12 - Rostrum of corpus callosum
13 - Optic chiasma in suprasellar cisterna
14 - Anterior clinoid process
15 - Temporal lobe
16 - Pituitary gland in sella turcica
17 - Internal carotid artery (intracavernous part)
18 - Internal carotid artery in carotid canal and groove

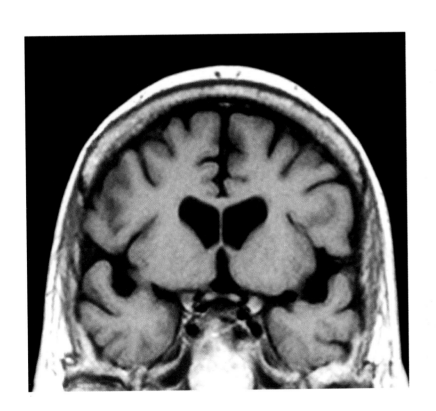

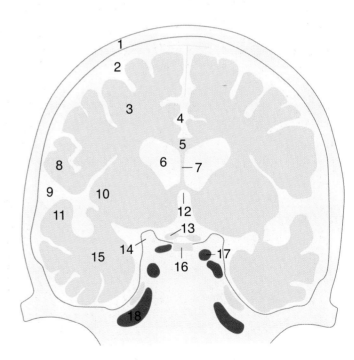

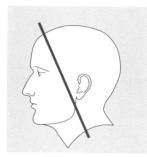

Coronal MR of brain

1 - Skull bone
2 - Subdural and subarachnoid spaces
3 - Frontal lobe
4 - Falx cerebri
5 - Corpus callosum
6 - Frontal horn of lateral ventricle
7 - Frontal operculum
8 - Lateral (Sylvian) sulcus
9 - Insula
10 - Septa pellucida
11 - Column of fornix

12 - Triangular recess of third ventricle
13 - Anterior commissure
14 - Temporal operculum
15 - Optic tract
16 - Optic recess of third ventricle
17 - Pituitary stalk in suprasellar cisterna
18 - Temporal lobe
19 - Trigeminal ganglion in Meckel's cave
20 - Internal carotid artery

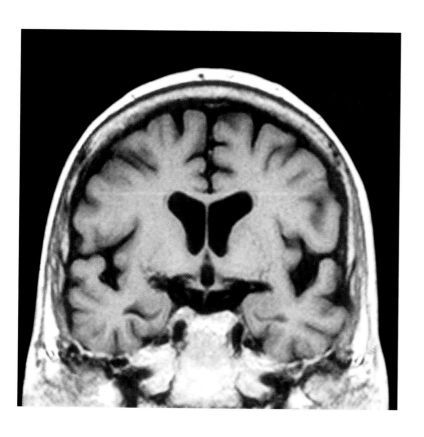

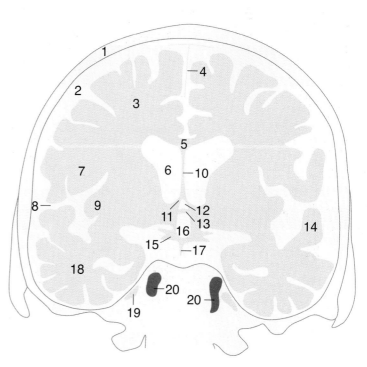

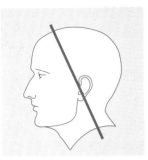

Coronal MR of brain

1 - Skull bone
2 - Subdural and subarachnoid spaces
3 - Falx cerebri
4 - Lateral ventricle
5 - Septa pellucida
6 - Frontal operculum
7 - Lateral (Sylvian) sulcus
8 - Temporal operculum
9 - Insula
10 - Choroid plexus of lateral ventricle

11 - Fornices
12 - Interventricular foramen (of Monro)
13 - Third ventricle
14 - Temporal lobe
15 - Collateral eminence
16 - Pes hippocampi
17 - Pons
18 - Basilar artery
19 - Temporal horn of lateral ventricle
20 - Collateral sulcus

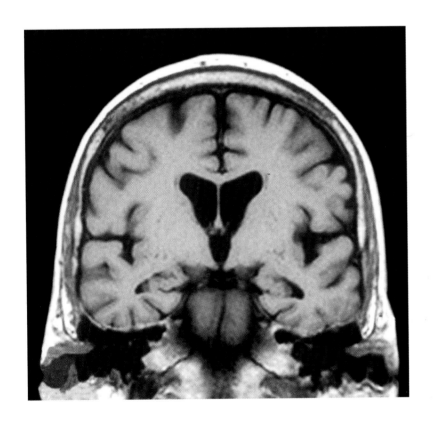

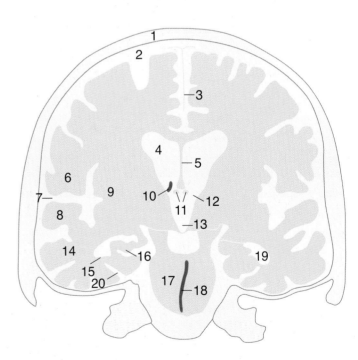

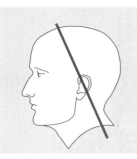

Coronal MR of brain

1 - Skull bone
2 - Subdural and subarachnoid spaces
3 - Superior sagittal sinus
4 - Falx cerebri
5 - Lateral ventricle
6 - Septa pellucida
7 - Lateral (Sylvian) sulcus
8 - Insula
9 - Choroid plexus of lateral ventricle
10 - Fornices
11 - Tela choroidea of third ventricle
12 - Third ventricle
13 - Thalamus
14 - Temporal lobe
15 - Hippocampus (Ammon's horn)
16 - Fimbria of hippocampus
17 - Interpeduncular fossa
18 - Choroid plexus in the temporal horn of lateral ventricle
19 - Temporal horn of lateral ventricle
20 - Hippocampal sulcus
21 - Pons
22 - Parahippocampal gyrus
23 - Collateral sulcus
24 - Medulla oblongata

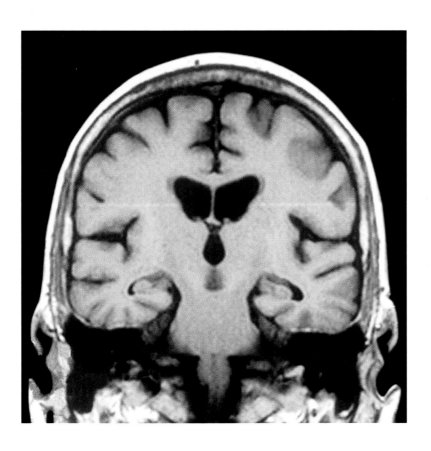

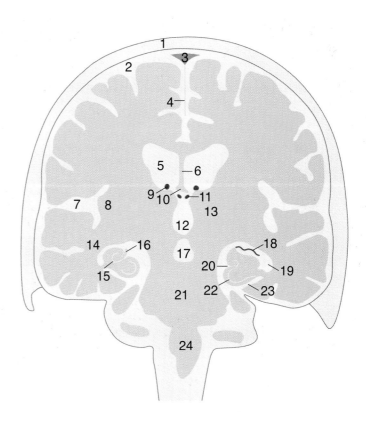

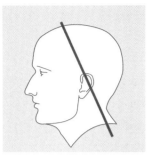

Coronal MR of brain

1 - Skull bone
2 - Subdural and subarachnoid spaces
3 - Superior sagittal sinus
4 - Falx cerebri
5 - Corpus callosum
6 - Lateral ventricle
7 - Fornix
8 - Choroidal fissure
9 - Choroid plexus of lateral ventricle
10 - Lateral (Sylvian) sulcus
11 - Thalamus
12 - Temporal lobe
13 - Hypothalamic sulcus
14 - Third ventricle
15 - Hypothalamus
16 - Subiculum
17 - Hippocampus (Ammon's horn)
18 - Fimbria of hippocampus
19 - Temporal horn of lateral ventricle
20 - Middle cerebellar peduncle
21 - Pontine raphe
22 - Medulla oblongata
23 - Superior temporal gyrus
24 - Middle temporal gyrus
25 - Inferior temporal gyrus
26 - Occipito-temporal gyrus

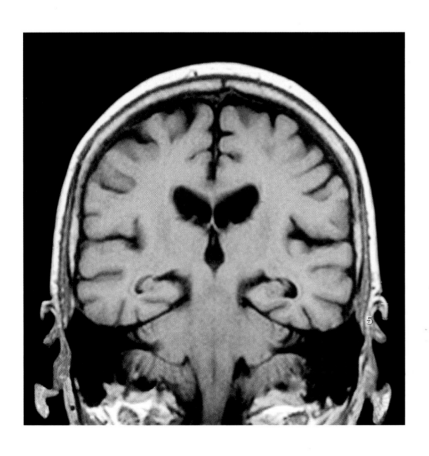

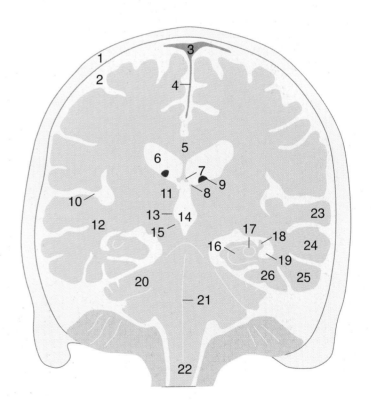

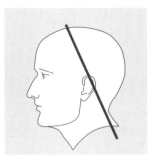

Coronal MR of brain

1 - Skull bone
2 - Subdural space
3 - Superior sagittal sinus and dura mater
4 - Subarachnoid space
5 - Falx cerebri
6 - Parietal lobe
7 - Body of lateral ventricle
8 - Crus of fornix
9 - Choroid plexus
10 - Pineal body and suprapineal recess
11 - Pulvinar of thalamus
12 - Temporal lobe
13 - Superior colliculus
14 - Inferior colliculus
15 - Temporal horn of lateral ventricle
16 - Superior cerebellar peduncle
17 - Fourth ventricle
18 - Tentorium cerebelli
19 - Vermis of cerebellum
20 - Hemisphere of cerebellum

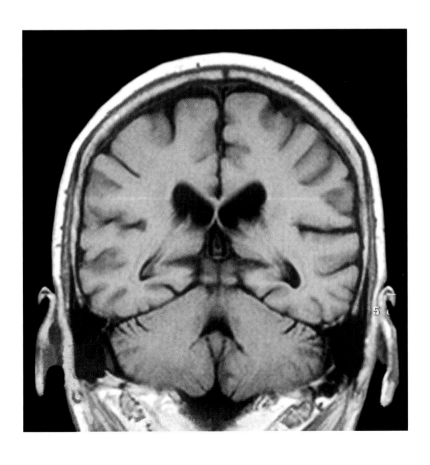

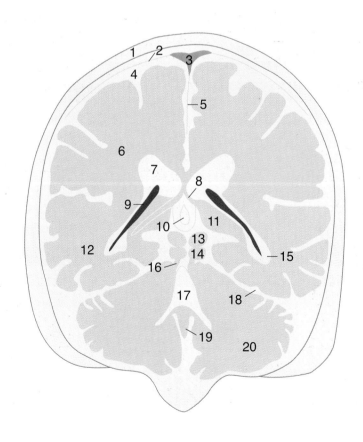

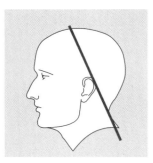

Coronal MR of brain

1 - Skull bone
2 - Superior sagittal sinus
3 - Dura mater
4 - Falx cerebri
5 - Parietal lobe
6 - Body of lateral ventricle
7 - Splenium of corpus callosum
8 - Choroid plexus (glomus choroideum) of lateral ventricle

9 - Temporal lobe
10 - Temporal horn of lateral ventricle
11 - Tentorium cerebelli
12 - Vermis of cerebellum
13 - Hemisphere of cerebellum
14 - Vallecula

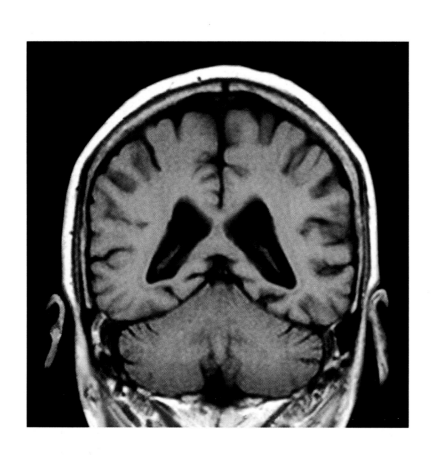

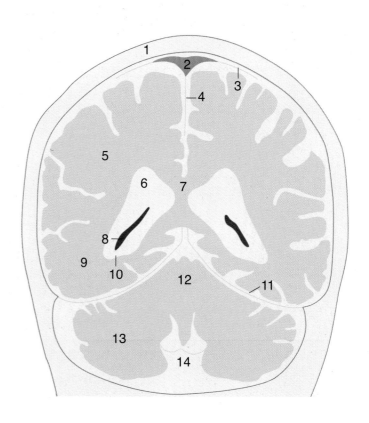

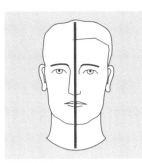

Sagittal MR of sella

1 - Frontal lobe
2 - Corpus callosum, rostrum
3 - Corpus callosum, genu
4 - Corpus callosum, body (trunk)
5 - Corpus callosum, splenium
6 - Septum pellucidum
7 - Fornix
8 - Internal cerebral vein
9 - Great cerebral vein (of Galen)
10 - Straight sinus
11 - Optic chiasma
12 - Thalamus
13 - Mamillary body
14 - Interpeduncular fossa and cistern
15 - Habenular commissure
16 - Posterior commissure
17 - Cerebral aqueduct
18 - Mesencephalon
19 - Tectum (corpora quadrigemina)
20 - Nasal cavity (septum)
21 - Sphenoidal sinus
22 - Clivus
23 - Pons
24 - Fourth ventricle
25 - Cerebellum
26 - Nasopharynx
27 - Medulla oblongata
28 - Oral cavity
29 - Soft palate
30 - Dens of axis
31 - Spinal cord

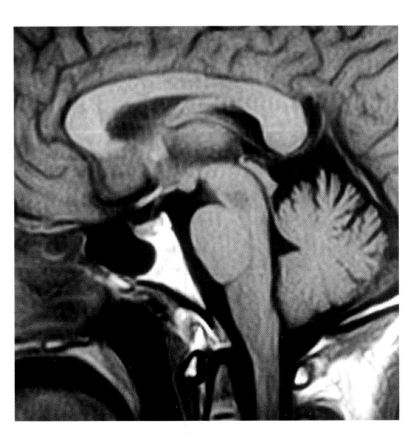

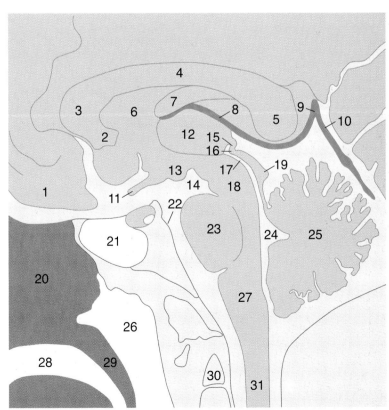

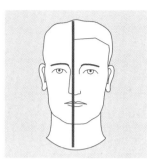

Sagittal MR of sella

1 - Frontal lobe
2 - Cingulate gyrus
3 - Corpus callosum, genu
4 - Corpus callosum, body (trunk)
5 - Corpus callosum, splenium
6 - Septum pellucidum
7 - Fornix
8 - Internal cerebral vein
9 - Thalamus
10 - Optic chiasma
11 - Lamina terminalis
12 - Optic recess
13 - Mamillary body
14 - Third ventricle
15 - Mesencephalon
16 - Superior colliculus

17 - Inferior colliculus
18 - Tentorium cerebelli
19 - Anterior lobe of pituitary gland
20 - Posterior lobe of pituitary gland
21 - Interpeduncular fossa and cistern
22 - Pons
23 - Fourth ventricle
24 - Cerebellum
25 - Nasal cavity (septum)
26 - Sphenoidal sinus
27 - Clivus
28 - Nasopharynx
29 - Soft palate
30 - Cerebellomedullary cistern (cisterna magna)

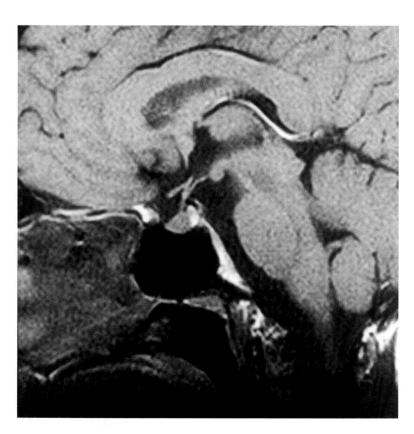

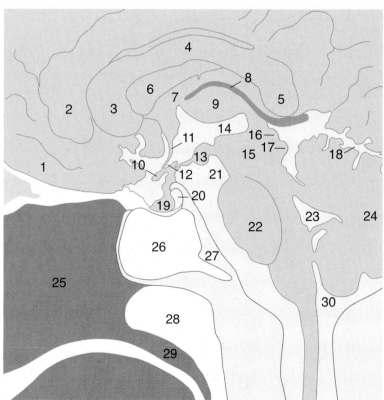

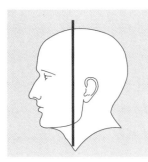

Coronal MR of sella

1 - Corpus callosum
2 - Frontal horn of lateral ventricle
3 - Septum pellucidum
4 - Vein of septum pellucidum
5 - Optic recess of third ventricle
6 - Optic chiasma
7 - Stalk of pituitary gland
8 - Posterior clinoid process
9 - Trigeminal cave (of Meckel)

10 - Pituitary gland (posterior lobe)
11 - Internal carotid artery
12 - Cavernous sinus
13 - Sphenoidal sinus
14 - Roof of pharynx
15 - Nasopharynx
16 - Pharyngeal opening of auditory tube (Rosenmuller's fossa)
17 - Lateral pterygoid muscle

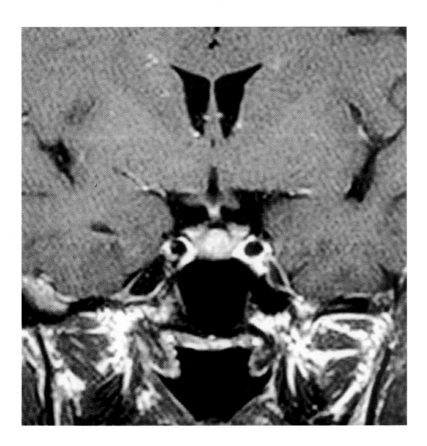

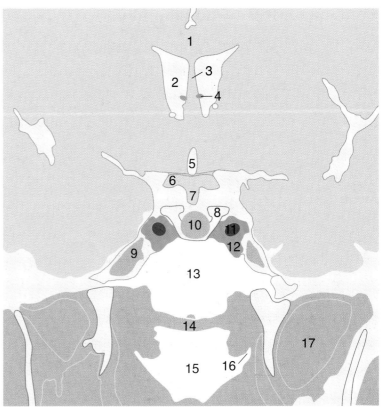

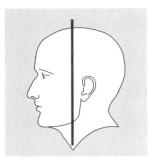

Coronal MR of sella

1 - Corpus callosum
2 - Frontal horn of lateral
    ventricle
3 - Septum pellucidum
4 - Interventricular foramen
    (of Monro)
5 - Third ventricle
6 - Floor of the third
    ventricle
7 - Optic tract
8 - Trigeminal cave
    (of Meckel)

9 - Dorsum sellae
10 - Sphenoidal sinus
11 - Internal carotid artery
12 - Roof of pharynx
13 - Nasopharynx
14 - Pterygoid process
15 - Lateral pterygoid muscle
16 - Pharyngeal opening of
    auditory tube
    (Rosenmuller's fossa)

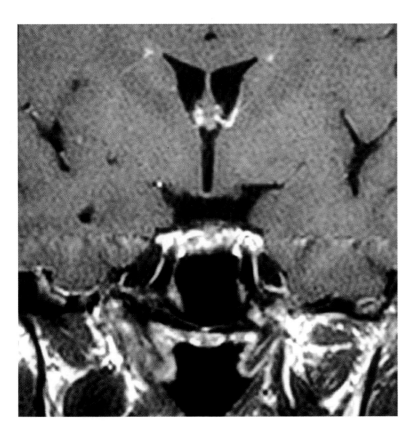

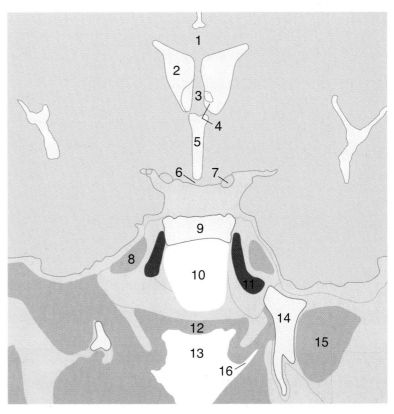

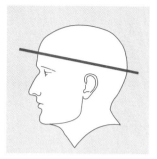

Axial MR of internal capsule

1 - Subcutaneous fat
2 - Longitudinal cerebral fissure
3 - Frontal horn of lateral ventricle
4 - Frontal operculum
5 - Temporal operculum
6 - Lateral (Sylvian) sulcus
7 - Insula
8 - Extreme capsule
9 - Claustrum
10 - External capsule
11 - Lentiform nucleus (putamen)
12 - Head of caudate nucleus
13 - Thalamus

14 - Internal capsule (anterior limb)
15 - Internal capsule (genu)
16 - Internal capsule (posterior limb)
17 - Corpus callosum (rostrum)
18 - Pericallosal cisterna
19 - Columns of fornix
20 - Third ventricle and internal cerebral veins
21 - Corpus callosum (splenium)
22 - Lateral ventricle
23 - Occipital lobe
24 - Superior sagittal sinus
25 - Subcallosal area

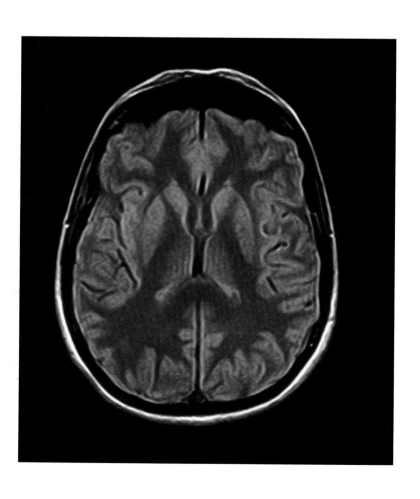

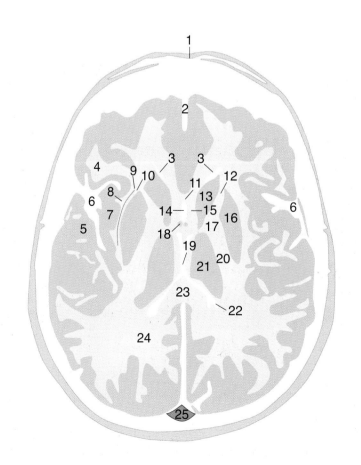

HEAD

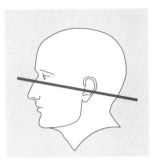

T2-weighted axial MR of the brain, facial and vestibulocochlear nerves

1 - Nasal cavity
2 - Eyeball
3 - Orbital fat
4 - Ethmoidal air cells
5 - Sphenoidal sinus
6 - Temporal lobe
7 - Internal carotid artery
8 - Basilar artery in prepontine cistern
9 - Petrous temporal bone
10 - Cochlea
11 - Vestibule and semicircular canals

12 - Facial nerve
13 - Vestibulocochlear nerve
14 - Internal acoustic meatus with evagination of subarachnoid space
15 - External acoustic meatus
16 - Cerebellar hemisphere
17 - Lateral recess of fourth ventricle
18 - Fourth ventricle
19 - Cerebellar vermis
20 - Sigmoid recess

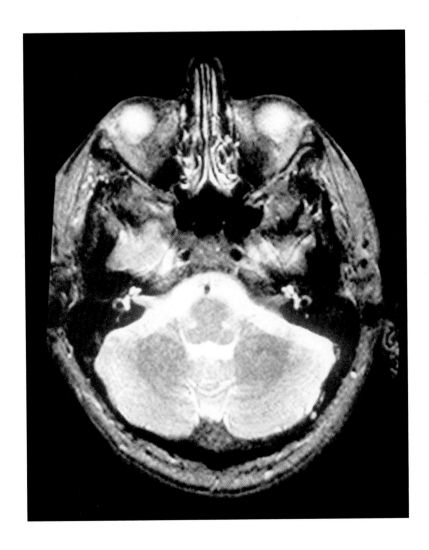

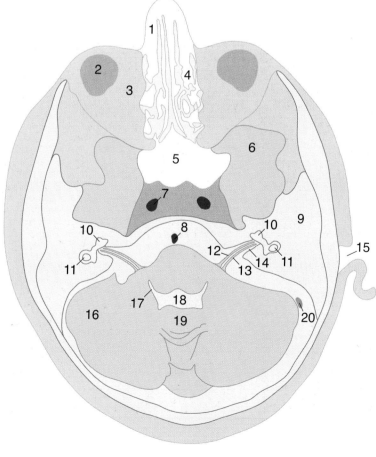

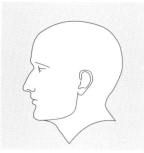

Arterial circle of Willis, CT angiography, 3D SSD reconstruction

1 - Anterior cerebral artery
2 - Anterior communicating
    artery (distended)
3 - Internal carotid artery
4 - Middle cerebral artery

5 - Posterior communicating
    artery
6 - Posterior cerebral artery
7 - Basilar artery

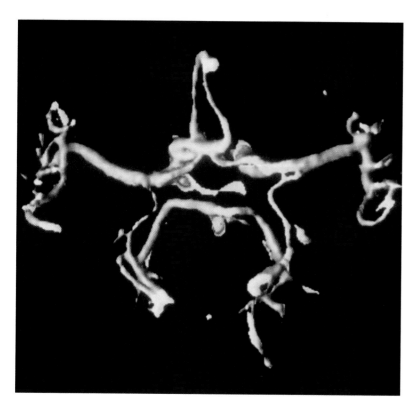

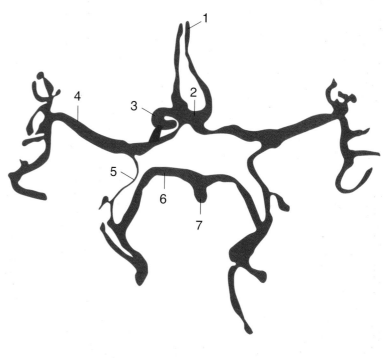

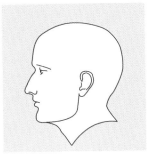

Internal carotid artery, digital subtraction arteriogram, lateral view

I. *Branches of the anterior cerebral artery*
1 - Frontal internal medial artery
2 - Frontal internal posterior artery
3 - Central artery
4 - Calloso-marginal artery
5 - Pericallosal artery
6 - Frontopolar artery
7 - Orbitofrontal artery
8 - Frontobasal artery
9 - Anterior cerebral artery

II. *Branches of the middle cerebral artery*
10 - Anterior and middle temporal arteries

11 - Posterior temporal artery
12 - Middle cerebral artery

III. *Branches of the internal carotid artery*
13 - Anterior choroid artery
14 - Ophthalmic artery
15 - Carotid syphon
16 - Internal carotid artery

IV. *Branches of external carotid artery*
17 - Superficial temporal artery
18 - Ascending palatine artery (from facial artery)
19 - Facial artery
20 - Occipital artery
21 - External carotid artery

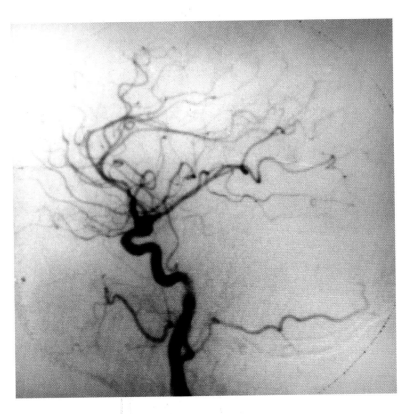

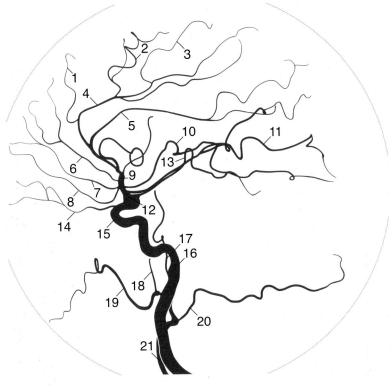

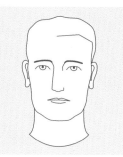

Internal carotid arteriogram, anteroposterior view

I. *Branches of the anterior cerebral artery*
1 - Pericallosal artery
2 - Callosomarginal artery
3 - Post-communicating portion of anterior cerebral artery
4 - Pre-communicating portion of anterior cerebral artery

II. *Branches of the middle cerebral artery*
5 - Posterior parietal branches
6 - Opercular portion
7 - Insular portion
8 - Sphenoid portion

III. *Parts of the internal carotid artery*
9 - Carotid syphon
10 - Petrous portion
11 - Cervical portion

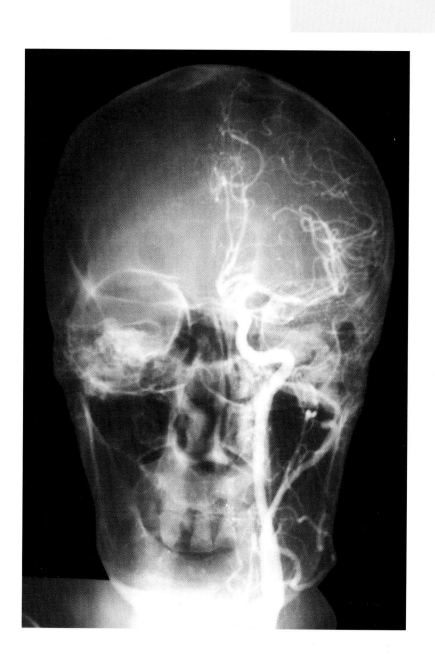

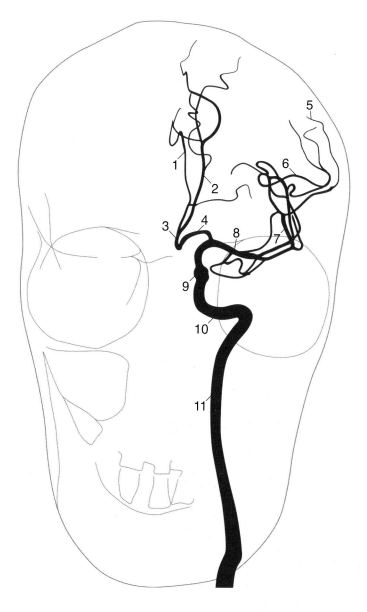

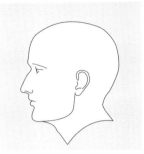

Angiogram of vertebral artery, lateral view

I. Branches of the basilar artery

1 - Parieto-occipital branches

2 - Right posterior cerebral artery

3 - Perforating thalamic artery

4 - Left posterior cerebral artery

5 - Internal occipital (calcarine) artery

6 - Superior cerebellar artery

7 - Inferior anterior cerebellar artery

8 - Basilar artery

II. Branches and portions of vertebral artery

9 - Inferior posterior cerebellar artery

10 - Loop between the transverse foramina of atlas and axis

11 - Ascending part

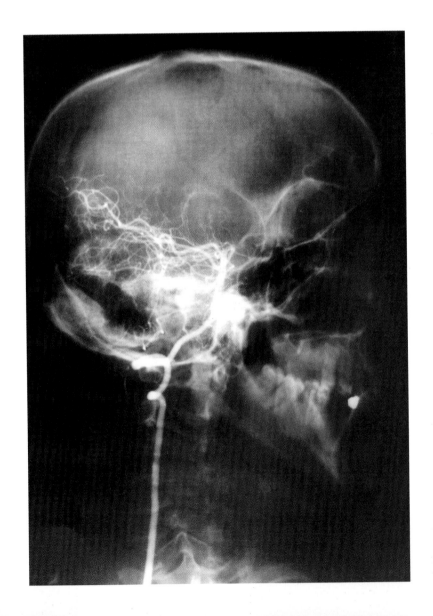

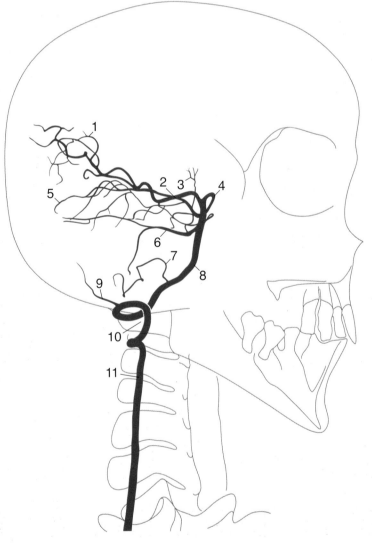

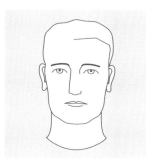

Angiogram of vertebral artery, anteroposterior view

I. Branches of the basilar artery

1 - Occipital branches
2 - Superior cerebellar artery
3 - Perforating thalamic branches
4 - Posterior cerebral artery
5 - Basilar artery
6 - Anterior inferior cerebellar artery

II. Branches and portions of the vertebral artery

7 - Posterior inferior cerebellar artery
8 - Intracranial part of vertebral artery
9 - Loop between transverse foramina of atlas and axis
10 - Ascending part of vertebral artery

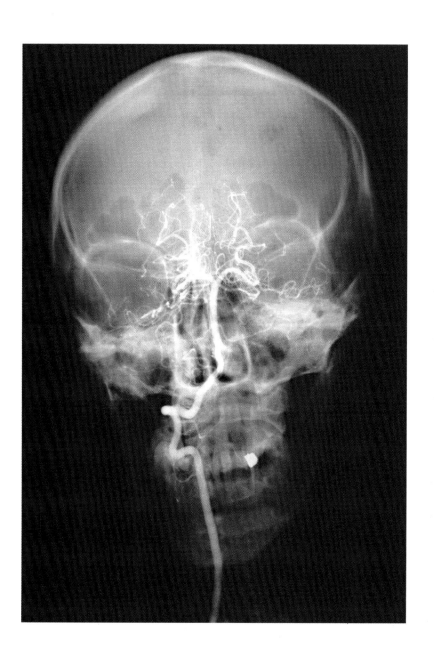

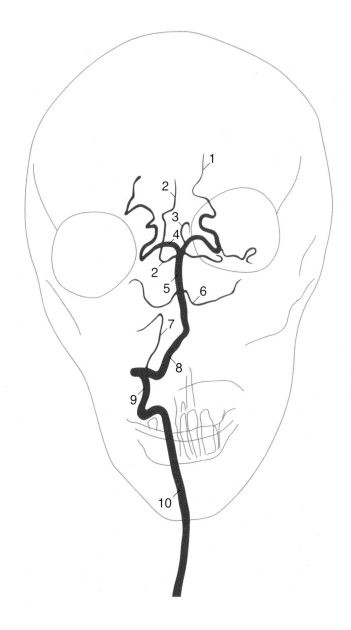

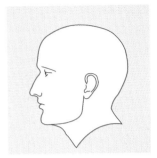

Intracranial veins and venous sinuses, digital subtraction venogram, early phase, lateral view

1 - Superior sagittal sinus
2 - Superficial cerebral veins
3 - Dorsal vein of corpus callosum
4 - Vein of septum pellucidum
5 - Thalamostriate vein
6 - Internal cerebral vein

7 - Great cerebral vein (of Galen)
8 - Basal vein (of Rosenthal)
9 - Straight sinus
10 - Temporo-occipital veins (vein of Labbé)
11 - Confluence of sinuses

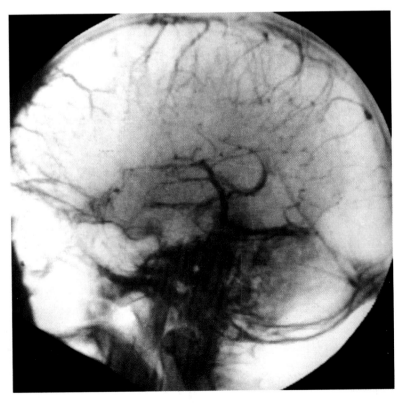

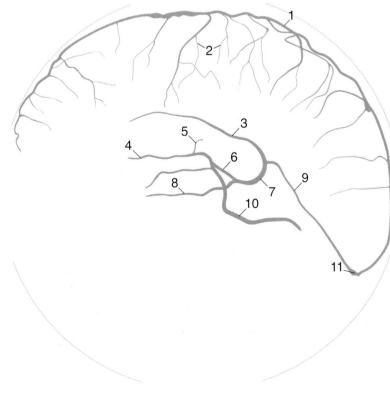

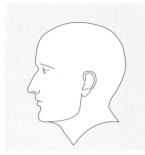

Intracranial veins and venous sinuses, digital subtraction venogram, late phase, lateral view

1 - Superior sagittal sinus
2 - Superficial cerebral veins
3 - Dorsal vein of corpus callosum
4 - Vein of septum pellucidum
5 - Thalamostriate vein
6 - Internal cerebral vein
7 - Great cerebral vein (of Galen)

8 - Basal vein (of Rosenthal)
9 - Temporo-occipital veins (vein of Labbé)
10 - Straight sinus
11 - Confluence of sinuses
12 - Transverse sinus
13 - Sigmoid sinus
14 - Internal jugular vein

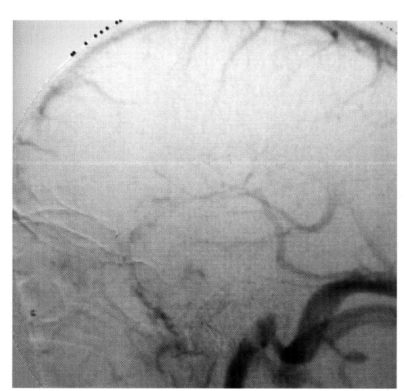

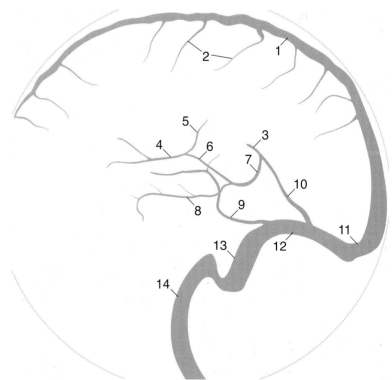

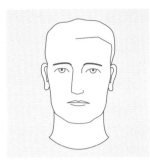

Intracranial veins and venous sinuses, digital subtraction venogram, late phase, anteroposterior view

1 - Superior sagittal sinus
2 - Superficial cerebral veins
3 - Confluence of sinuses
4 - Transverse sinus
5 - Sigmoid sinus
6 - Jugular bulb
7 - Internal jugular vein

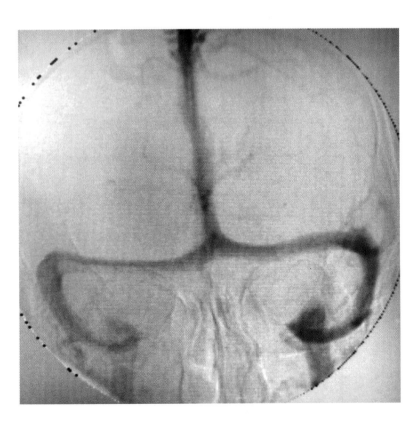
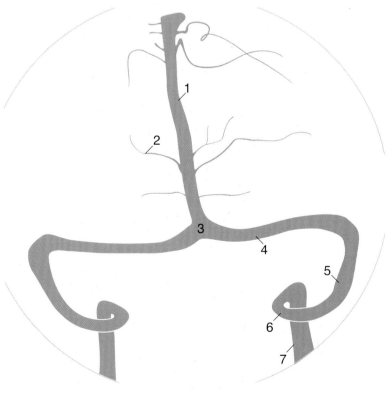

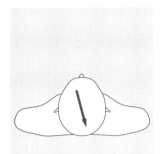

Ultrasonograms of infant brain
A – oblique sagittal view, B – midsagittal view.

1 - Frontal lobe
2 - Insular gyri
3 - Parietal lobe
4 - Temporal lobe
5 - Cingulate sulcus
6 - Cingulate gyrus
7 - Genu of corpus callosum
8 - Septum pellucidum and vein of septum pellucidum
9 - Body (trunk) of corpus callosum
10 - Splenium of corpus callosum

11 - Fornix
12 - Third ventricle
13 - Thalamus
14 - Pituitary gland
15 - Interpeduncular fossa
16 - Cerebral aqueduct
17 - Tectum of mesencephalon
18 - Pons
19 - Fourth ventricle
20 - Cerebellum
21 - Tentorium cerebelli
22 - Medulla oblongata

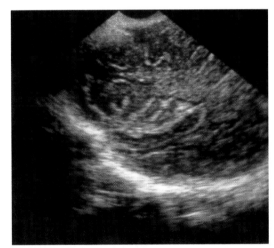
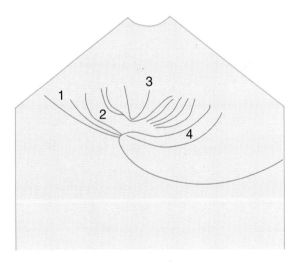
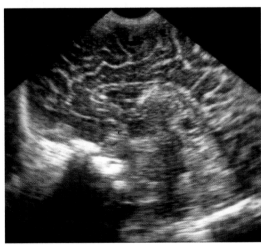
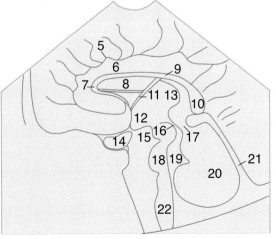

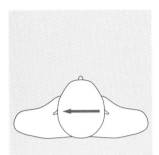

Ultrasonograms of infant brain
A – oblique coronal section through the body of lateral ventricle, B – oblique coronal section through the temporal horn of lateral ventricle.

1 - Falx cerebri
2 - Choroid plexus of lateral ventricle
3 - Cerebral hemisphere
4 - Cerebellum
5 - Corpus callosum
6 - Lateral ventricle

7 - Choroid plexus of lateral ventricle
8 - Thalamus
9 - Brainstem
10 - Choroid plexus of temporal horn

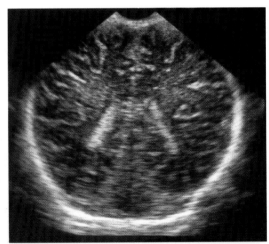

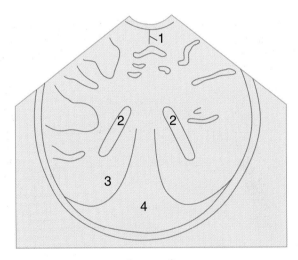

A

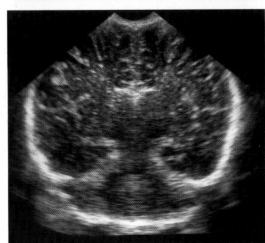

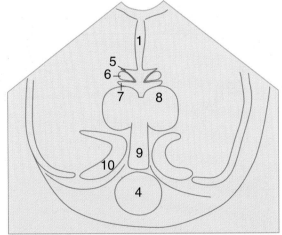

B

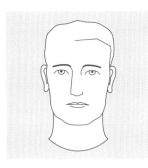

Perfusion SPECT study of the brain
A – colour-coded axial image at the level of the thalamus,
B – midsagittal image.
The radiopharmacon is accumulated in amounts proportional
to the vascular perfusion of brain tissue. Highest level of
perfusion (marked by red colour) is observed in the gray
matter. Low perfusion is marked by blue colour.

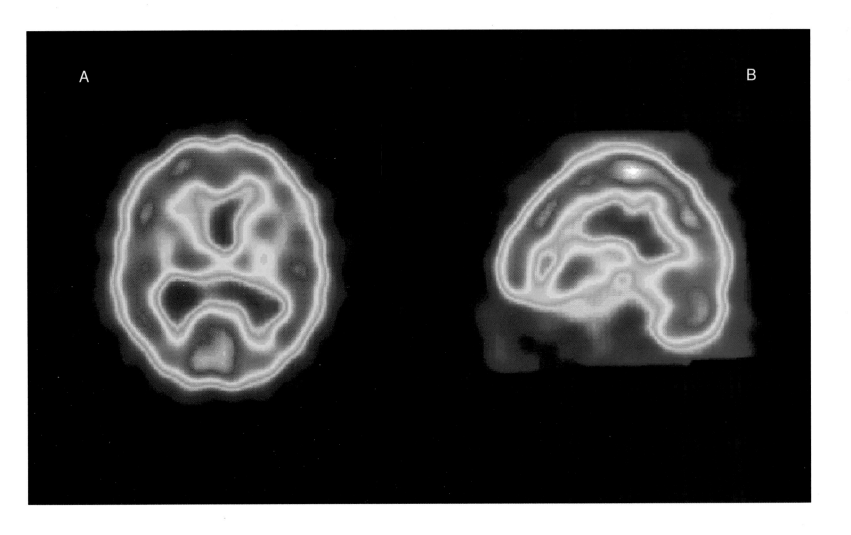

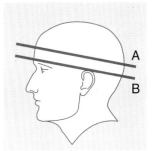

Visual cortical areas of the brain, axial view
Red: area V1 (striate cortex), yellow: area V2. Based on cytoarchitectonic maps superimposed over MR templates, standardised by computer (Roland et al., in: Human Brain Mapping, 1993). With the permission of Balazs Gulyas, Karolinska Institute, Stockholm. The images were made with the help of K. Amounts, B. Gulyas, J. Larsson, A. Malikovic, P.E. Roland and K. Zilles.

A

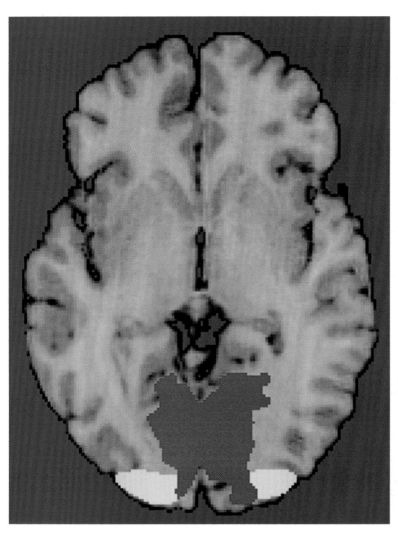

B

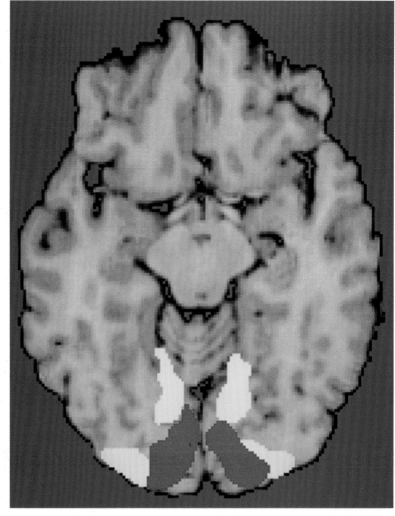

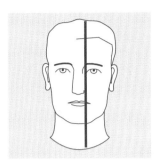

Visual cortical areas of the brain, midsagittal view
Red: area V1 (striate cortex), yellow: area V2. Based on cytoarchitectonic maps superimposed over MR templates, standardised by computer (Roland et al., in: Human Brain Mapping, 1993). With the permission of Balazs Gulyas, Karolinska Institute, Stockholm. The images were made with the help of K. Amounts, B. Gulyas, J. Larsson, A. Malikovic, P.E. Roland and K. Zilles.

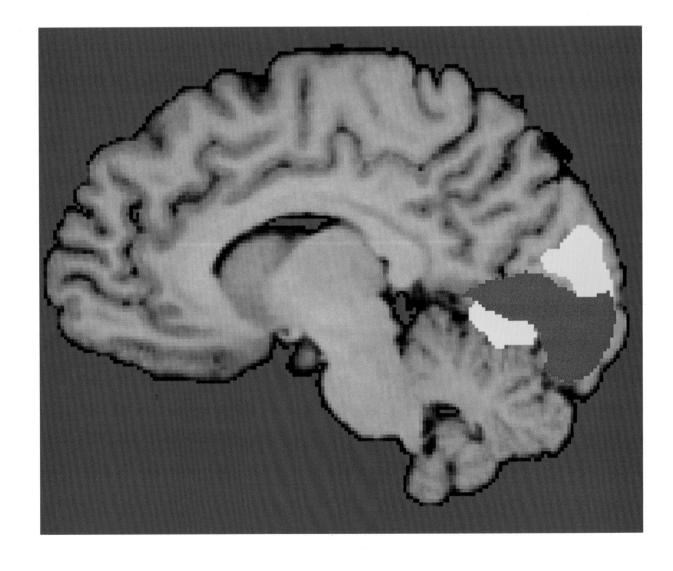

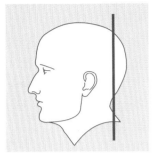

Visual cortical areas of the brain and PET activation, coronal view

A – image without PET activation, B – image with PET activation. Red: area V1 (striate cortex), yellow: area V2, blue – activation in V1 by form stimulation (associated with the central field of vision), green – similar activation in V2. Based on cytoarchitectonic maps superimposed over MR templates, standardised by computer (Roland et al., in: Human Brain Mapping, 1993). With the permission of Balazs Gulyas, Karolinska Institute, Stockholm. The images were made with the help of K. Amounts, B. Gulyas, J. Larsson, A. Malikovic, P.E. Roland and K. Zilles. PET activation was measured by perfusion tracer (butanol) as described by Gulyas et al. (1998), Human Brain Mapping 6: 115-127.

A

B

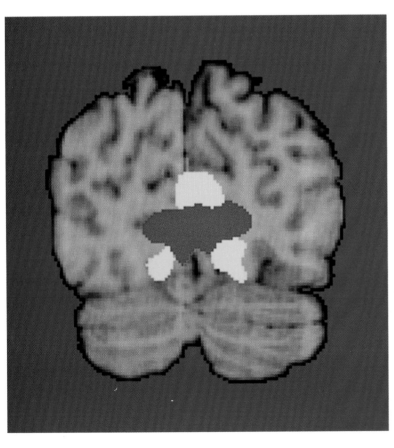
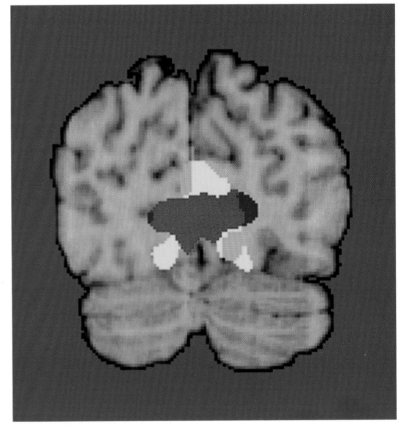

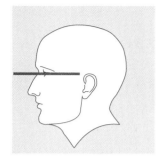

Axial MR of the orbit

1 - Iris
2 - Zygomatic bone
3 - Lens
4 - Ciliary body
    (ciliary muscle)
5 - Medial check ligament
6 - Eyeball (vitreous body)
7 - Rectus lateralis muscle
8 - Optic nerve
9 - Rectus medialis muscle
10 - Orbital lamina
11 - Orbital fat
12 - Ethmoidal air cells

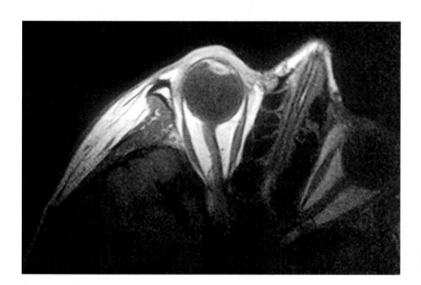

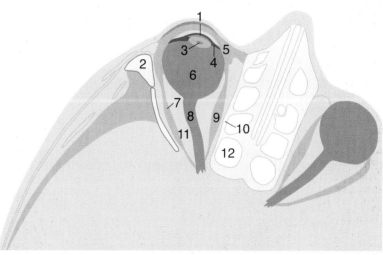

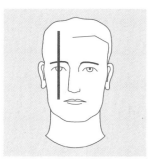

Sagittal MR of the orbit

1 - Frontal bone	8 - Anterior chamber of eye
2 - Brain	9 - Lens
3 - Upper eyelid	10 - Ciliary body
4 - Tarsus	11 - Vitreous body
5 - Tendon of levator palpebrae superioris muscle	12 - Orbital fat pad
	13 - Lower eyelid
6 - Rectus superior and levator palpebrae superioris muscles	14 - Rectus inferior muscle
	15 - Orbicularis oculi muscle
	16 - Obliquus inferior muscle
7 - Optic nerve	17 - Maxillary sinus

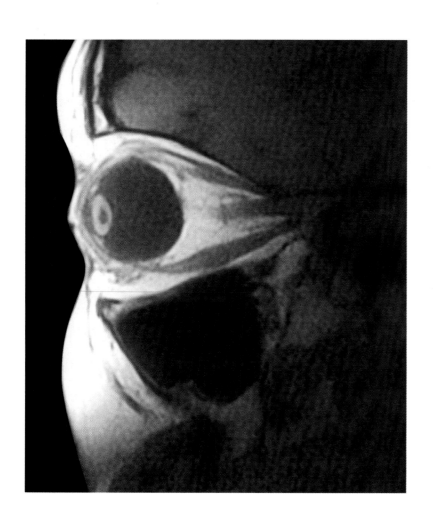

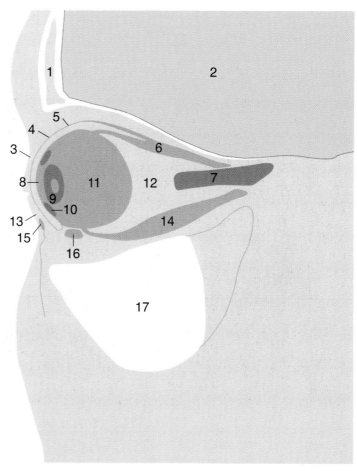

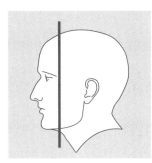

Coronal MR of the orbit

1 - Temporalis muscle
2 - Rectus lateralis muscle
3 - Rectus superior and levator palpebrae superioris muscles
4 - Optic nerve
5 - Orbital fat pad
6 - Obliquus superior muscle
7 - Ethmoidal air cells
8 - Rectus inferior muscle

9 - Rectus medialis muscle
10 - Zygomatic arch
11 - Maxillary sinus
12 - Middle nasal concha (turbinate)
13 - Inferior nasal concha (turbinate)
14 - Nasal septum
15 - Hard palate

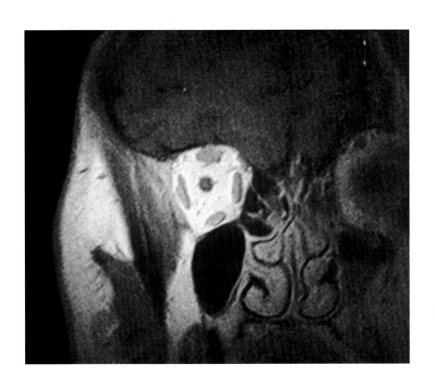

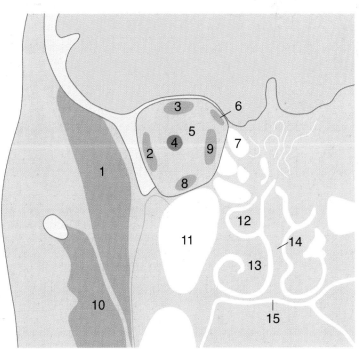

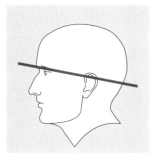

Axial CT of petrous temporal

1 - Head of mandible
2 - Foramen spinosum
3 - Sphenoidal sinus (partitioned)
4 - Nasal cavity
5 - External acoustic meatus
6 - Malleus
7 - Incus

8 - Pyramidal eminence
9 - Cochlea
10 - Internal acoustic meatus
11 - Mastoid air cells
12 - Facial nerve canal
13 - Vestibule
14 - Posterior semicircular canal

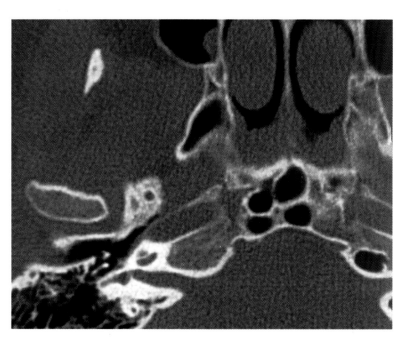

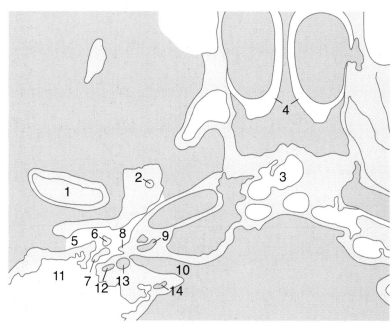

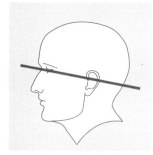

Axial CT of petrous temporal

1 - Head of mandible
2 - Foramen spinosum
3 - Auditory (Eustachian) tube
4 - Sphenoidal sinus
5 - Nasal cavity
6 - Tympanic cavity
7 - Malleus

8 - Incus
9 - Vestibule
10 - Cochlea
11 - Internal acoustic meatus
12 - Mastoid air cells
13 - Lateral semicircular canal
14 - Posterior semicircular canal

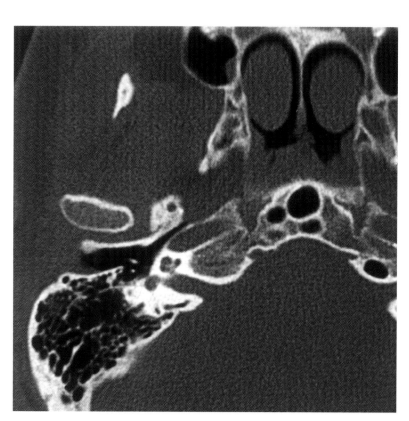
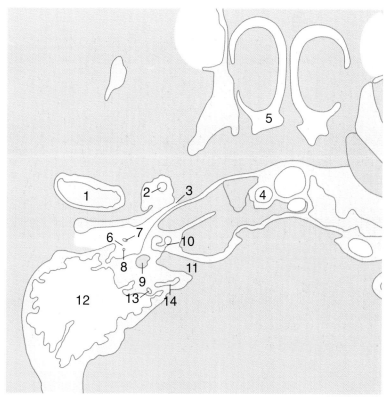

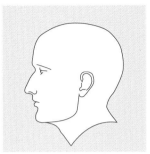

Facial skeleton, 3D CT SSD reconstruction, lateral view

1 - Orbit
2 - Zygomatic bone
3 - Zygomatic arch
4 - Temporal fossa
5 - External acoustic meatus
6 - Mastoid process
7 - Anterior nasal spine
8 - Alveolar process
    of maxilla
9 - Coronoid process
    of mandible
10 - Condylar process
    of mandible

11 - Ramus of mandible
12 - Inferior dental arch
13 - Mental foramen
14 - Body of mandible
15 - Angle of mandible
16 - Body of cervical vertebra III
17 - Spinous process
18 - Mental protuberance
19 - Body of hyoid bone
20 - Greater cornu (horn)
    of hyoid bone

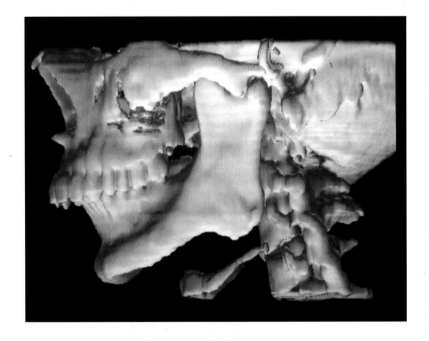

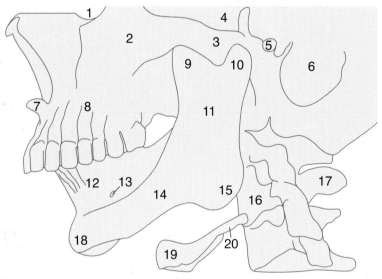

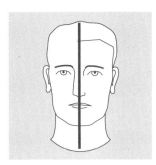

Sagittal MR of nasal and oral cavities, and the pharynx

1 - Scalp
2 - Skull bone
3 - Subarachnoid space
4 - Brain (gyri)
5 - Frontal sinus
6 - Ethmoidal air cells
7 - Sphenoethmoid recess
8 - Pituitary gland
9 - Sphenoidal sinus
10 - Superior nasal concha
11 - Middle nasal concha
12 - Inferior nasal concha
13 - Nasal vestibule
14 - Upper lip
15 - Oral vestibule and incisor teeth
16 - Hard palate
17 - Soft palate
18 - Nasopharynx
19 - Uvula
20 - Lower lip
21 - Mandible
22 - Tongue, genioglossus muscle
23 - Vallecula
24 - Oropharynx
25 - Epiglottis
26 - Geniohyoid muscle
27 - Laryngopharynx

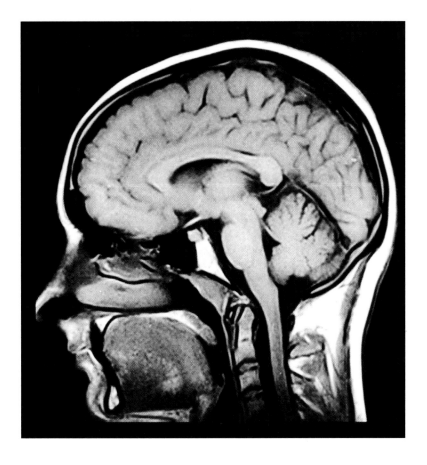

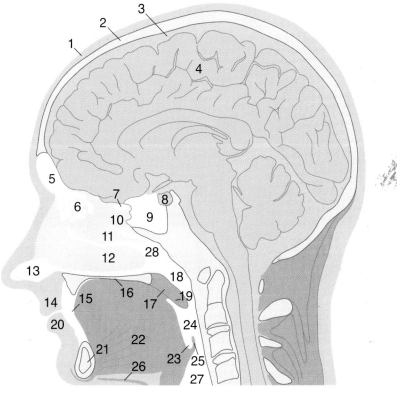

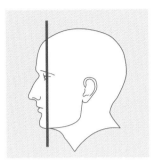

Coronal CT of head

1 - Brain
2 - Frontal sinus
　　(heavily extended)
3 - Crista galli
4 - Eyeball
5 - Orbital fat
6 - Perpendicular lamina
　　of ethmoid
7 - Orbital lamina of ethmoid
8 - Nasal septum
9 - Body of maxilla
10 - Inferior nasal concha

11 - Inferior nasal meatus
12 - Maxillary sinus
　　 (of Highmore)
13 - Fat pad of Bichat
14 - Alveolar process
　　 of maxilla
15 - Hard palate
16 - Oral cavity
17 - Tongue
18 - Buccinator muscle
19 - Inferior dental arch

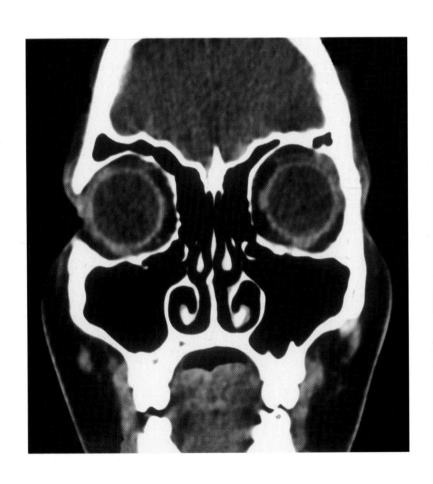

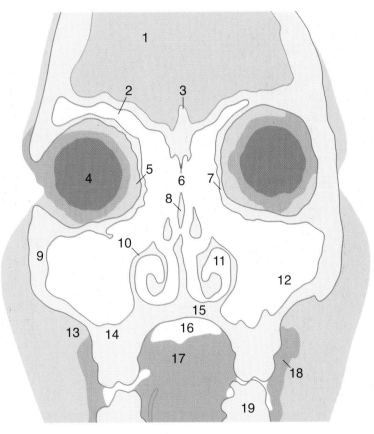

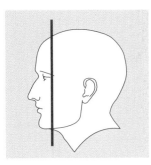

Coronal CT of head

1 - Frontal bone, squama
2 - Orbital part of frontal bone
3 - Brain
4 - Ethmoid bone, crista galli
5 - Obliquus superior muscle
6 - Rectus superior and levator palpebrae superioris muscles
7 - Rectus medialis muscle
8 - Optic nerve
9 - Rectus lateralis muscle
10 - Temporalis muscle
11 - Rectus inferior muscle
12 - Maxillary sinus
13 - Inferior nasal concha (turbinate)
14 - Nasal septum
15 - Masseter muscle
16 - Zygomatic arch
17 - Alveolar process of maxilla
18 - Hard palate
19 - Alveolar process of mandible
20 - Buccinator muscle
21 - Tongue

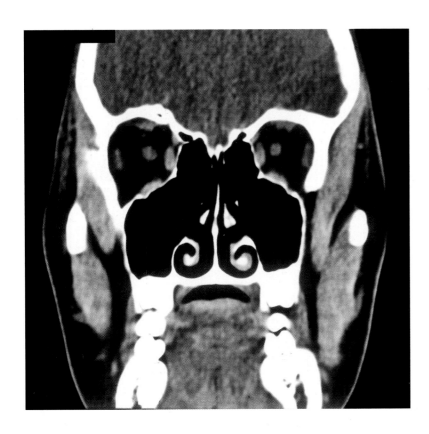

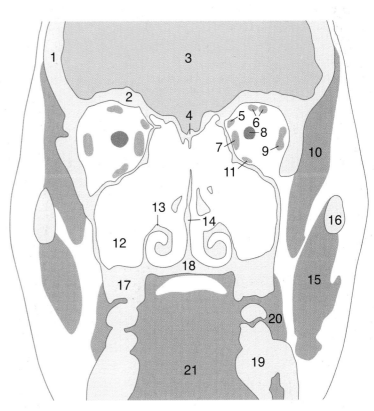

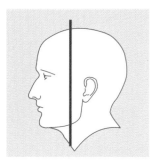

Coronal CT of head

1 - Ala major (greater wing) of sphenoid
2 - Sphenoidal sinus
3 - Brain
4 - Squamous part of temporal bone
5 - Temporalis muscle
6 - Infratemporal fossa
7 - Pterygoid process
8 - Vomer
9 - Nasopharynx
10 - Zygomatic arch
11 - Masseter muscle
12 - Mandible
13 - Hamulus of pterygoid process
14 - Soft palate
15 - Oral cavity
16 - Tongue

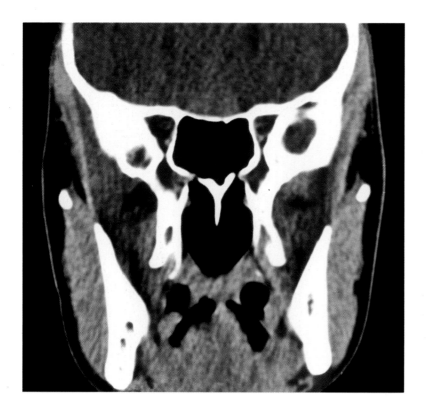

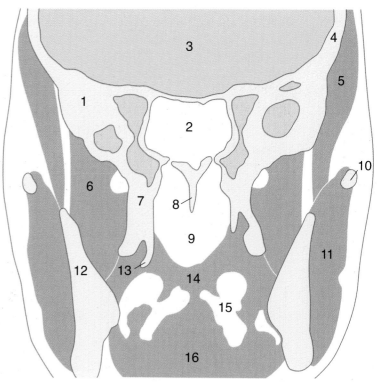

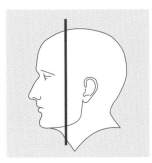

Coronal CT of head

1 - Temporalis muscle
2 - Ala major (greater wing) of sphenoid
3 - Brain
4 - Sphenoidal sinus
5 - Infratemporal fossa
6 - Lateral pterygoid muscle
7 - Pterygoid process
8 - Vomer
9 - Zygomatic arch
10 - Masseter muscle
11 - Mandible
12 - Medial pterygoid muscle
13 - Levator veli palatini muscle
14 - Tensor veli palatini muscle
15 - Nasopharynx
16 - Soft palate
17 - Palatine tonsil
18 - Uvula
19 - Oral cavity

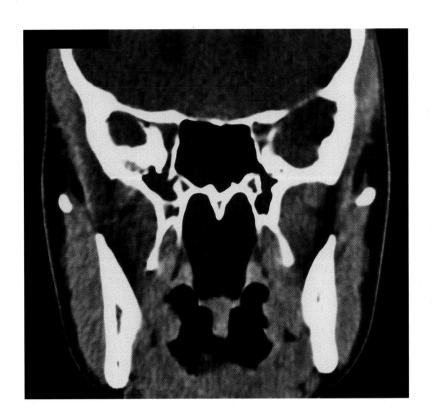

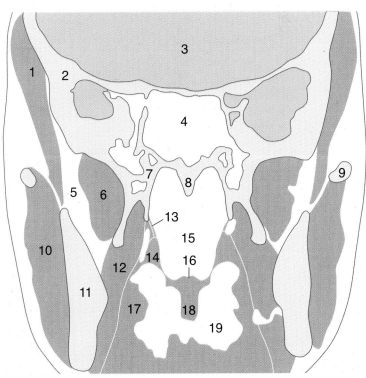

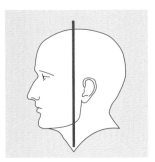

Coronal CT of head

1 - Brain
2 - Anterior clinoid process
3 - Sphenoidal sinus
4 - Pterygoid process
5 - Zygomatic arch
6 - Temporal bone, squama
7 - Temporalis muscle
8 - Masseter muscle
9 - Lateral pterygoid muscle
10 - Medial pterygoid muscle
11 - Parapharyngeal space
12 - Wall of pharynx
13 - Nasopharynx
14 - Torus tubarius
15 - Ramus of mandible
16 - Palatine tonsil
17 - Oropharynx

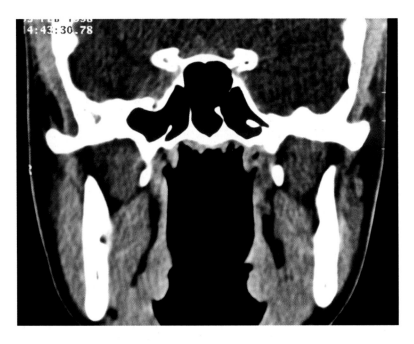

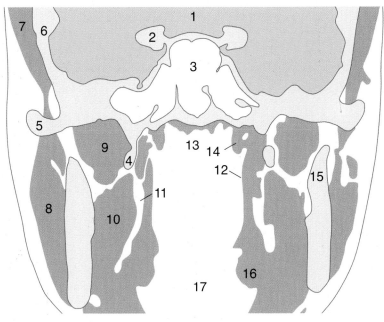

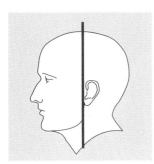

Coronal CT of head

1 - Temporalis muscle
2 - Brain
3 - Anterior clinoid process
4 - Body of sphenoid
5 - Temporomandibular joint
6 - Condylar process
    of mandible
7 - Ramus of mandible
8 - Lateral pterygoid muscle
9 - Parapharyngeal space

10 - Superior pharyngeal
      constrictor
11 - Posterior wall
      of nasopharynx
12 - Medial pterygoid muscle
13 - Nasopharynx
14 - Masseter muscle
15 - Oropharynx
16 - Mylohyoid muscle
17 - Digastric muscle

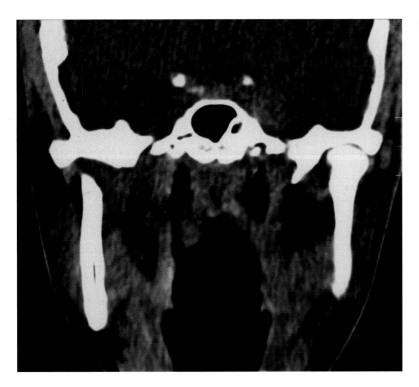

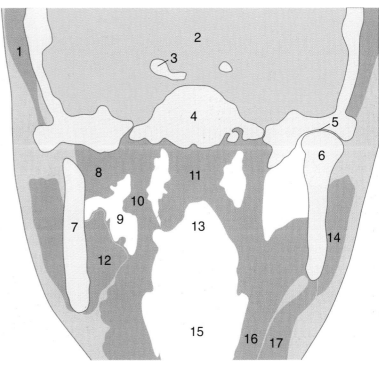

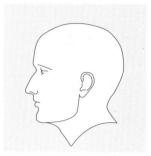

External carotid arteriogram, lateral view

1 - Parietal branch of
  superficial temporal artery
2 - Frontal branch of
  superficial temporal artery
3 - Superficial temporal
  artery
4 - Posterior auricular artery

5 - Maxillary artery
6 - Occipital artery
7 - Facial artery
8 - External carotid artery
9 - Superior thyroid artery
10 - Lingual artery
11 - Common carotid artery

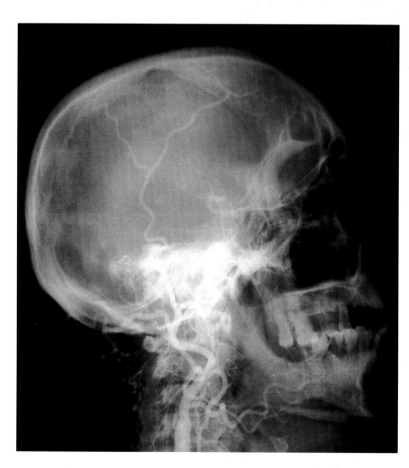

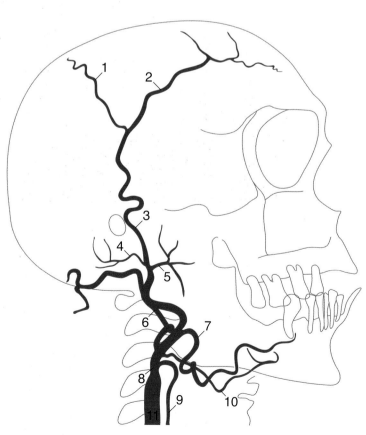

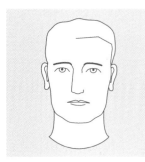

Deciduous teeth, orthopantomogram of 7-year-old child

1 - Maxillary sinus (of Highmore)
2 - Nasal cavity
3 - Condylar process of mandible
4 - Coronoid process of mandible
5 - Hard palate
6 - Second deciduous molar
7 - First deciduous molar
8 - Deciduous canine
9 - Third permanent molar (before eruption)
10 - Second permanent molar (before eruption)
11 - First permanent molar
12 - Second premolar (before eruption)
13 - First premolar (before eruption)
14 - Permanent canine (before eruption)
15 - Lateral permanent incisor
16 - Central permanent incisor
17 - Root canal
18 - Pulp cavity

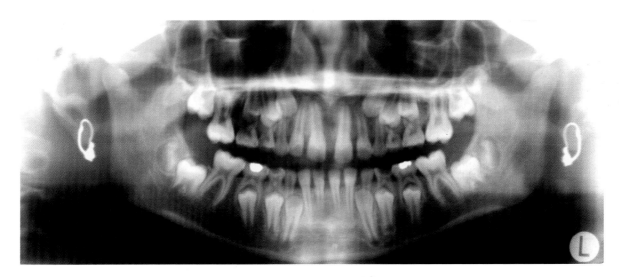

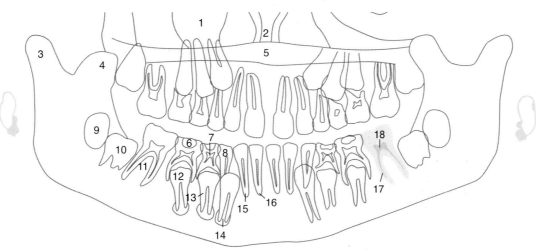

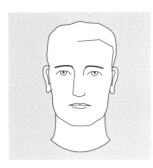

Permanent teeth, orthopantomogram of 19-year-old female

1 - Condylar process
    of mandible
2 - Coronoid process
    of mandible
3 - Right maxillary sinus
    (of Highmore)
4 - Nasal cavity
5 - Left maxillary sinus
    (of Highmore)
6 - Hard palate
7 - Third molar
8 - Second molar

9 - First molar
10 - Second premolar
11 - First premolar
12 - Canine
13 - Lateral incisor
14 - Central incisor
15 - Crown of tooth
16 - Pulp chamber
17 - Pulp horn
18 - Root of tooth
19 - Root canal
20 - Body of mandible

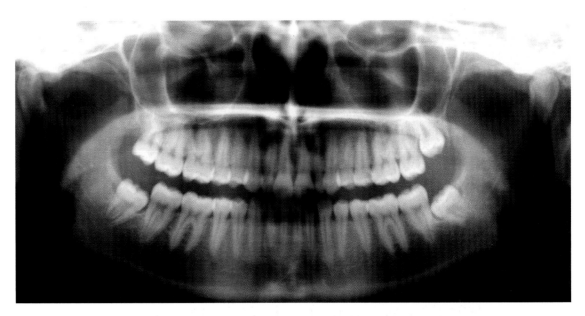

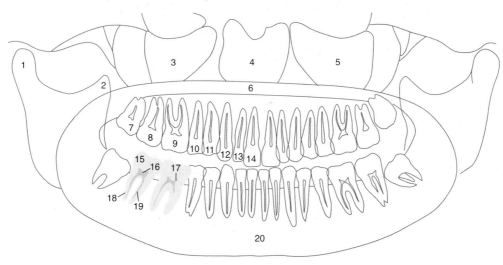

NECK

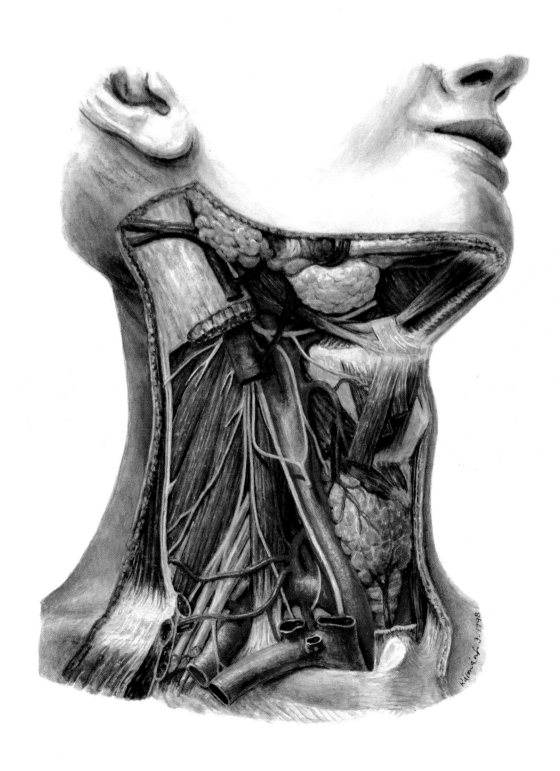

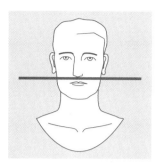

Axial MR of neck

1 - Superior dental arch
2 - Hard palate
3 - Masseter muscle
4 - Ramus of mandible
5 - Medial pterygoid muscle
6 - Soft palate
7 - Parotid gland (superficial lobe)
8 - External carotid artery
9 - Internal jugular vein
10 - Internal carotid artery
11 - Longus capitis and longus colli muscles
12 - Nasopharynx
13 - Retromandibular vein
14 - Vertebral artery
15 - Superior articular facet of atlas
16 - Dens (odontoid process) of axis
17 - Transverse ligament of atlas
18 - Spinal cord
19 - Lateral mass of atlas
20 - Posterior belly of digastric muscle
21 - Sternocleidomastoid and splenius capitis muscles
22 - Deep cervical artery and vein
23 - Rectus capitis posterior major and minor muscles
24 - Semispinalis capitis muscle

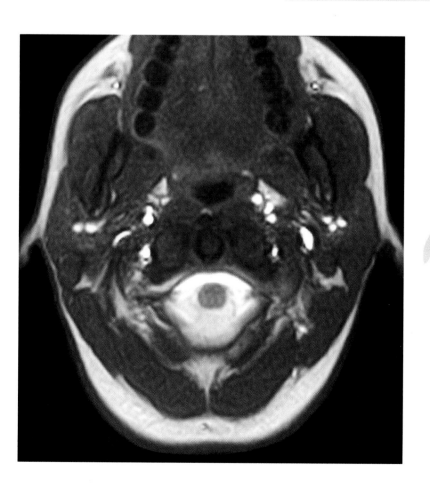

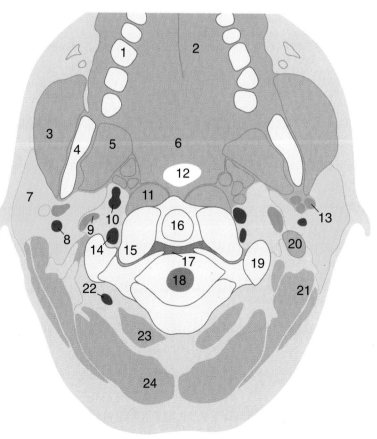

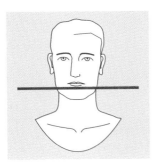

Axial CT of neck

1 - Mentalis muscle
2 - Depressor anguli oris muscle
3 - Mandible
4 - Mylohyoid muscle
5 - Hyoglossus muscle
6 - Genioglossus muscle
7 - Sublingual vein
8 - Submandibular gland
9 - Oropharynx
10 - Facial vein
11 - Platysma
12 - Posterior belly of digastric muscle
13 - Stylohyoid muscle
14 - External carotid artery
15 - Internal carotid artery
16 - Longus capitis and longus colli muscles
17 - Retromandibular vein
18 - Sternocleidomastoid muscle
19 - External jugular vein
20 - Internal jugular vein
21 - Cervical vertebra
22 - Levator scapulae muscle
23 - Longissimus capitis and cervicis muscles
24 - Semispinalis capitis muscle
25 - Semispinalis cervicis muscle
26 - Splenius capitis muscle
27 - Trapezius muscle

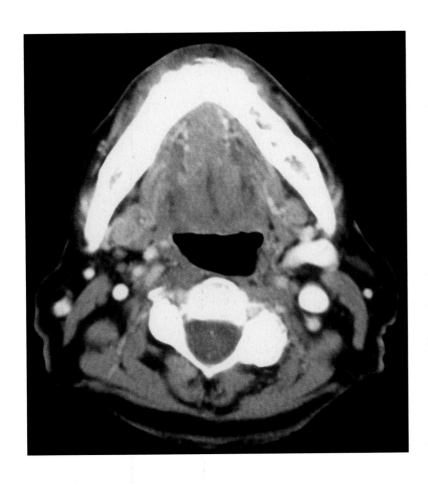

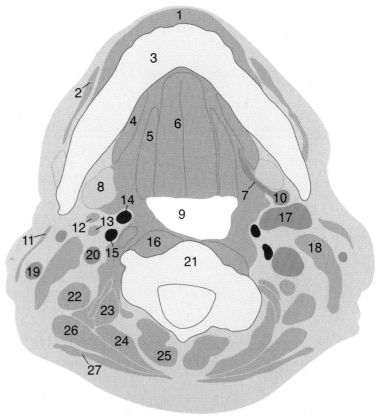

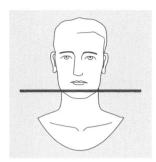

Axial CT of neck

1 - Mentalis muscle
2 - Depressor anguli oris muscle
3 - Mandible
4 - Mylohyoid muscle
5 - Sublingual vein in lateral lingual groove
6 - Genioglossus muscle
7 - Hyoglossus muscle
8 - Submandibular gland
9 - Facial vein
10 - External carotid artery
11 - Oropharynx
12 - Facial artery
13 - Confluence of veins leading to internal jugular vein
14 - Platysma
15 - Internal jugular vein
16 - Stylohyoid muscle
17 - Internal carotid artery
18 - Longus capitis and longus colli muscles
19 - Sternocleidomastoid muscle
20 - External jugular vein
21 - Levator scapulae muscle
22 - Deep cervical artery
23 - Semispinalis cervicis muscle
24 - Semispinalis capitis muscle
25 - Splenius capitis muscle
26 - Trapezius muscle

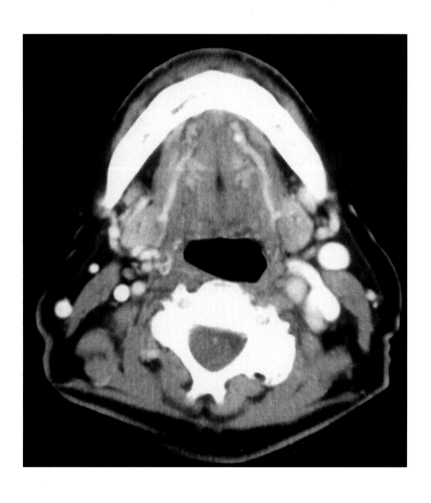

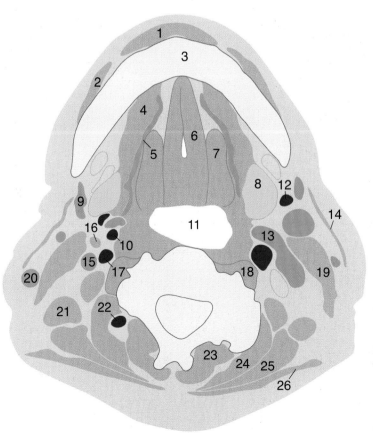

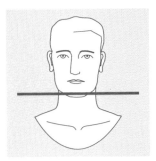

Axial CT of neck

1 - Mandible
2 - Mylohyoid muscle
3 - Hyoglossus muscle
4 - Genioglossus muscle
5 - Lingual artery
6 - Submandibular gland
7 - Platysma
8 - Facial vein
9 - External carotid artery
10 - Oropharynx
11 - Hyoid bone
12 - Superior cornu of thyroid cartilage
13 - Internal carotid artery
14 - Internal jugular vein
15 - Sternocleidomastoid muscle
16 - External jugular vein
17 - Scalenus anterior muscle
18 - Scalenus medius muscle
19 - Vertebral artery
20 - Retropharyngeal space
21 - Longus capitis and longus colli muscles
22 - Scalenus posterior muscle
23 - Levator scapulae muscle
24 - Splenius capitis muscle
25 - Trapezius muscle
26 - Longissimus capitis, cervicis and semispinalis capitis muscles
27 - Semispinalis cervicis muscle
28 - Nuchal ligament

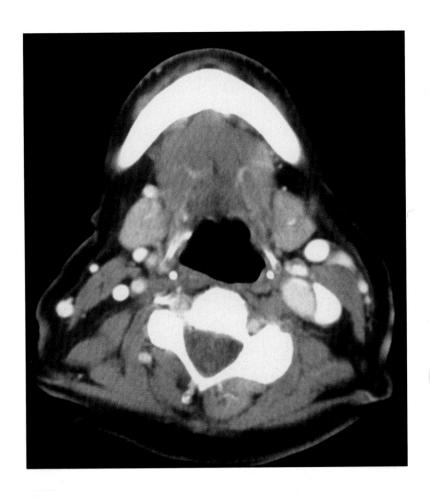

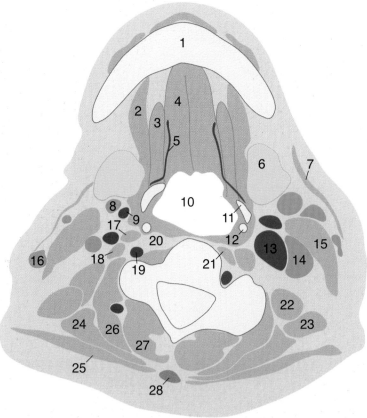

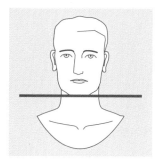

Axial CT of neck

1 - Mandible
2 - Anterior belly of digastric muscle
3 - Submental artery
4 - Mylohyoid and geniohyoid muscles
5 - Body of hyoid bone
6 - Submandibular gland
7 - Vallecula
8 - Middle glosso-epiglottic fold
9 - Root of tongue
10 - Superior cornu of thyroid cartilage
11 - External carotid artery
12 - Sternocleidomastoid muscle
13 - External jugular vein
14 - Internal jugular vein
15 - Internal carotid artery
16 - Retropharyngeal space
17 - Scalenus muscles
18 - Levator scapulae muscle
19 - Trapezius muscle
20 - Splenius capitis muscle
21 - Semispinalis capitis, and longissimus capitis and cervicis muscles
22 - Semispinalis cervicis muscle
23 - Nuchal ligament
24 - Bifid spinous process of cervical vertebra IV

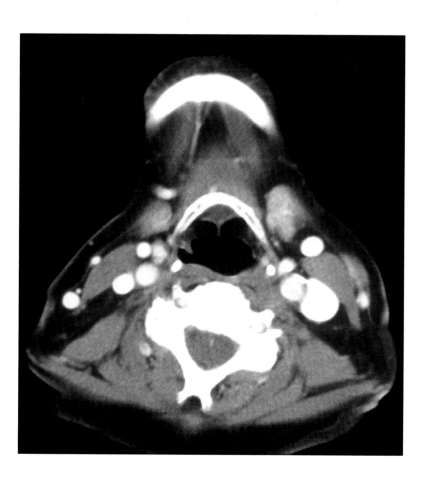

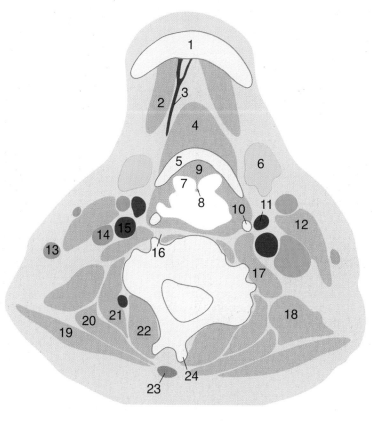

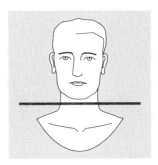

Axial CT of neck

1 - Anterior jugular vein
2 - Infrahyoid muscles
3 - Thyrohyoid membrane
4 - Pre-epiglottic fat
5 - Epiglottis
6 - Cuneiform cartilage
7 - Corniculate cartilage
8 - Thyroid cartilage
9 - External carotid artery
10 - Sternocleidomastoid muscle

11 - External jugular vein
12 - Internal jugular vein
13 - Internal carotid artery
14 - Cervical vertebra V
15 - Vertebral artery
16 - Scalenus medius muscle
17 - Levator scapulae muscle
18 - Erector spinae muscle

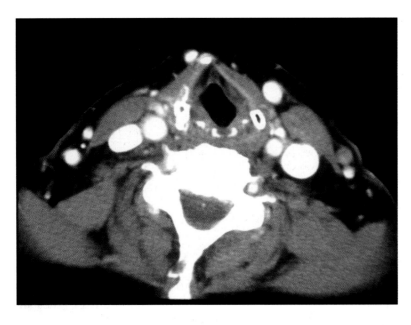

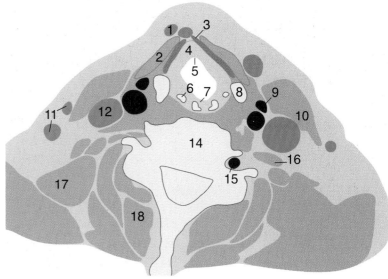

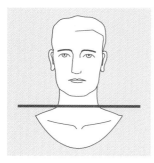

Axial CT of neck

1 - Anterior jugular vein
2 - Thyroid cartilage
3 - Laryngeal vestibule
4 - Common facial vein
5 - Sternocleidomastoid muscle
6 - Thyroid gland
7 - Arytenoid cartilage
8 - Superior thyroid artery
9 - Common carotid artery
10 - Internal jugular vein
11 - External jugular vein
12 - Scalenus medius muscle
13 - Laryngopharynx
14 - Scalenus posterior muscle
15 - Vertebral artery
16 - Levator scapulae muscle
17 - Longissimus cervicis muscle
18 - Semispinalis muscle
19 - Erector spinae muscle
20 - Splenius capitis muscle
21 - Deep cervical vessels

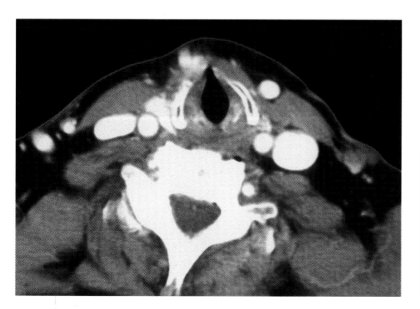

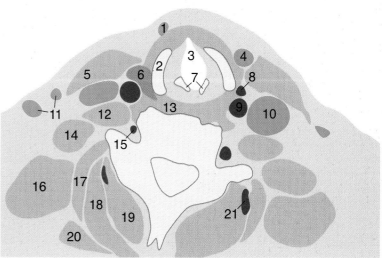

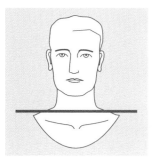

Axial CT of neck

1 - Anterior jugular vein
2 - Wall of trachea and infrahyoid muscles
3 - Thyroid gland
4 - Tracheal lumen (subglottic)
5 - Inferior laryngeal artery
6 - Sternocleidomastoid muscle, sternal head
7 - External jugular vein
8 - Internal jugular vein
9 - Scalenus anterior muscle
10 - Common carotid artery
11 - Oesophagus
12 - Longus colli muscle
13 - Vertebral artery
14 - Scalenus anterior muscle
15 - Sternocleidomastoid muscle, clavicular head
16 - Scalenus medius muscle
17 - Scalenus posterior muscle
18 - Levator scapulae muscle
19 - Erector spinae muscle
20 - Lamina and spinous process of thoracic vertebra I
21 - Rib I

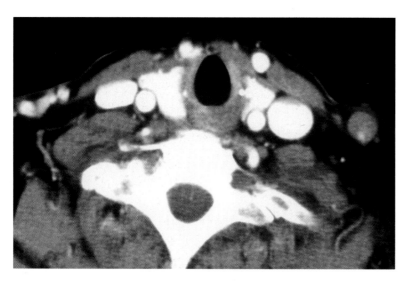

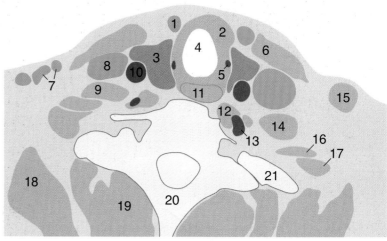

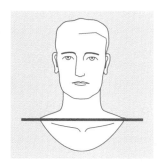

Axial CT of neck

1 - Anterior jugular vein
2 - Trachea
3 - Sternocleidomastoid
    muscle, sternal head
4 - Internal jugular vein
5 - Common carotid artery
6 - Thyroid gland
7 - Oesophagus
8 - Sternocleidomastoid
    muscle, clavicular head

 9 - Vertebral artery
10 - Vertebral vein
11 - Scalenus anterior muscle
12 - Scalenus medius muscle
13 - Scalenus posterior muscle
14 - Levator scapulae muscle
15 - Erector spinae muscle
16 - Thoracic vertebra I
17 - Rib I
18 - Rib II

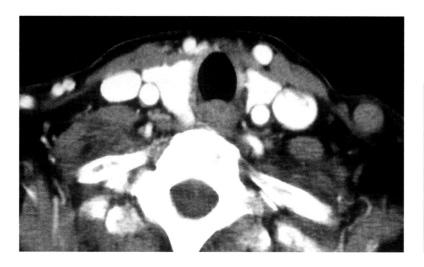

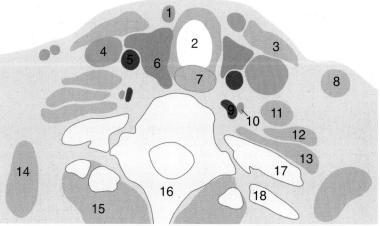

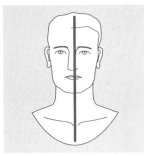

Sagittal MR of the head and the neck (craniocervical junction)

1 - Brain, frontal lobe
2 - Corpus callosum
3 - Ethmoidal air cells
4 - Pituitary gland in sella turcica
5 - Third ventricle
6 - Nasal cavity
7 - Sphenoidal sinus
8 - Interpeduncular fossa
9 - Cerebral aqueduct, mesencephalon
10 - Nasopharynx

11 - Clivus
12 - Pons
13 - Fourth ventricle
14 - Soft palate
15 - Anterior arch of atlas
16 - Membrana tectoria
17 - Dens axis
18 - Medulla oblongata
19 - Posterior arch of atlas
20 - Rectus capitis posterior minor muscle
21 - Semispinalis capitis muscle
22 - Oropharynx
23 - Posterior longitudinal ligament

24 - Spinous process of axis
25 - Suboccipital fat
26 - Laryngopharynx
27 - Anterior longitudinal ligament
28 - Spinal cord
29 - Ligamenta flava
30 - Semispinalis cervicis muscle
31 - Nuchal ligament
32 - Spinous process of cervical vertebra VII (prominens)
33 - Trachea
34 - Thecal sac
35 - Erector spinae muscle

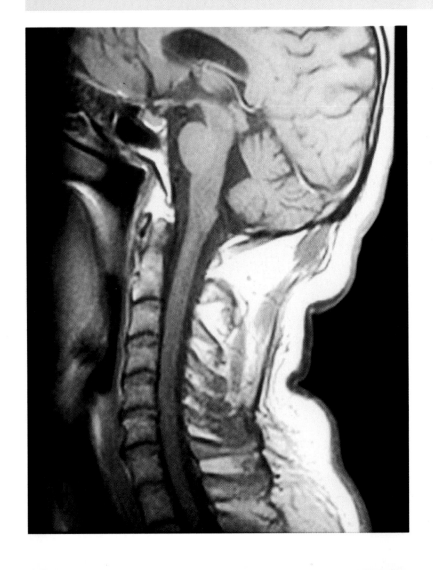

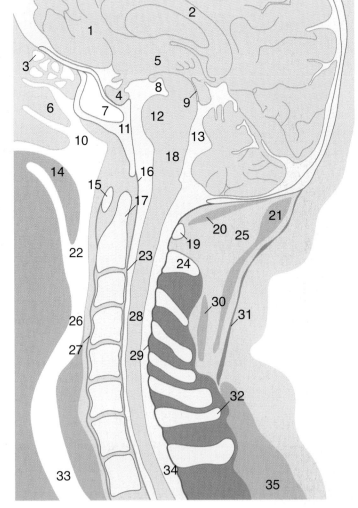

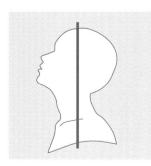

Coronal MR of neck

1 - Brain, parietal lobe
2 - Brain, temporal lobe
3 - Nasopharynx
4 - Ramus of mandible
5 - Right common carotid artery
6 - Cervical vertebrae
7 - Left internal carotid artery
8 - External jugular vein
9 - Internal jugular vein
10 - Right subclavian artery
11 - Scalenus anterior, insertion
12 - Trachea
13 - Left common carotid artery
14 - Right subclavian vein
15 - Right brachiocephalic vein
16 - Left brachiocephalic vein
17 - Left subclavian vein
18 - Superior vena cava
19 - Arch of aorta
20 - Main pulmonary artery
21 - Ascending aorta
22 - Heart
23 - Lung

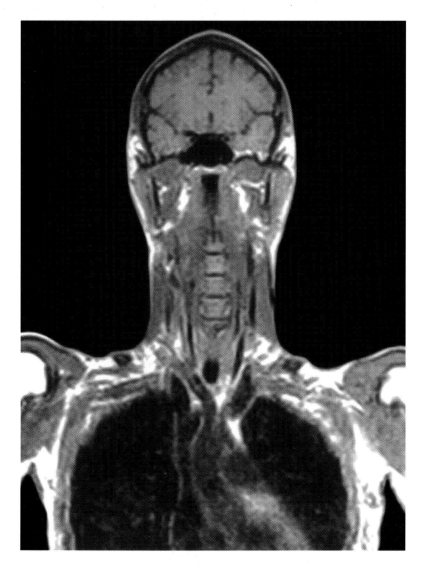

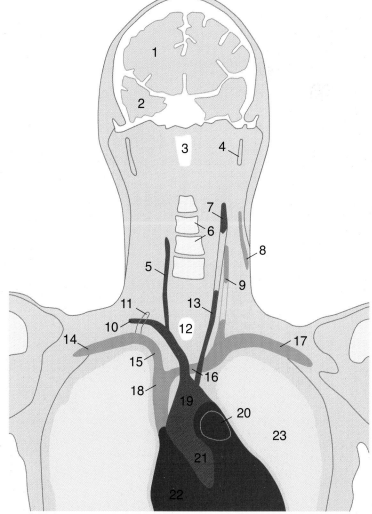

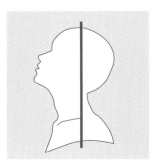

Coronal MR of neck

1 - Brain
2 - Retromandibular vein
3 - Sternocleidomastoid muscle
4 - Cervical vertebra
5 - Internal carotid artery
6 - Scalenus anterior muscle
7 - Humerus, glenohumeral joint
8 - Right subclavian artery
9 - Vertebral artery
10 - Superior vena cava
11 - Brachiocephalic artery
12 - Left common carotid artery
13 - Arch of aorta
14 - Ascending aorta
15 - Right atrium
16 - Left ventricle

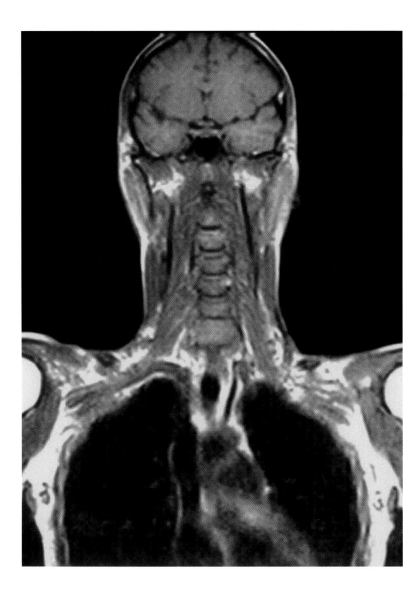

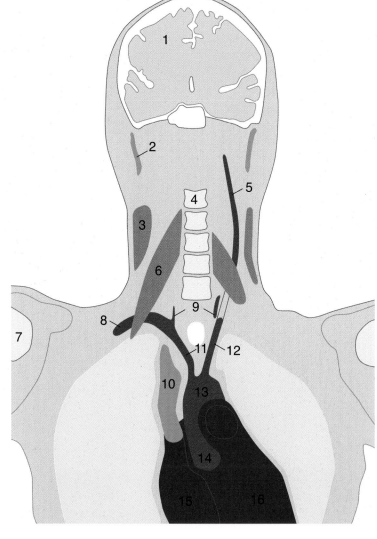

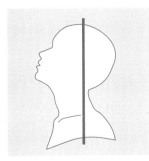

Coronal MR of neck

1 - Brain
2 - Right vertebral artery
3 - Left vertebral artery
4 - Right internal carotid artery
5 - Left internal carotid artery
6 - Dens axis
7 - Vertebral artery in foramina transversaria
8 - Cervical vertebra IV
9 - Scalenus medius and posterior muscles
10 - Sternocleidomastoid muscle
11 - Trachea
12 - Left subclavian artery
13 - Arch of aorta
14 - Main pulmonary artery
15 - Heart

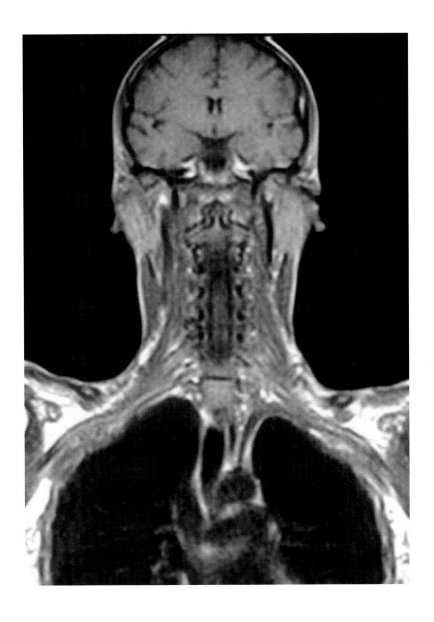

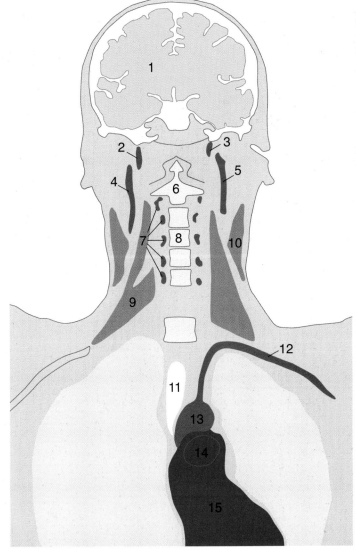

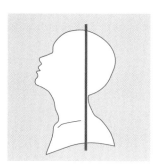

Coronal MR of neck

1 - Brain
2 - Cerebellum
3 - Rectus capitis posterior major and minor muscles
4 - Obliquus capitis inferior muscle
5 - Splenius capitis and semispinalis capitis muscles
6 - Spinous process of axis
7 - Multifidus muscles
8 - Spinal canal
9 - Lung
10 - Hilum of lung
11 - Arch of aorta
12 - Descending thoracic aorta

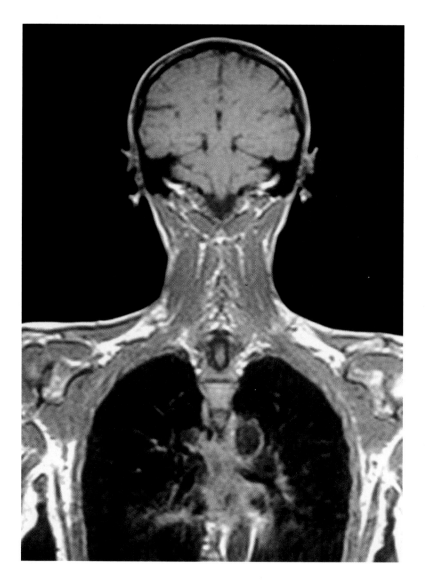

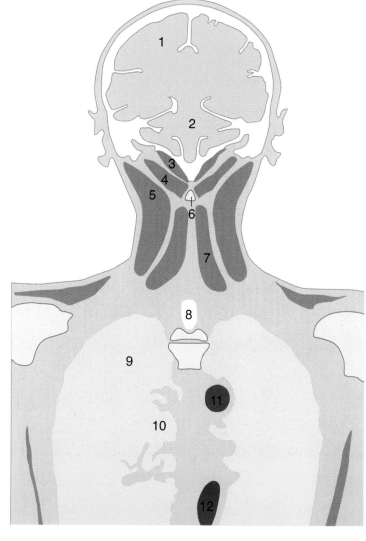

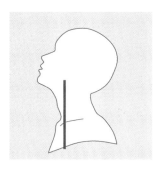

Coronal MR of larynx

1 - Laryngeal vestibule
2 - Laryngeal sinus and saccule
3 - Vocal fold

4 - Cricoid cartilage
5 - Infraglottic cavity
6 - Clavicle

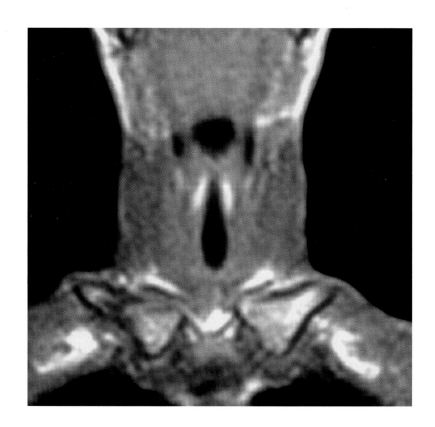

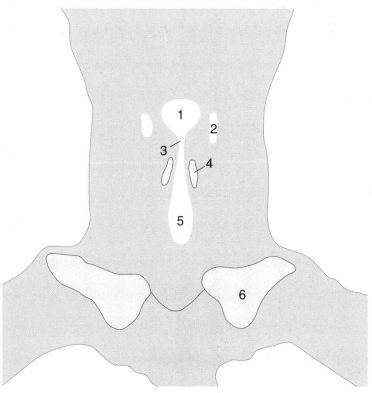

THORAX

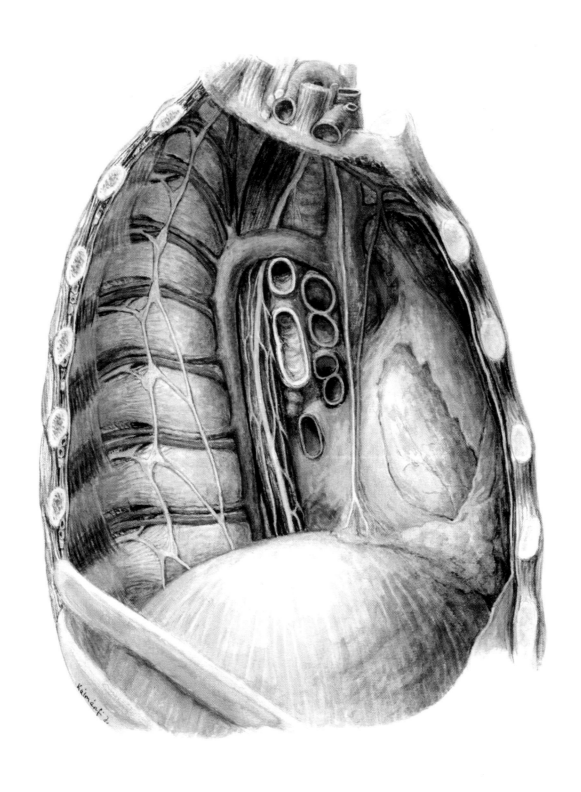

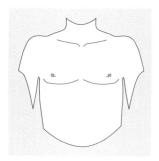

3D CT-SSD reconstruction of osseous thorax, left anterior oblique view

1 - Clavicle
2 - Sternoclavicular joint
3 - Rib I
4 - Scapula
5 - Manubrium of sternum

6 - Body of sternum
7 - Xiphoid process
8 - Costal cartilage
   (partially calcified)
9 - Vertebral column

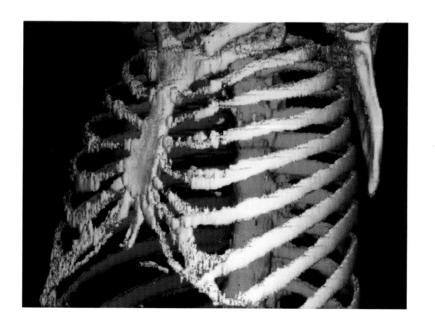

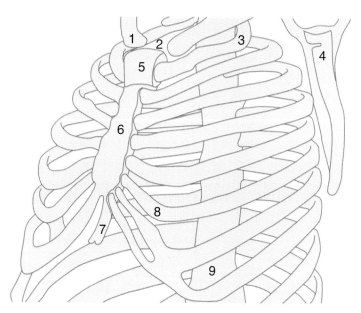

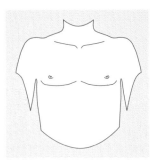

3D CT-SSD reconstruction of osseous thorax, inferior dorsal view

1 - Acromion
2 - Spine of scapula
3 - Spinous process
    of vertebra
4 - Glenoid process
    of scapula
5 - Costotransversal joint
6 - Infraspinous fossa

7 - Rib
8 - Floating rib
9 - Articular process
    of vertebra
10 - Vertebral canal
11 - Body of vertebra
12 - Sternum
13 - Xiphoid process

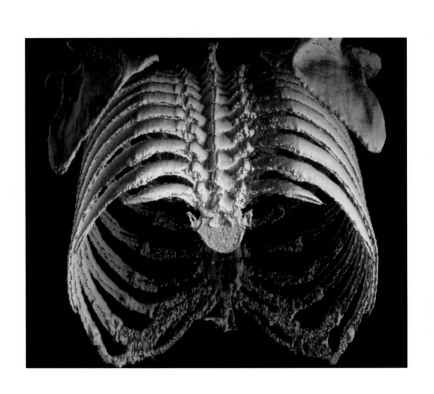

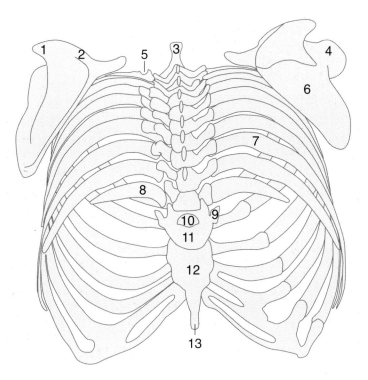

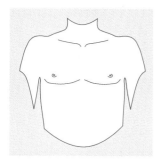

3D CT-SSD reconstruction of osseous thorax, left dorsal view

1 - Supraspinous fossa
2 - Spine of scapula
3 - Infraspinous fossa
4 - Spinous process
    of vertebra

5 - Costotransversal joint
6 - Arch of vertebra
7 - Costal cartilage
8 - Costal angle

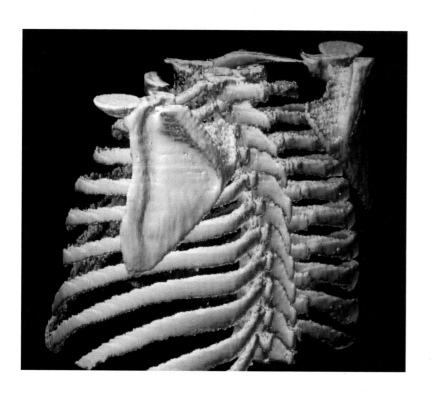

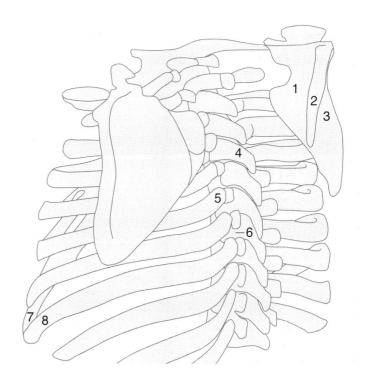

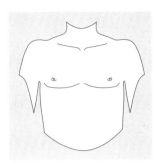

X-ray of thorax, postero-anterior view

1 - Clavicle
2 - Vertebral column
3 - Intercostal space
4 - Ribs
5 - Pulmonary hilum
6 - Left atrium
7 - Aortic knuckle
8 - Pulmonary trunk
9 - Left auricle

10 - Right atrium
11 - Left ventricle
12 - Right ventricle
13 - Left cardiophrenic angle
14 - Diaphragm
15 - Air bubble of stomach
16 - Costodiaphragmatic recess (left costophrenic angle)

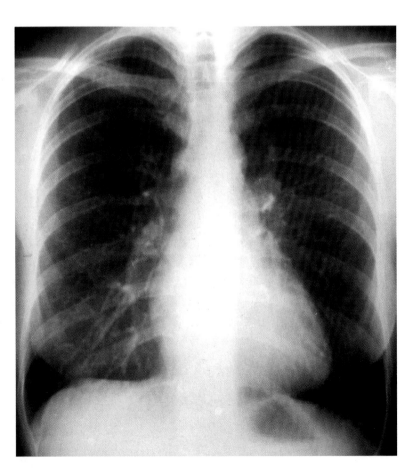

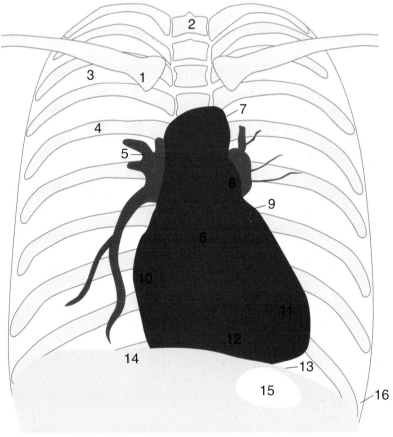

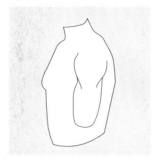

X-ray of thorax, lateral view

1 - Vertebral column
2 - Trachea
3 - Manubrium of sternum
4 - Ascending aorta
5 - Pulmonary artery (right)
6 - Retrosternal space
7 - Main bronchus

8 - Anterior aspect of right ventricle
9 - Body of sternum
10 - Posterior aspect of left atrium
11 - Descending thoracic aorta
12 - Diaphragm

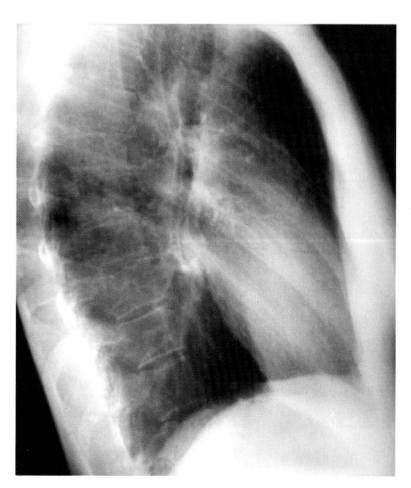

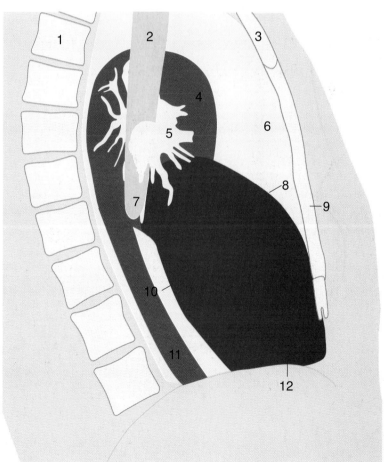

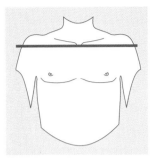

Axial CT of thorax

1 - Pectoralis major muscle
2 - Sternum
3 - Sternoclavicular joint
4 - Clavicle
5 - Pectoralis minor muscle
6 - Rib I
7 - Right brachiocephalic vein/internal jugular vein confluence
8 - Right common carotid artery
9 - Thyroid (retrosternal extension)
10 - Trachea
11 - Left brachiocephalic vein
12 - Left common carotid artery
13 - Lung
14 - Right subclavian artery
15 - Oesophagus
16 - Left subclavian artery
17 - Latissimus dorsi muscle
18 - Subscapularis muscle
19 - Serratus anterior muscle
20 - Thoracic vertebra
21 - Infraspinatus muscle
22 - Scapular spine
23 - Supraspinatus muscle
24 - Rhomboid muscles
25 - Erector spinae muscle
26 - Trapezius muscle

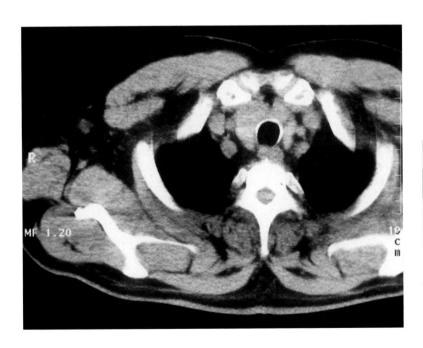

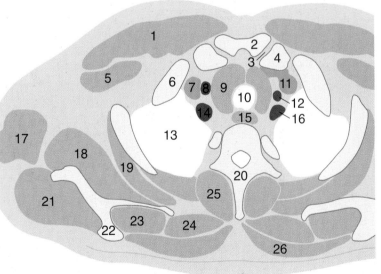

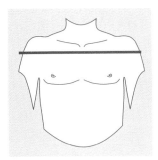

Axial CT of thorax

1 - Pectoralis major muscle
2 - Sternum
3 - Pectoralis minor muscle
4 - Right brachiocephalic vein
5 - Right common carotid artery
6 - Left brachiocephalic vein
7 - Left common carotid artery
8 - Right subclavian artery
9 - Trachea

10 - Oesophagus
11 - Left subclavian artery
12 - Latissimus dorsi muscle
13 - Subscapularis muscle
14 - Serratus anterior muscle
15 - Thoracic vertebra
16 - Infraspinatus muscle
17 - Scapular spine
18 - Supraspinatus muscle
19 - Rhomboid muscles
20 - Trapezius muscle
21 - Erector spinae muscle

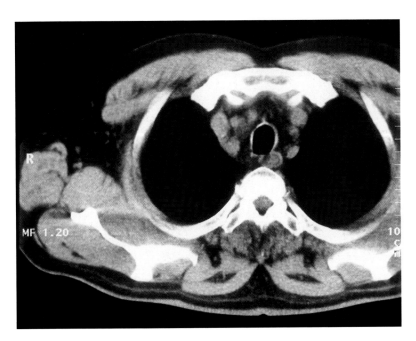

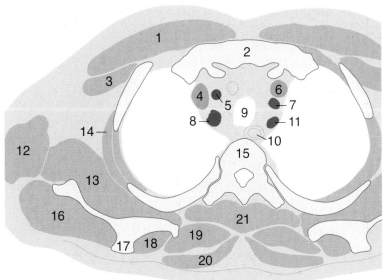

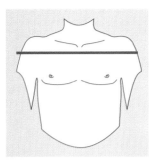

Axial CT of thorax

1 - Pectoralis major muscle
2 - Sternum
3 - Pectoralis minor muscle
4 - Right brachiocephalic vein
5 - Left brachiocephalic vein
6 - Brachiocephalic artery
7 - Left common carotid artery
8 - Trachea
9 - Oesophagus
10 - Left subclavian artery

11 - Latissimus dorsi muscle
12 - Teres major muscle
13 - Rib
14 - Thoracic vertebra
15 - Subscapularis muscle
16 - Erector spinae muscle
17 - Rhomboid muscles
18 - Infraspinatus muscle
19 - Scapular spine
20 - Supraspinatus muscle
21 - Trapezius muscle

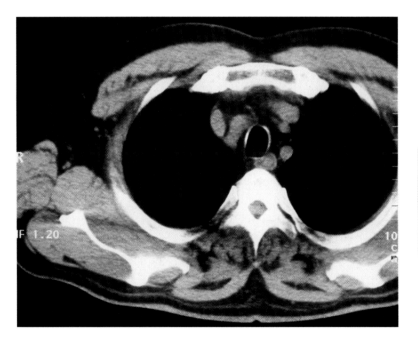

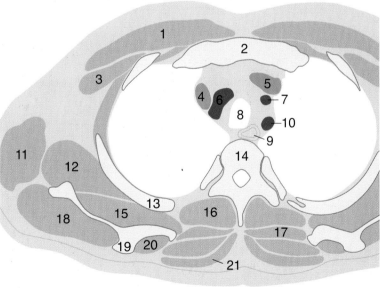

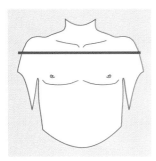

Axial CT of thorax

1 - Pectoralis major muscle
2 - Sternum
3 - Pectoralis minor muscle
4 - Left brachiocephalic vein
5 - Right brachiocephalic vein
6 - Brachiocephalic artery
7 - Left common carotid artery
8 - Trachea
9 - Left subclavian artery
10 - Oesophagus
11 - Latissimus dorsi muscle
12 - Teres major muscle
13 - Subscapularis muscle
14 - Serratus anterior muscle
15 - Teres minor muscle
16 - Infraspinatus muscle
17 - Scapula
18 - Rhomboid muscles
19 - Trapezius muscle
20 - Erector spinae muscle

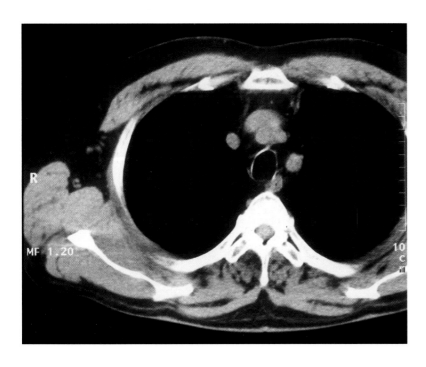

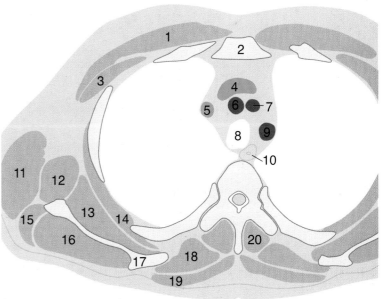

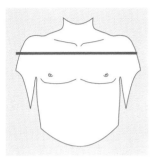

Axial CT of thorax

1 - Pectoralis major muscle
2 - Sternum
3 - Pectoralis minor muscle
4 - Superior mediastinum, thymic residue
5 - Left brachiocephalic vein
6 - Superior vena cava
7 - Arch of aorta
8 - Azygos vein
9 - Trachea
10 - Oesophagus
11 - Latissimus dorsi muscle
12 - Subscapularis muscle
13 - Infraspinatus muscle
14 - Rhomboid muscles
15 - Trapezius muscle
16 - Erector spinae muscle
17 - Thoracic vertebra
18 - Scapula

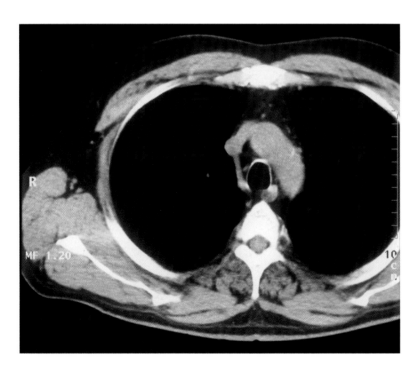

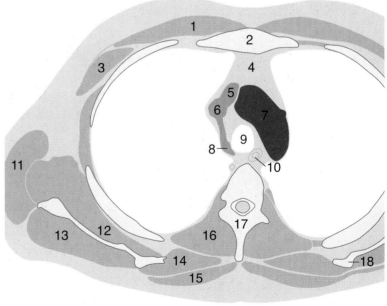

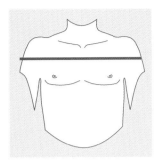

Axial CT of thorax

1 - Pectoralis major muscle
2 - Sternum
3 - Rib
4 - Superior mediastinum, thymic residue
5 - Ascending aorta
6 - Superior vena cava
7 - Reflexion of pericardium
8 - Left pulmonary artery
9 - Bifurcation of trachea (carina)
10 - Oesophagus

11 - Azygos vein
12 - Descending thoracic aorta
13 - Latissimus dorsi muscle
14 - Teres major muscle
15 - Subscapularis muscle
16 - Scapula
17 - Infraspinatus muscle
18 - Rhomboid muscles
19 - Trapezius muscle
20 - Erector spinae muscle
21 - Arch of vertebra

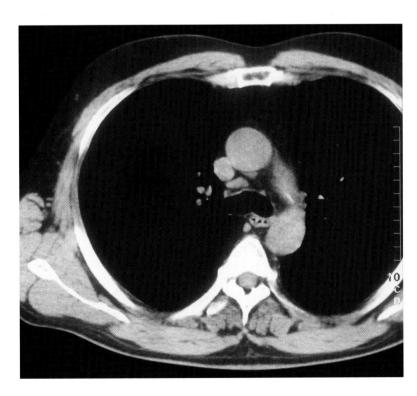

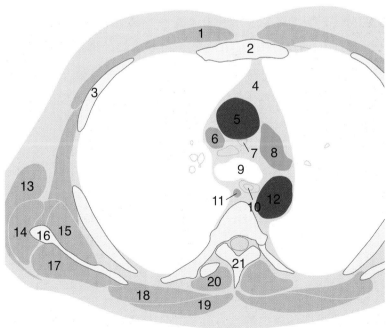

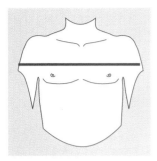

Axial CT of thorax

1 - Sternum
2 - Mediastinal pleura
3 - Ascending aorta
4 - Pulmonary trunk
5 - Serratus anterior muscle
6 - Right upper pulmonary vein
7 - Superior vena cava
8 - Right pulmonary artery
9 - Left pulmonary artery
10 - Right bronchus intermedius
11 - Left principal bronchus
12 - Latissimus dorsi muscle
13 - Azygos vein
14 - Oesophagus
15 - Descending thoracic aorta
16 - Teres major muscle
17 - Scapula
18 - Subscapularis muscle
19 - Infraspinatus muscle
20 - Rhomboid muscles
21 - Intervertebral foramen
22 - Thoracic vertebra
23 - Spinal cord
24 - Erector spinae muscle
25 - Trapezius muscle

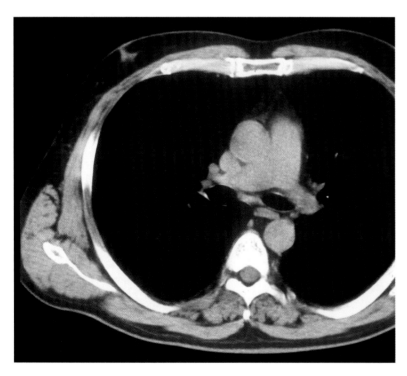

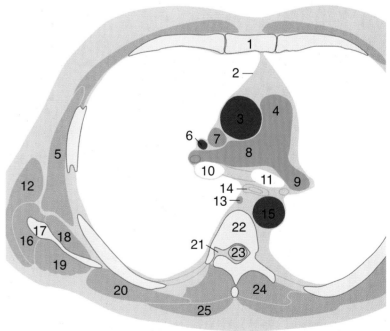

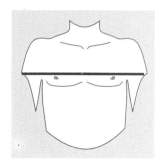

Axial CT of thorax

1 - Sternum
2 - Ascending aorta
3 - Pulmonary trunk
(conus arteriosus)
4 - Right pulmonary artery
5 - Left upper pulmonary
vein
6 - Serratus anterior muscle
7 - Right bronchus
intermedius
8 - Left main bronchus
9 - Oesophagus

10 - Left basal pulmonary
artery
11 - Latissimus dorsi muscle
12 - Azygos vein
13 - Descending thoracic aorta
14 - Scapula
15 - Teres major muscle
16 - Rhomboid muscles
17 - Thoracic vertebra
18 - Erector spinae muscle
19 - Trapezius muscle

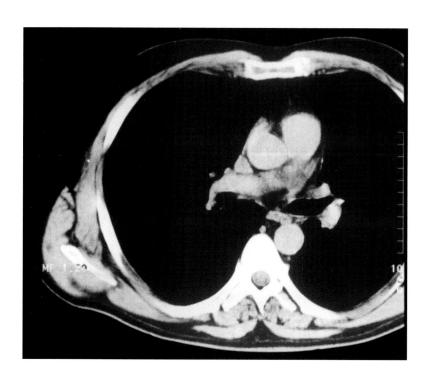

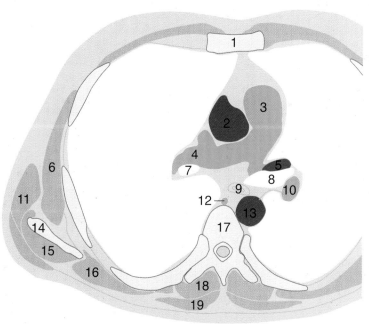

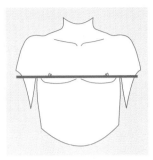

Axial CT of thorax

1 - Internal thoracic vessels
2 - Right atrium (appendage)
3 - Right ventricular outflow tract
4 - Superior vena cava
5 - Ascending aorta
6 - Serratus anterior muscle
7 - Right lower lobe bronchus
8 - Right upper pulmonary vein

9 - Left atrium
10 - Oesophagus
11 - Azygos vein
12 - Descending thoracic aorta
13 - Thoracic vertebra
14 - Latissimus dorsi muscle
15 - Scapula
16 - Rhomboid muscles
17 - Erector spinae muscle
18 - Trapezius muscle

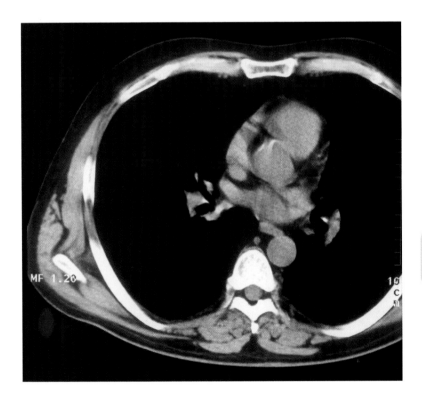

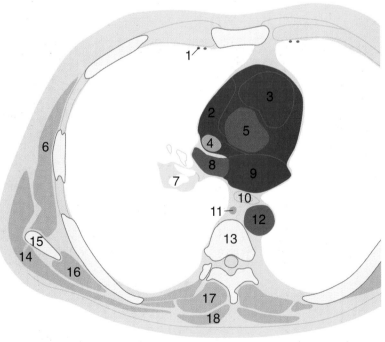

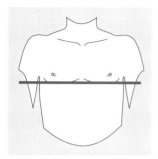

Axial CT of thorax

1 - Costal cartilages
2 - Xiphoid process
3 - Serratus anterior muscle
4 - Lung (middle lobe)
5 - Right ventricle
6 - Right atrium
7 - Left ventricle

8 - Left atrium
9 - Oesophagus
10 - Descending thoracic aorta
11 - Latissimus dorsi muscle
12 - Thoracic vertebra
13 - Erector spinae muscle
14 - Trapezius muscle

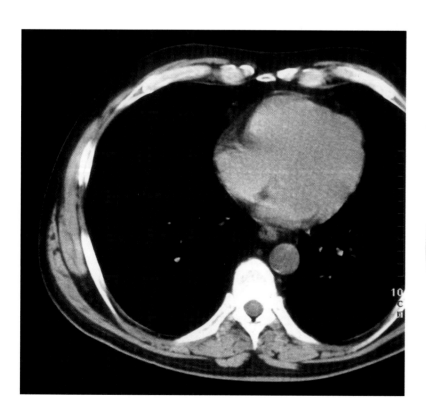

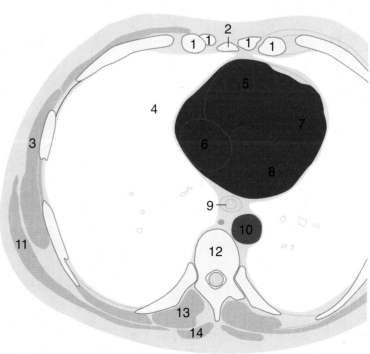

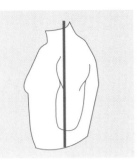

Coronal MR of thorax

1 - Trachea
2 - Left common carotid artery
3 - Brachiocephalic trunk
4 - Left subclavian artery
5 - Superior vena cava
6 - Aortic knuckle
7 - Ascending aorta
8 - Pulmonary trunk
9 - Right ventricle
10 - Muscular interventricular septum
11 - Left ventricle
12 - Wall of left ventricle
13 - Diaphragm

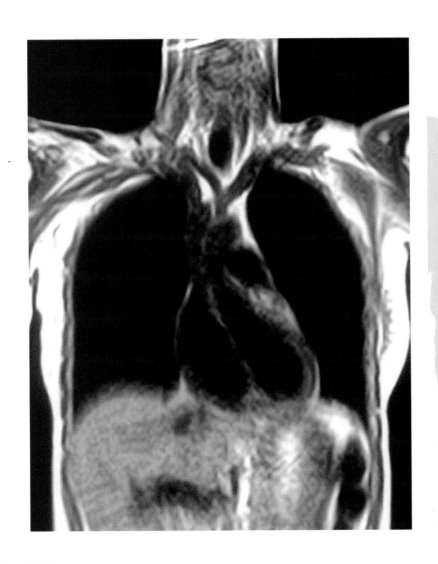

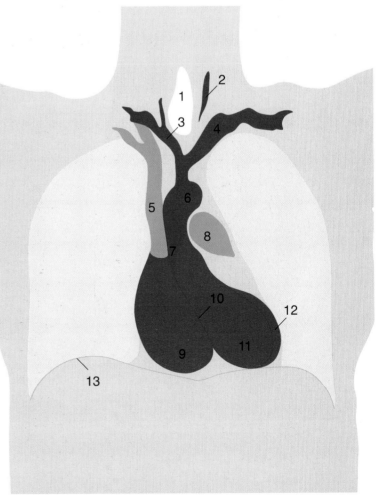

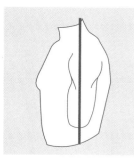

Coronal MR of thorax

1 - Cervical spine
2 - Trachea
3 - Aortic knuckle
4 - Right pulmonary artery
5 - Left pulmonary artery
6 - Left atrium

7 - Right atrium
8 - Left ventricular wall
9 - Left ventricular cavity
10 - Diaphragm
11 - Inferior vena cava
12 - Descending aorta

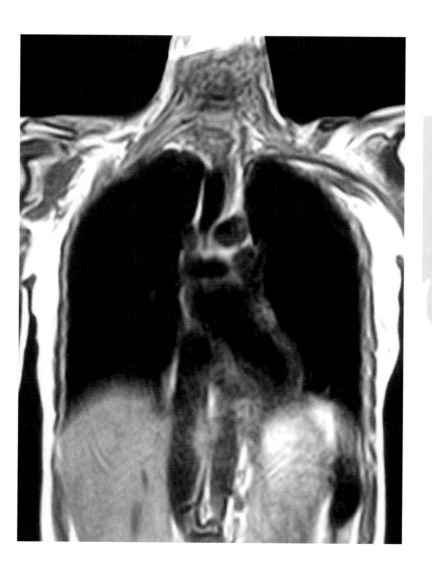

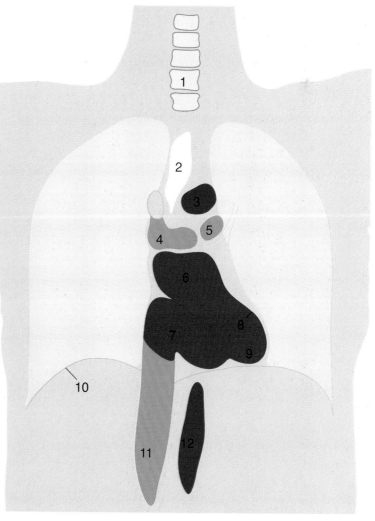

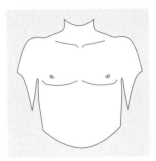

3-D reconstruction CT of bronchial tree
A - coronal section plane, B - head view (craniocaudal aspect).

1 - Trachea
2 - Right main bronchus
3 - Left main bronchus
4 - Bronchus intermedius
5 - Left superior lobar
    bronchus
6 - Left inferior lobar
    bronchus

7 - Segmental bronchus
8 - Secondary branches
    of bronchi
9 - Tertiary branches
    of bronchi
10 - Carina in tracheal
     bifurcation

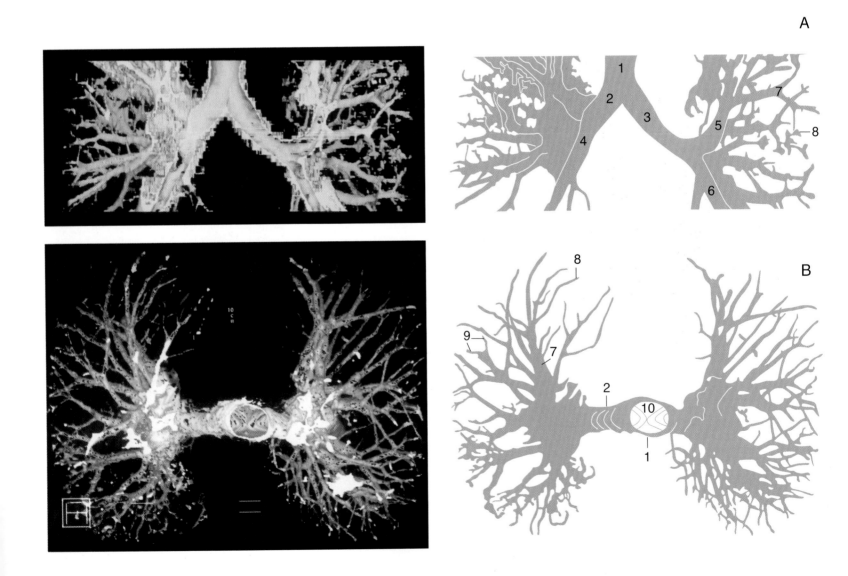

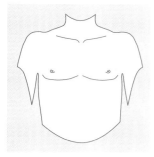

Bronchogram of right lung, anteroposterior view

1 - Trachea
2 - Apical segmental bronchus of upper lobe
3 - Right principal bronchus
4 - Posterior segmental bronchus of upper lobe
5 - Superior lobar bronchus
6 - Anterior segmental bronchus of upper lobe
7 - Bronchus intermedius (right bronchus)
8 - Medial segmental bronchus of middle lobe
9 - Lateral segmental bronchus of middle lobe
10 - Inferior lobar bronchus
11 - Lateral basal segmental bronchus of lower lobe
12 - Medial basal segmental bronchus of lower lobe
13 - Posterior basal segmental bronchus of lower lobe
14 - Anterior basal segmental bronchus of lower lobe

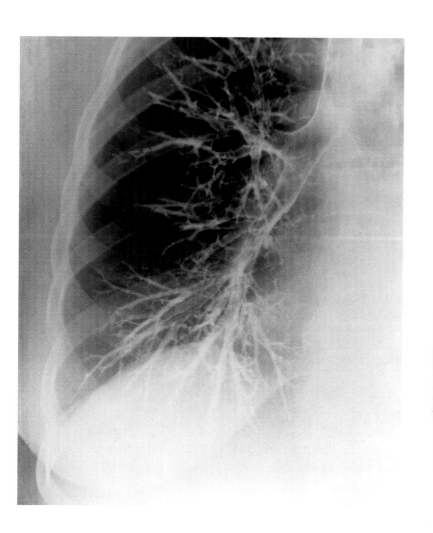

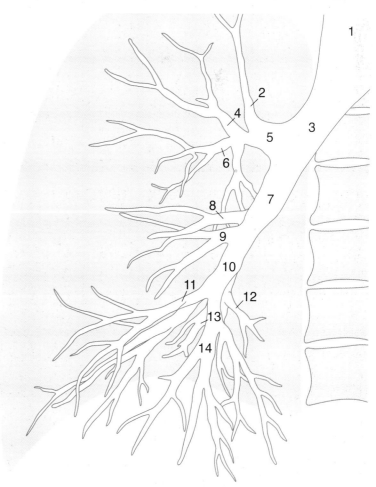

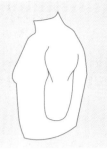

Bronchogram of right lung, lateral view

1 - Right principal bronchus
2 - Apical segmental bronchus of upper lobe
3 - Posterior segmental bronchus of upper lobe
4 - Anterior segmental bronchus of upper lobe
5 - Bronchus intermedius (right bronchus)
6 - Apical segmental bronchus of lower lobe
7 - Inferior lobar bronchus
8 - Middle lobar bronchus
9 - Lateral segmental bronchus of middle lobe
10 - Posterior basal segmental bronchus of lower lobe
11 - Anterior basal segmental bronchus of lower lobe
12 - Medial segmental bronchus of middle lobe
13 - Lateral basal segmental bronchus of lower lobe
14 - Medial basal segmental bronchus of lower lobe

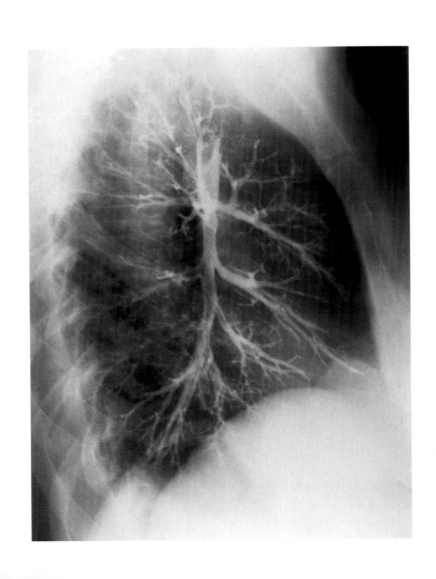

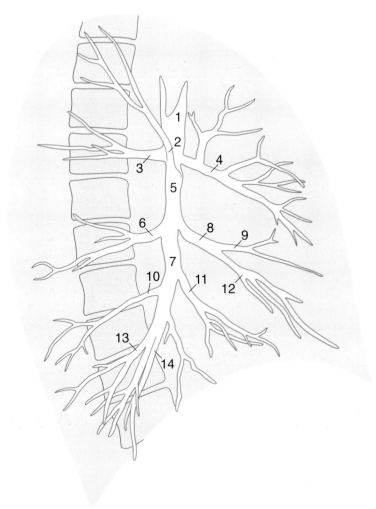

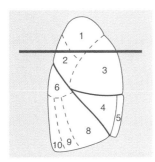

Segmental anatomy of lungs, axial CT
Bronchopulmonary segments are indicated by traditional numbering, other structures by letters troughout the entire series (pp. 145-152).

1 - Apical of upper lobe
2 - Posterior of upper lobe
3 - Anterior of upper lobe
4 - Lateral of middle lobe (right lung), superior lingular (left lung)
5 - Medial of middle lobe (right lung), inferior lingular (left lung)

6 - Apical of lower lobe
7 - Medial basal of lower lobe (inconspicuous in the left lung)
8 - Anterior basal of lower lobe
9 - Lateral basal of lower lobe
10 - Posterior basal of lower lobe
a - Trachea

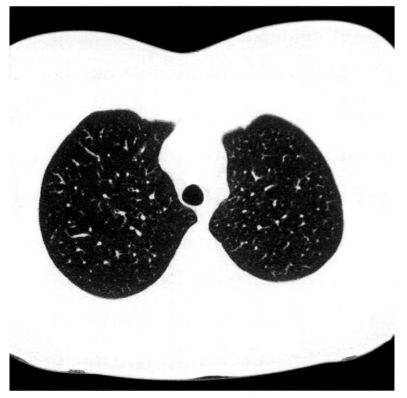

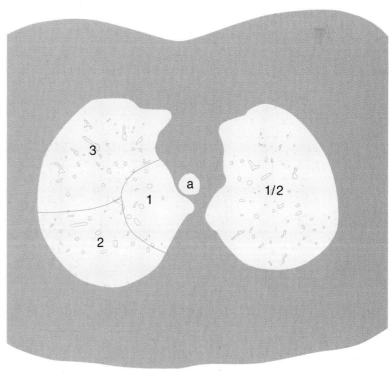

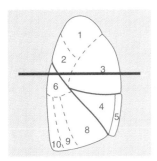

Segmental anatomy of lungs, axial CT
Bronchopulmonary segments are indicated by traditional numbering, other structures by letters troughout the entire series (pp. 145-152).

1 - Apical of upper lobe
2 - Posterior of upper lobe
3 - Anterior of upper lobe
4 - Lateral of middle lobe (right lung), superior lingular (left lung)
5 - Medial of middle lobe (right lung), inferior lingular (left lung)
6 - Apical of lower lobe

7 - Medial basal of lower lobe (inconspicuous in the left lung)
8 - Anterior basal of lower lobe
9 - Lateral basal of lower lobe
10 - Posterior basal of lower lobe
a - Trachea
b - Oblique fissure of right lung
c - Oblique fissure of left lung

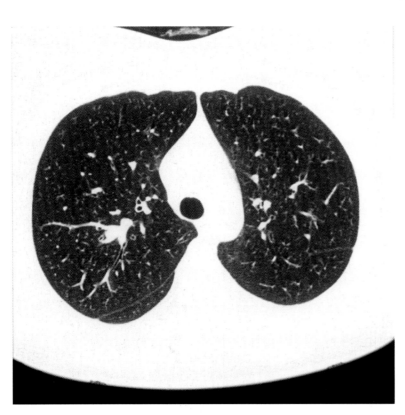

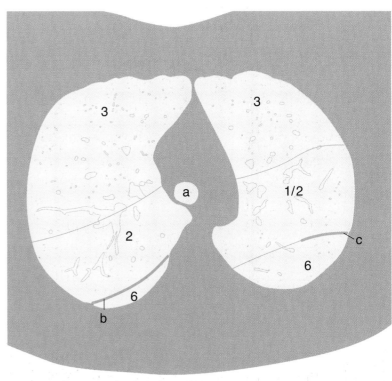

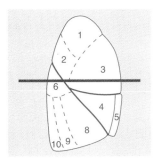

Segmental anatomy of lungs, axial CT

Bronchopulmonary segments are indicated by traditional numbering, other structures by letters troughout the entire series (pp. 145-152).

1 - Apical of upper lobe
2 - Posterior of upper lobe
3 - Anterior of upper lobe
4 - Lateral of middle lobe (right lung), superior lingular (left lung)
5 - Medial of middle lobe (right lung), inferior lingular (left lung)
6 - Apical of lower lobe
7 - Medial basal of lower lobe (inconspicuous in the left lung)

8 - Anterior basal of lower lobe
9 - Lateral basal of lower lobe
10 - Posterior basal of lower lobe
b - Oblique fissure of right lung
c - Oblique fissure of left lung
d - Right main bronchus
e - Left main bronchus
f - Right pulmonary hilum
g - Left pulmonary hilum

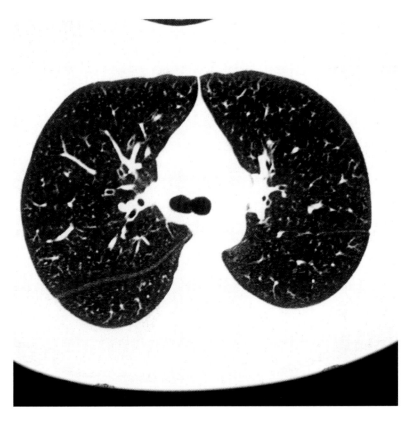

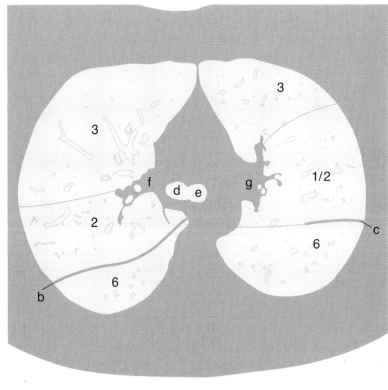

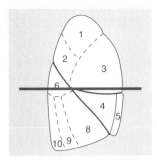

Segmental anatomy of lungs, axial CT

Bronchopulmonary segments are indicated by traditional numbering, other structures by letters troughout the entire series (pp. 145-152).

1 - Apical of upper lobe
2 - Posterior of upper lobe
3 - Anterior of upper lobe
4 - Lateral of middle lobe (right lung), superior lingular (left lung)
5 - Medial of middle lobe (right lung), inferior lingular (left lung)
6 - Apical of lower lobe
7 - Medial basal of lower lobe (inconspicuous in the left lung)

8 - Anterior basal of lower lobe
9 - Lateral basal of lower lobe
10 - Posterior basal of lower lobe
b - Oblique fissure of right lung
c - Oblique fissure of left lung
d - Right main bronchus
e - Left main bronchus
f - Right pulmonary hilum
g - Left pulmonary hilum

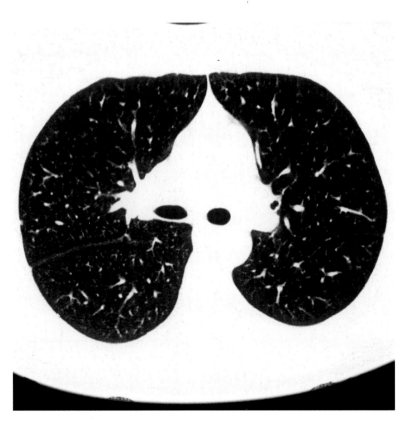

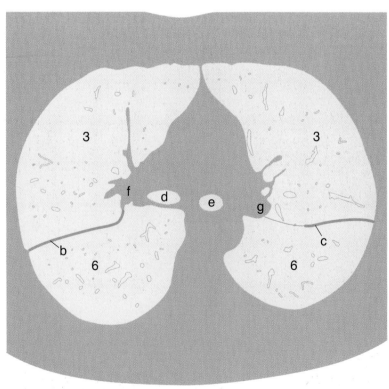

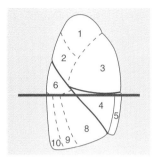

Segmental anatomy of lungs, axial CT

Bronchopulmonary segments are indicated by traditional numbering, other structures by letters troughout the entire series (pp. 145-152).

1 - Apical of upper lobe
2 - Posterior of upper lobe
3 - Anterior of upper lobe
4 - Lateral of middle lobe (right lung), superior lingular (left lung)
5 - Medial of middle lobe (right lung), inferior lingular (left lung)
6 - Apical of lower lobe
7 - Medial basal of lower lobe (inconspicuous in the left lung)

8 - Anterior basal of lower lobe
9 - Lateral basal of lower lobe
10 - Posterior basal of lower lobe
b - Oblique fissure of right lung
c - Oblique fissure of left lung
d - Right main bronchus
e - Left main bronchus
f - Right pulmonary hilum
g - Left pulmonary hilum

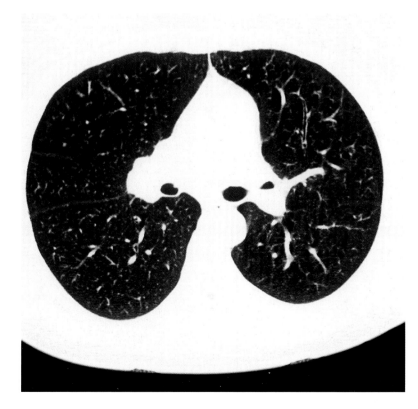

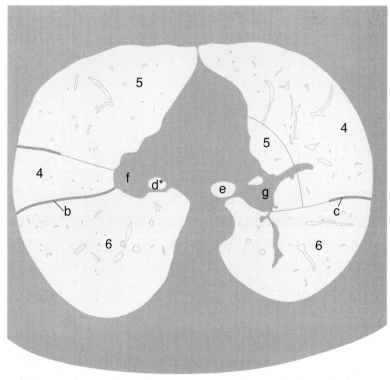

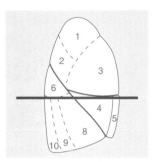

Segmental anatomy of lungs, axial CT

Bronchopulmonary segments are indicated by traditional numbering, other structures by letters troughout the entire series (pp. 145-152).

1 - Apical of upper lobe
2 - Posterior of upper lobe
3 - Anterior of upper lobe
4 - Lateral of middle lobe (right lung), superior lingular (left lung)
5 - Medial of middle lobe (right lung), inferior lingular (left lung)
6 - Apical of lower lobe

7 - Medial basal of lower lobe (inconspicuous in the left lung)
8 - Anterior basal of lower lobe
9 - Lateral basal of lower lobe
10 - Posterior basal of lower lobe
b - Oblique fissure of right lung
c - Oblique fissure of left lung

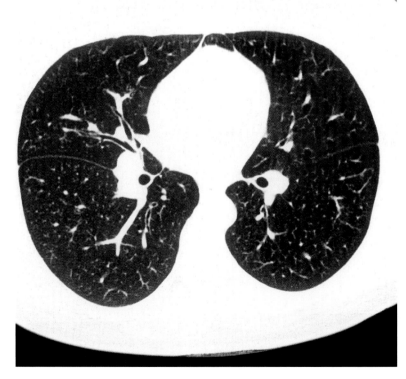

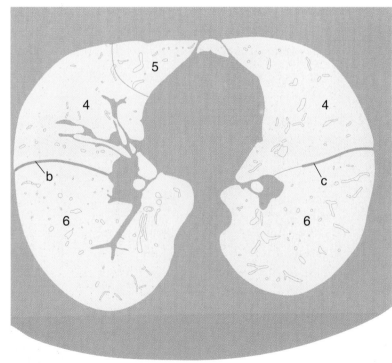

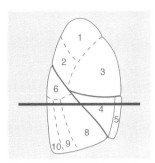

Segmental anatomy of lungs, axial CT

Bronchopulmonary segments are indicated by traditional numbering, other structures by letters troughout the entire series (pp. 145-152).

1 - Apical of upper lobe
2 - Posterior of upper lobe
3 - Anterior of upper lobe
4 - Lateral of middle lobe (right lung), superior lingular (left lung)
5 - Medial of middle lobe (right lung), inferior lingular (left lung)
6 - Apical of lower lobe
7 - Medial basal of lower lobe (inconspicuous in the left lung)
8 - Anterior basal of lower lobe
9 - Lateral basal of lower lobe
10 - Posterior basal of lower lobe
b - Oblique fissure of right lung
c - Oblique fissure of left lung
h - Heart

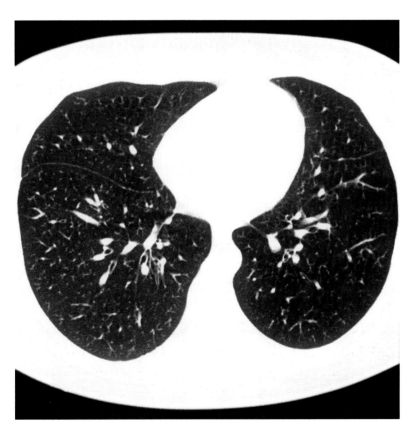

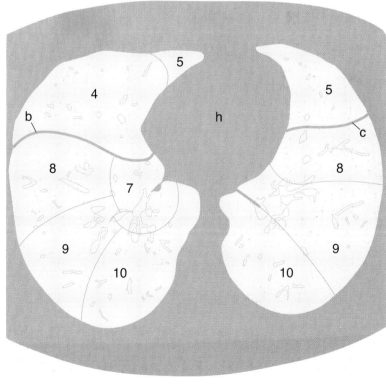

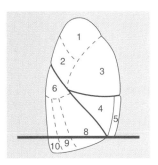

Segmental anatomy of lungs, axial CT

Bronchopulmonary segments are indicated by traditional numbering, other structures by letters troughout the entire series (pp. 145-152).

1 - Apical of upper lobe
2 - Posterior of upper lobe
3 - Anterior of upper lobe
4 - Lateral of middle lobe
    (right lung), superior
    lingular (left lung)
5 - Medial of middle lobe
    (right lung), inferior
    lingular (left lung)
6 - Apical of lower lobe

7 - Medial basal of lower lobe
    (inconspicuous in the
    left lung)
8 - Anterior basal of lower lobe
9 - Lateral basal of lower lobe
10 - Posterior basal of lower lobe
b - Oblique fissure of right lung
c - Oblique fissure of left lung
h - Heart
i - Diaphragm

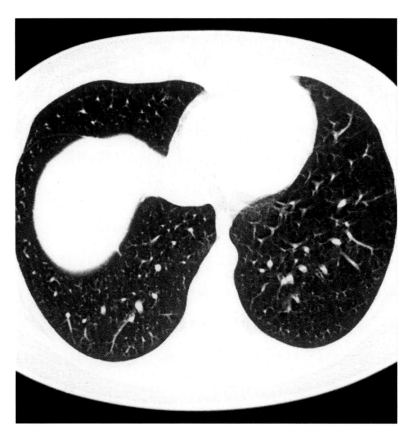

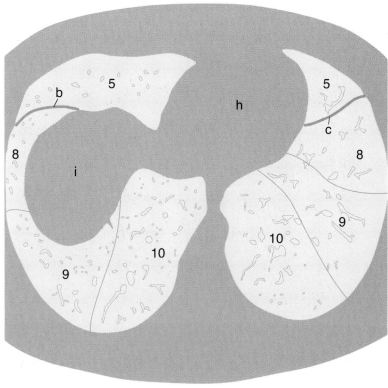

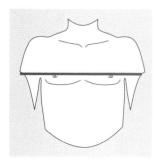

High resolution axial CT of lungs at the level of pulmonary hilum

1 - Costal cartilage IV
2 - Rib V
3 - Heart and pericardium
4 - Rib VI
5 - Middle lobar bronchus and artery
6 - Rib VII
7 - Pulmonary artery

8 - Inferior lobar bronchus and artery
9 - Oesophagus
10 - Azygos vein
11 - Aorta
12 - Hemiazygos vein
13 - Rib VIII
14 - Thoracic vertebra VIII

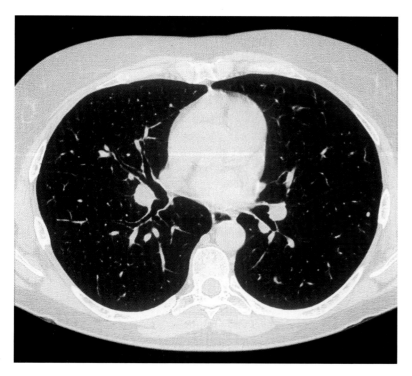

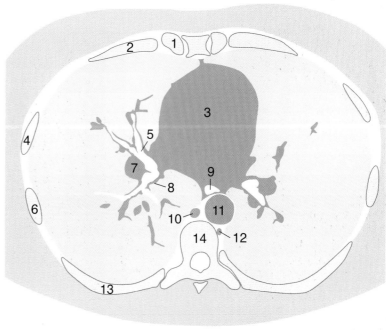

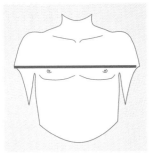

High resolution axial CT of right pulmonary hilum, enlarged view

1 - Heart
2 - Medial segmental bronchus of middle lobe
3 - Lateral segmental bronchus of middle lobe
4 - Middle lobar bronchus
5 - Inferior lobar bronchus
6 - Anterior basal segmental bronchus of inferior lobe
7 - Medial basal segmental bronchus of inferior lobe
8 - Oblique fissure

9 - Middle lobe
10 - Inferior lobe
11 - Medial segmental artery of middle lobe
12 - Lateral segmental artery of middle lobe
13 - Pulmonary artery
14 - Anterior basal segmental artery of inferior lobe
15 - Mediobasal segmental artery of inferior lobe
16 - Spine

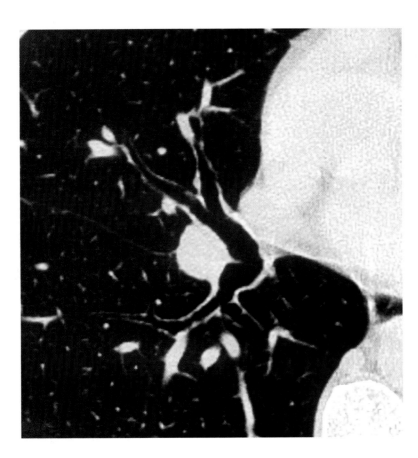

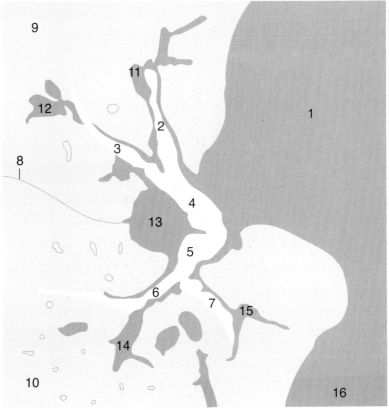

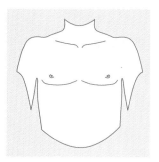

High resolution CT of lung parenchyma

1 - Heart
2 - Oblique fissure
3 - Parenchyma of lung
4 - Lobar bronchus, cross section

5 - Lobar artery, cross section
6 - Spine

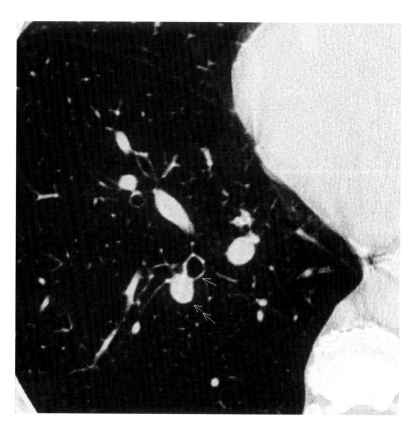

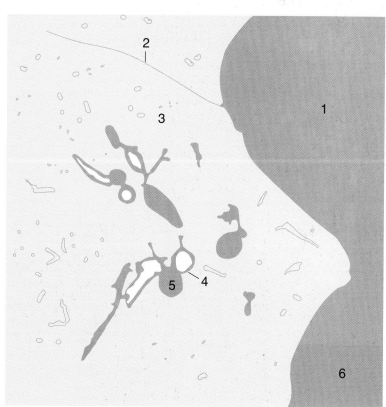

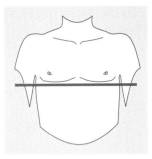

Axial CT of heart

1 - Sternum
2 - Costal cartilage
3 - Pericardium
4 - Pulmonary trunk
5 - Right atrium
6 - Interatrial septum
7 - Ascending aorta
8 - Left coronary (anterior descending) artery
9 - Left atrium

10 - Right pulmonary vein
11 - Right inferior lobar bronchus
12 - Right pulmonary artery
13 - Left inferior lobar artery
14 - Oesophagus
15 - Aorta
16 - Azygos vein
17 - Vertebra

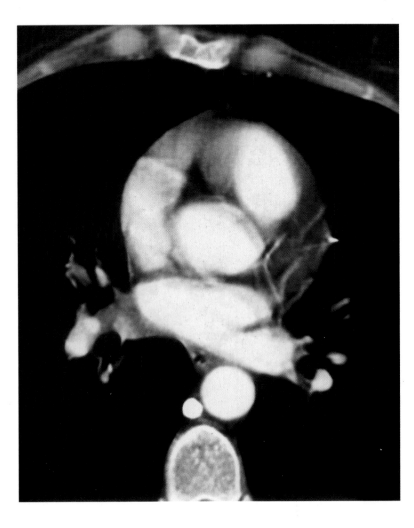

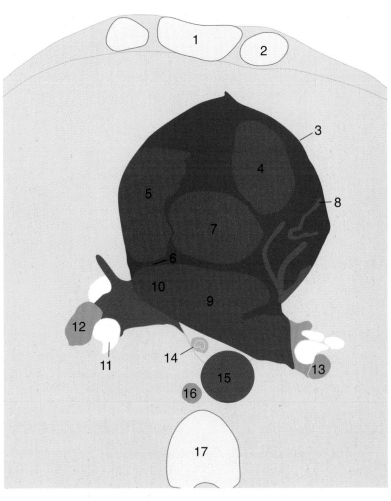

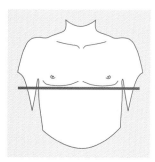

Axial CT of heart

1 - Sternum
2 - Costal cartilage
3 - Pericardium
4 - Right ventricle
5 - Right main coronary artery
6 - Right atrium
7 - Left ventricle

8 - Left atrium
9 - Right lower pulmonary veins
10 - Oesophagus
11 - Aorta
12 - Azygos vein
13 - Vertebra

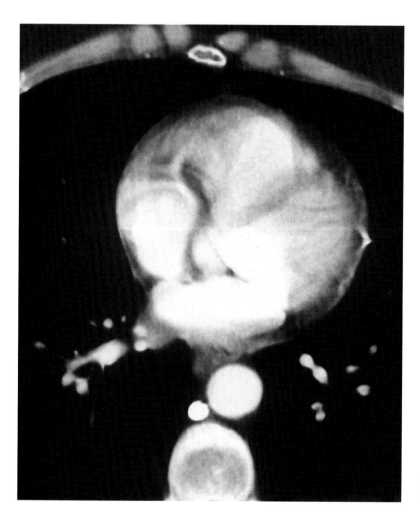

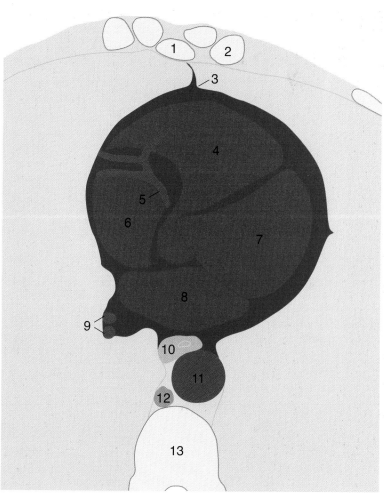

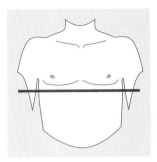

Axial CT of heart

1 - Sternum
2 - Costal cartilage
3 - Pericardium
4 - Right ventricular cavity
5 - Left ventricular cavity
6 - Muscular interventricular
    septum

7 - Right atrium
8 - Inferior vena cava
9 - Oesophagus
10 - Aorta
11 - Azygos vein
12 - Hemiazygos vein
13 - Vertebra

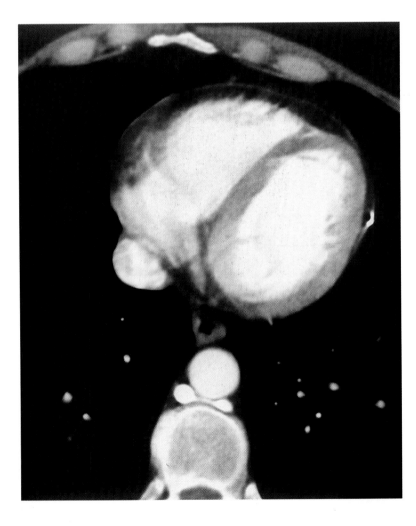

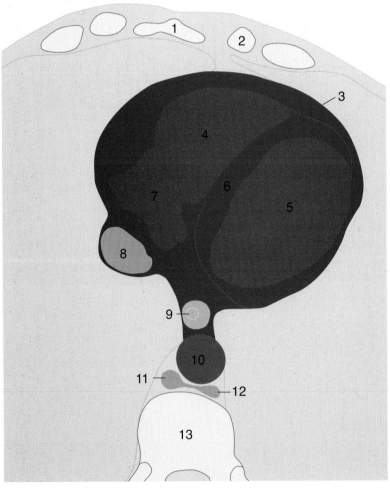

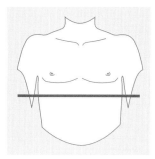

Axial CT of heart

1 - Sternum	9 - Inferior vena cava
2 - Costal cartilage	10 - Oesophagus
3 - Pericardium	11 - Aorta
4 - Right ventricle	12 - Azygos vein
5 - Muscular interventricular septum	13 - Hemiazygos vein
6 - Left ventricle	14 - Posterior intercostal vein
7 - Right atrium	15 - Vertebra
8 - Muscular wall of left ventricle	

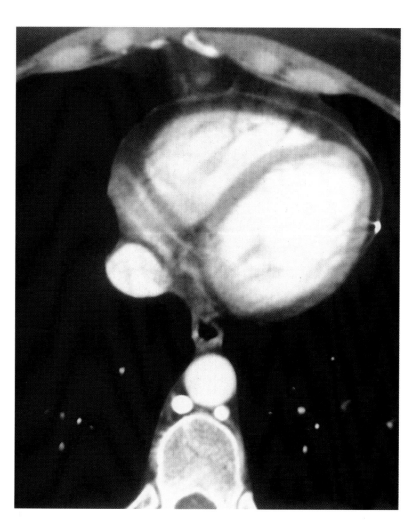

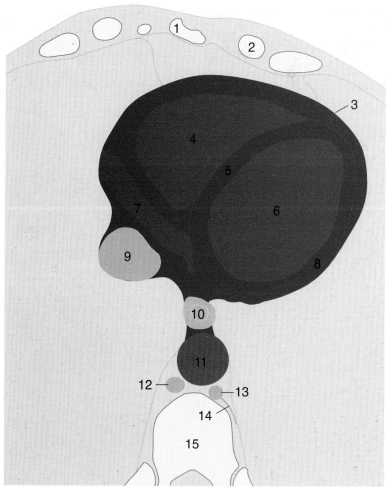

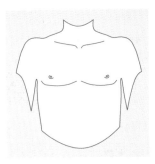

Angiocardiograms
A - left ventricle in systolic phase, B - left ventricle in diastolic phase.

1 - Ascending aorta
2 - Catheter
3 - Left (obtuse) margin
4 - Interventricular septum
5 - Apex of heart
6 - Diaphragm

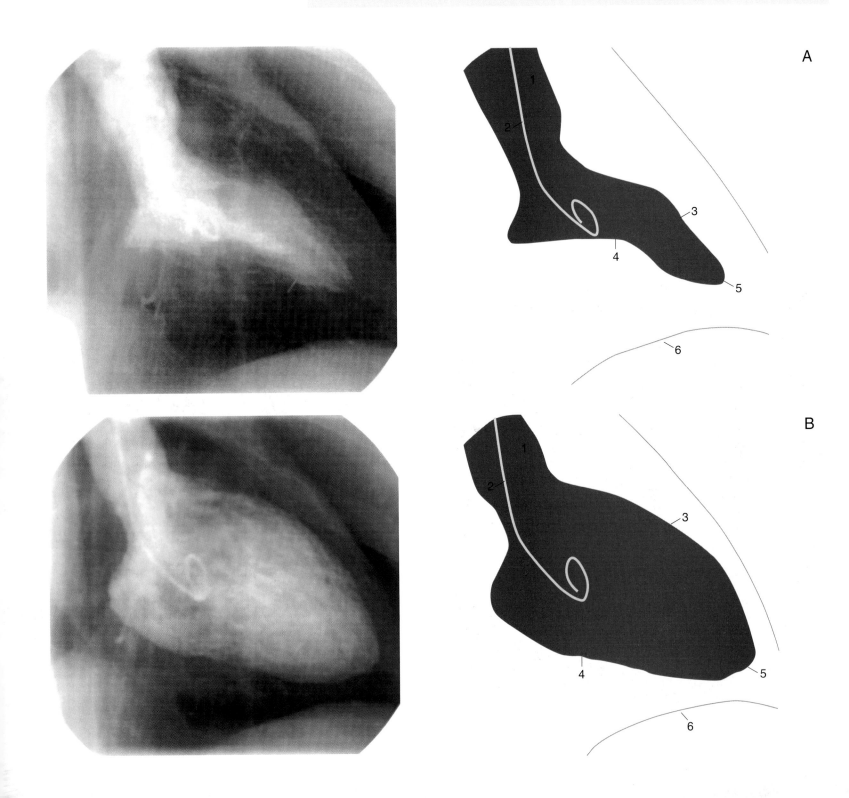

A

B

Angiocardiogram of left coronary artery, anterior aspect

1 - Catheter
2 - Left main coronary artery
3 - Obtuse marginals
4 - Anterior descending
   (interventricular) artery
5 - Circumflex artery

6 - Vertebral column
7 - Diagonal branch
8 - Pacemaker in the right
   atrium with tip in right
   ventricle

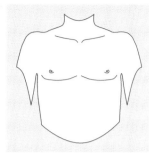

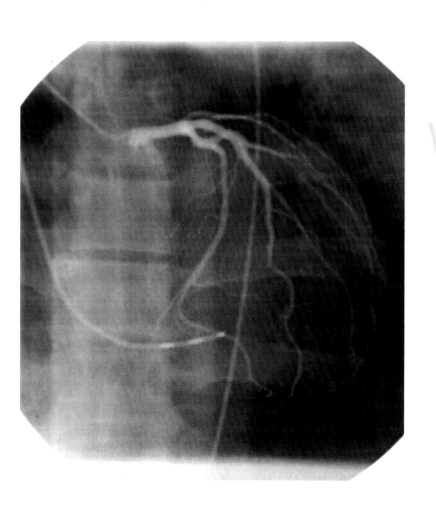

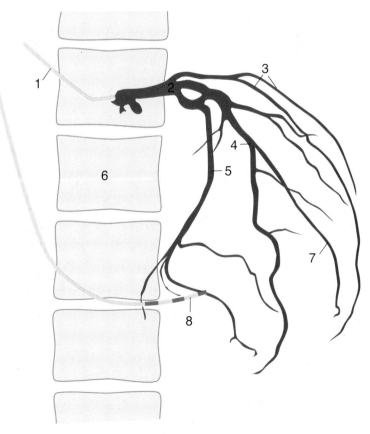

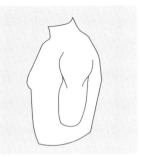

Angiocardiogram of left coronary artery, lateral aspect

1 - Catheter
2 - Anterior descending
    (interventricular) artery
3 - Left main coronary artery
    seen end on
4 - Circumflex artery
5 - Sternum

6 - Diagonal branches
7 - Posterolateral branch
8 - Obtuse marginals
9 - Pacemaker in the right
    atrium with tip in right
    ventricle

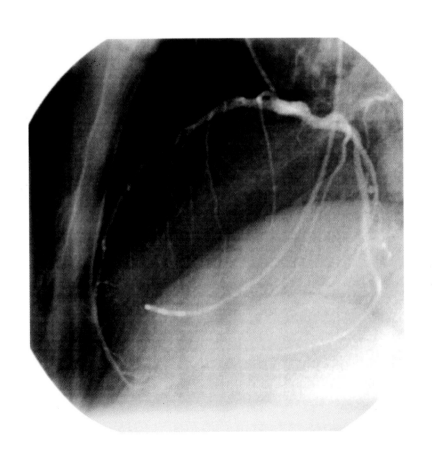

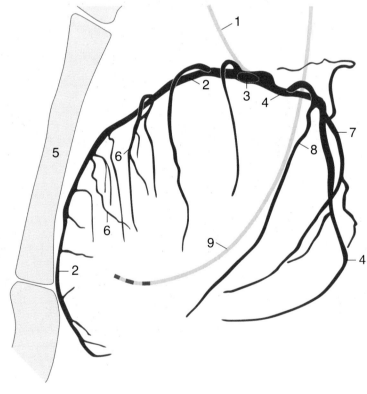

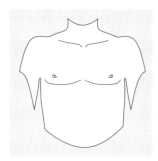

Angiocardiogram of right coronary artery, apical aspect

1 - Sinus artery
2 - Catheter
3 - Right coronary artery
4 - Right ventricular branch

5 - Vertebral column
6 - Posterolateral branch
7 - Posterior descending
    (interventricular) artery

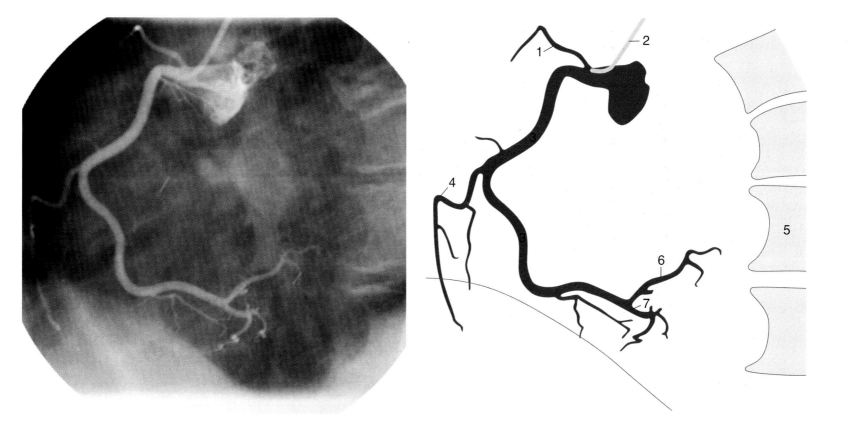

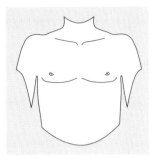

Angiocardiography. Bioprosthesis in the mitral (bicuspid) valve, left anterior oblique aspect

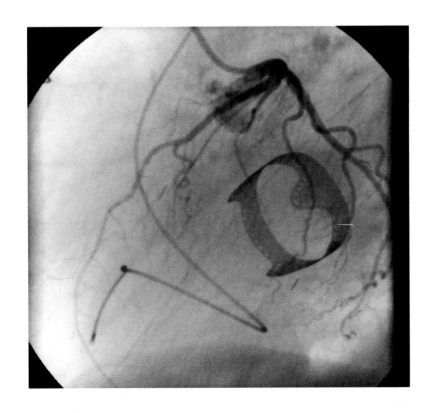

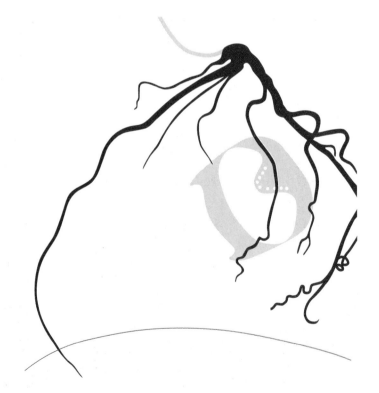

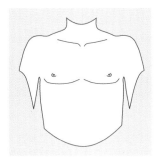

Angiocardiography. Artificial implant in the mitral (bicuspid) valve, closed state corresponding to systole

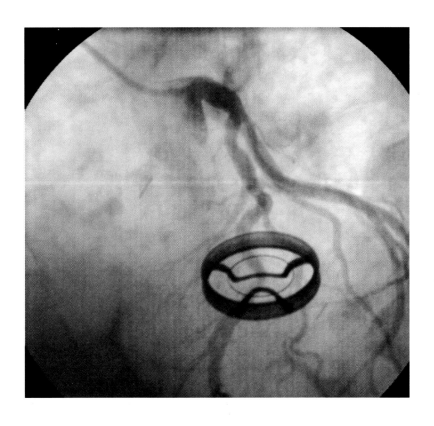

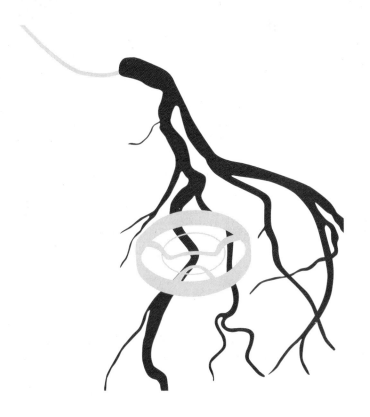

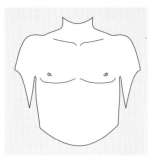

Artificial implant in the aortic valve, open state corresponding to systole

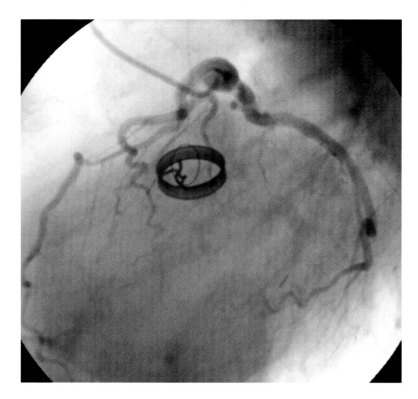

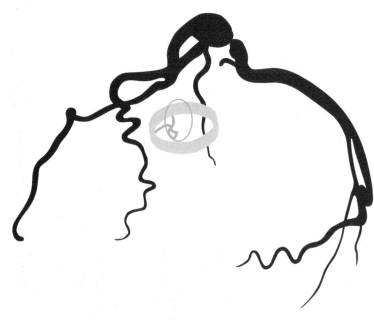

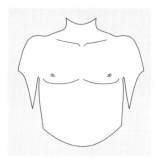

Coronary bypass (graft) in the right coronary artery
Arrows mark beginning and end of graft.

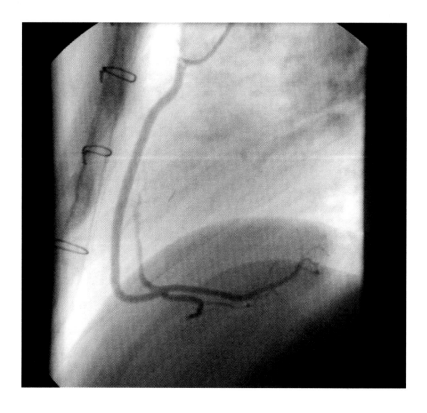

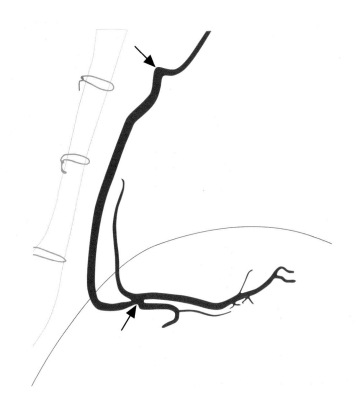

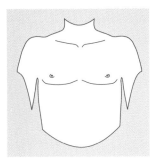

Ultrasound images of heart (echocardiogram)

A - long axis of left ventricle, B - aortic valve, C - the four chambers, D - left parasternal short axis, representing the mitral valve.

1 - Right ventricle
2 - Left ventricle
3 - Left ventricular outflow tract
4 - Aorta
5 - Left atrium
6 - Anterior leaflet of mitral valve
7 - Posterior leaflet of mitral valve
8 - Chordae tendineae
9 - Right atrium
10 - Interventicular septum

11 - Tricuspid valve
12 - Atrioventricular septum
13 - Mitral (bicuspid) valve
14 - Interatrial septum
15 - Right ventricular outflow tract
16 - Pulmonary artery
17 - Right coronary cusp of aortic valve
18 - Left coronary cusp of aortic valve
19 - Non-coronary cusp of aortic valve

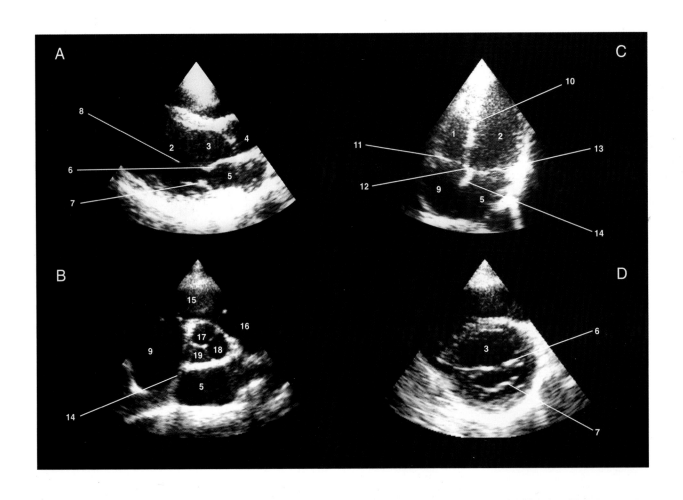

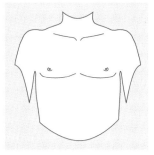

Branches of the aortic arch, angiogram, anteroposterior view

1 - Right common carotid artery
2 - Right vertebral artery
3 - Left common carotid artery
4 - Left vertebral artery
5 - Clavicle
6 - Costocervical trunk
7 - Right subclavian artery
8 - Thyrocervical trunk

9 - Brachiocephalic trunk
10 - Left subclavian artery
11 - Left axillary artery
12 - Right internal thoracic artery
13 - Aortic arch
14 - Ascending aorta
15 - Descending thoracic aorta

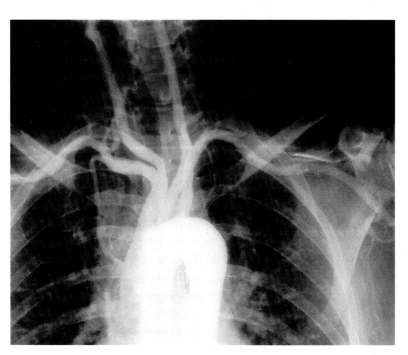

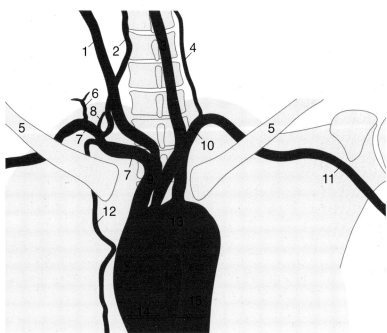

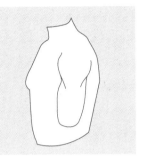

Thoracic part of oesophagus, barium swallow, lateral view

1 - Trachea
2 - Ascending aorta
3 - Impression of aortic arch
4 - Spine
5 - Impression of left main bronchus
6 - Left atrium of heart
7 - Cardiac impression

8 - Retrocardiac space
9 - Diaphragm
10 - Oesophageal opening (aperture) of diaphragm, oesophago-gastric junction
11 - Contrast medium in oesophagus

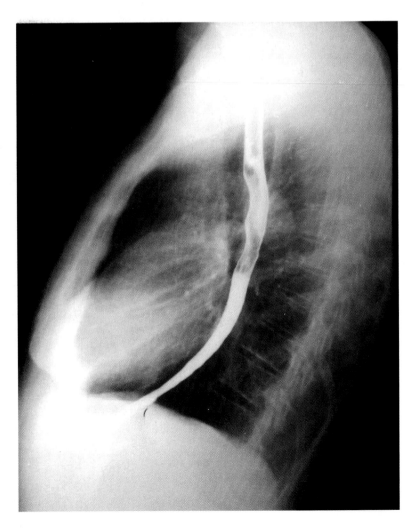

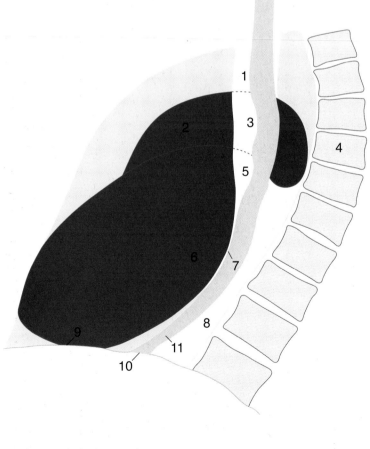

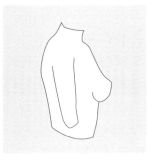

Breast, mammography, craniocaudal view

1 - Pectoralis major muscle
2 - Line of skin
3 - Suspensory ligaments
   (of Cooper)

4 - Subareolar area
5 - Nipple
6 - Mammary fat

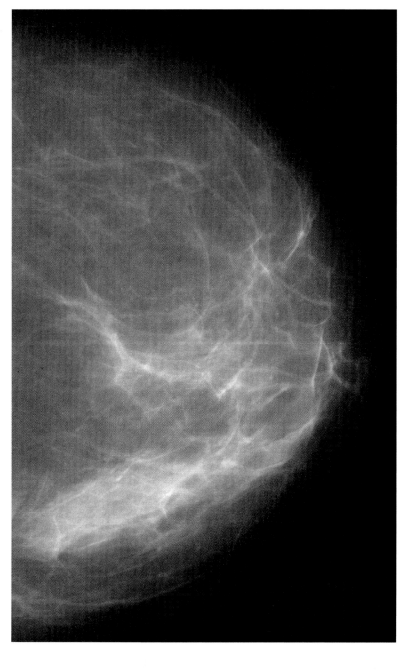

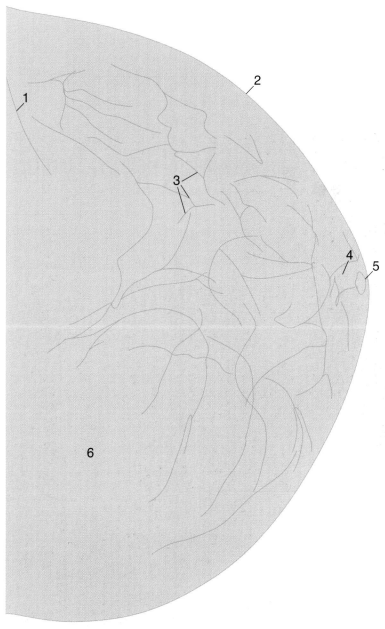

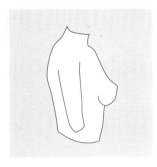

Breast, mammography, oblique view

1 - Pectoralis major muscle
2 - Line of skin
3 - Suspensory ligaments
   (of Cooper)
4 - Subareolar area
5 - Nipple
6 - Mammary fat
7 - Inframammary fold

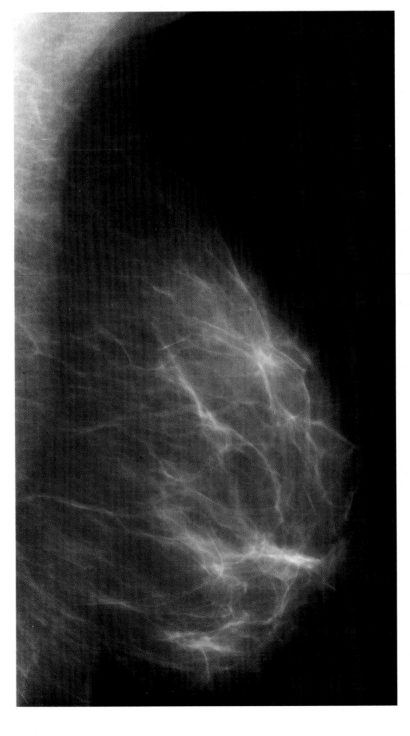

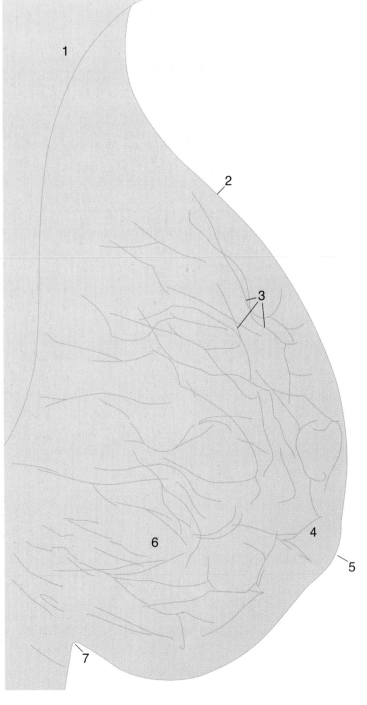

ABDOMEN

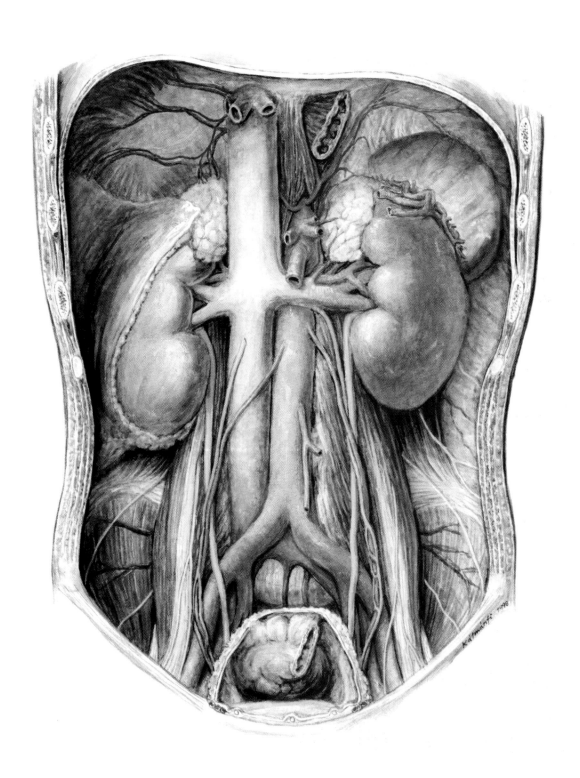

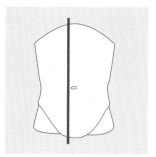

Parasagittal MR of body cavities

1 - Trachea
2 - Arch of aorta
3 - Ascending aorta
4 - Aorto-pulmonary window
5 - Sternum
6 - Descending aorta
7 - Right ventricle of heart
8 - Oesophagus in
   retrocardiac space
9 - Diaphragm
10 - Costal cartilage

11 - Liver
12 - Thoracic vertebra XII
13 - Inferior vena cava
14 - Transverse colon
15 - Rectus abdominis muscle
16 - Tendinous intersection
17 - Intestinal loops
18 - Sacrum
19 - Urinary bladder
20 - Rectum

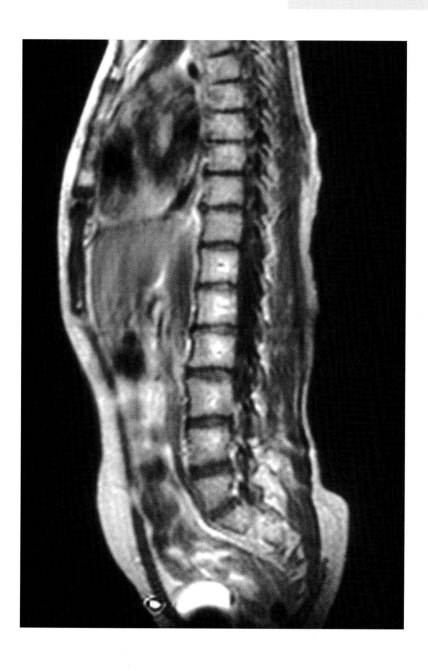

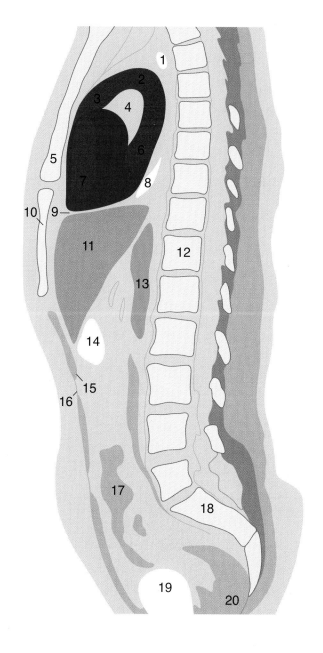

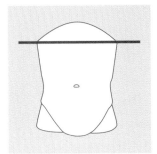

Axial CT of abdomen

1 - Rectus sheath and rectus
abdominis muscle
2 - Rib
3 - Liver
4 - Stomach
5 - Colon, splenic flexure
6 - Costodiaphragmatic
recess
7 - Hepatic veins
8 - Inferior vena cava

9 - Right crus of diaphragm
10 - Oesophagogastric
junction (cardia)
11 - Left subphrenic space
12 - Intercostal muscles
13 - Spleen
14 - Aorta
15 - Thoracic vertebra X
16 - Erector spinae muscle
17 - Latissimus dorsi muscle

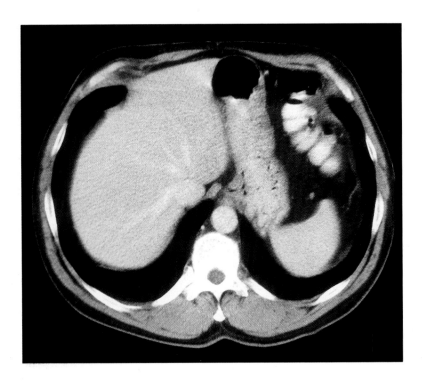

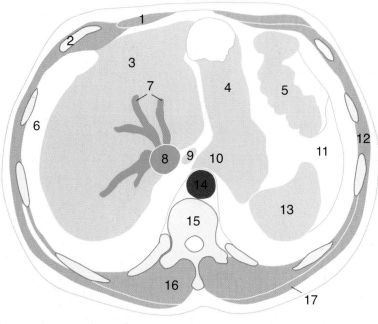

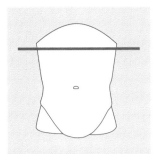

Axial CT of abdomen

1 - Linea alba
2 - Rectus sheath and rectus
    abdominis muscle
3 - Rib
4 - Liver
5 - Stomach
6 - Colon
7 - Hepatic veins
8 - Inferior vena cava

9 - Crura of diaphragm
    (forming median arcuate
    ligament)
10 - Left subphrenic space
11 - Spleen
12 - Aorta
13 - Thoracic vertebra XI
14 - Erector spinae muscle
15 - Latissimus dorsi muscle

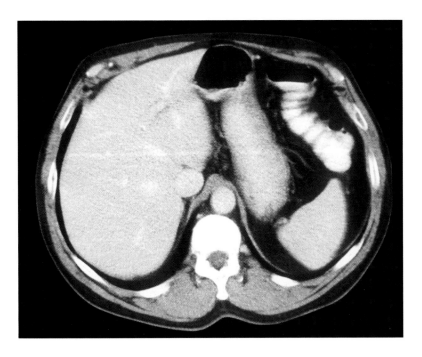

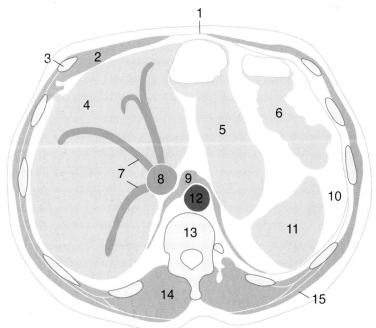

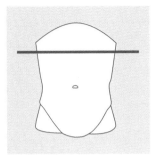

Axial CT of abdomen

1 - Rectus sheath and rectus abdominis muscle
2 - Rib
3 - Liver
4 - Stomach (air bubble and body)
5 - Colon
6 - Right adrenal gland
7 - Inferior vena cava
8 - Crura of diaphragm
9 - Aorta
10 - Left gastro-epiploic artery
11 - Spleen
12 - Thoracic vertebra XI
13 - Erector spinae muscle
14 - Latissimus dorsi muscle

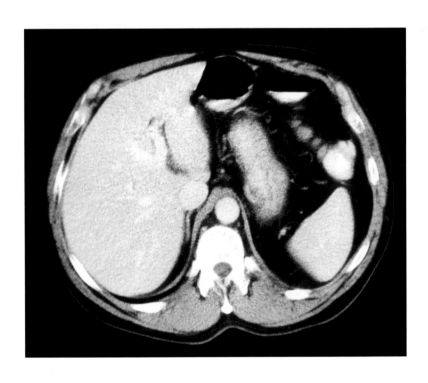

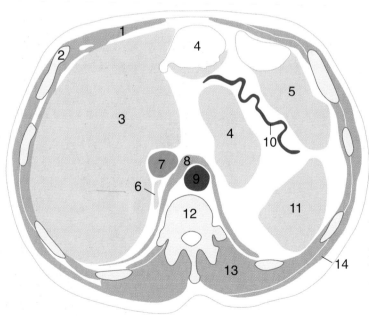

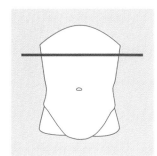

Axial CT of abdomen

1 - Rectus sheath and rectus abdominis muscle
2 - Rib
3 - Liver
4 - Stomach (body)
5 - Colon
6 - Falciform fissure, ligamentum teres
7 - Caudate lobe of liver
8 - Pancreas (body/tail)
9 - Jejunum
10 - Inferior vena cava
11 - Crus of diaphragm
12 - Splenic artery
13 - Spleen
14 - Right adrenal gland
15 - Thoracic vertebra XII
16 - Erector spinae muscle
17 - Latissimus dorsi muscle

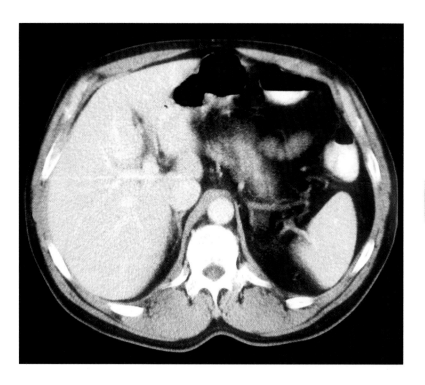

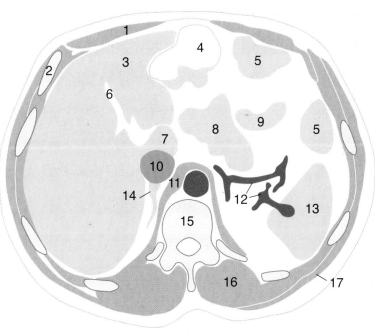

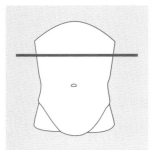

Axial CT of abdomen

1 - Rectus sheath
2 - Rib
3 - Liver
4 - Stomach
5 - Colon
6 - Ligamentum teres and falciform fissure
7 - Jejunum
8 - Body of pancreas
9 - Lobar branches of portal vein
10 - Caudate lobe of liver
11 - Inferior vena cava
12 - Coeliac trunk branching into hepatic and left gastric arteries
13 - Aorta
14 - Splenic artery
15 - Spleen
16 - Left adrenal gland
17 - Left kidney
18 - Right adrenal gland adjacent to the bare area of liver
19 - Thoracic vertebra XII
20 - Erector spinae muscle

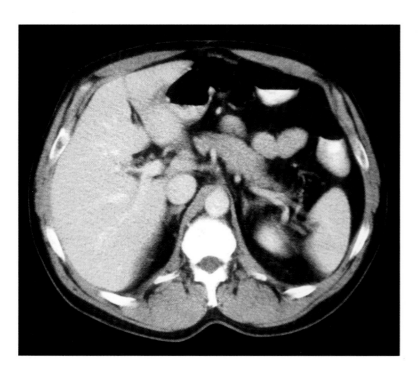

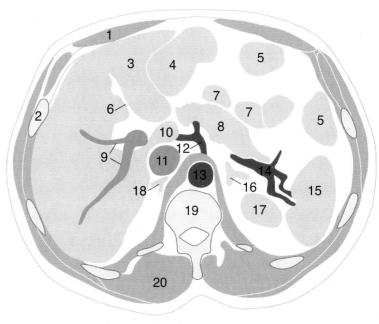

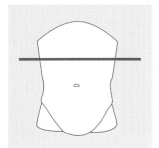

Axial CT of abdomen

1 - Rectus sheath and rectus abdominis muscle
2 - Rib
3 - Left lobe of liver, medial segment IV
4 - Left lobe of liver, lateral segments II-III
5 - Duodenal cap
6 - Stomach (antrum)
7 - Colon
8 - Hepatic artery
9 - Portal vein
10 - Neck of pancreas
11 - Jejunum
12 - Splenic vein
13 - Tail of pancreas
14 - Left adrenal gland
15 - Inferior vena cava
16 - Crus of diaphragm
17 - Superior mesenteric artery
18 - Aorta
19 - Thoracic vertebra XII
20 - Erector spinae muscle
21 - Left kidney
22 - Spleen

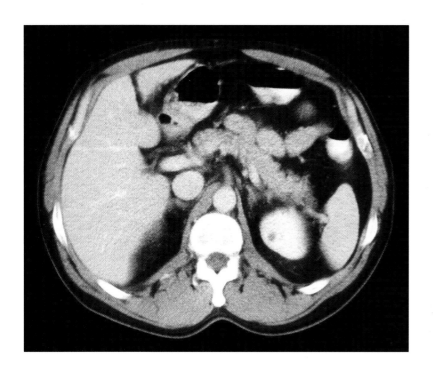

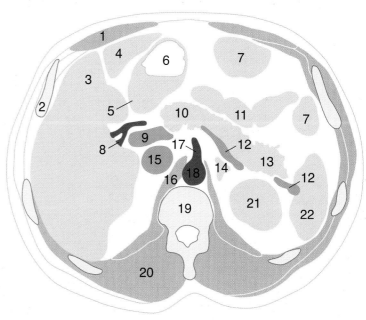

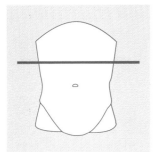

Axial CT of abdomen

1 - Linea alba
2 - Rectus sheath and rectus abdominis muscle
3 - Rib
4 - Right lobe of liver
5 - Left lobe of liver
6 - Colon
7 - Duodenum, pars superior (duodenal cap, first part)
8 - Splenic vein
9 - Jejunum
10 - Tail of pancreas

11 - Inferior vena cava
12 - Right crus of diaphragm
13 - Superior mesenteric artery
14 - Aorta
15 - Left kidney
16 - Spleen
17 - Right kidney
18 - Lumbar vertebra I
19 - Quadratus lumborum muscle
20 - Erector spinae muscle

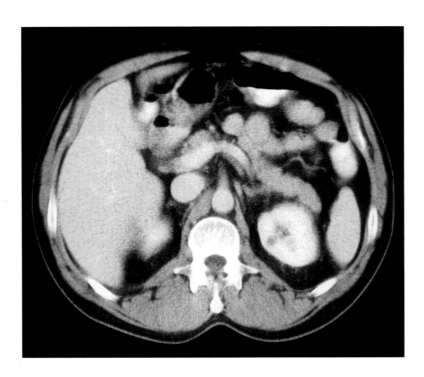
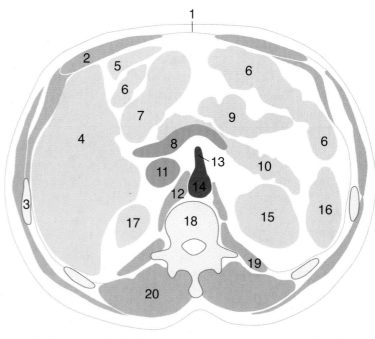

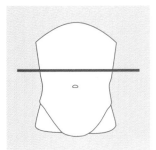

Axial CT of abdomen

1 - Linea alba
2 - Rectus sheath and rectus abdominis muscles
3 - Liver
4 - Gall bladder
5 - Transverse colon
6 - Anterolateral abdominal muscles
7 - Duodenum, pars descendens (second part)
8 - Jejunum
9 - Tail of pancreas
10 - Head of pancreas
11 - Superior mesenteric vein
12 - Superior mesenteric artery
13 - Aorta
14 - Inferior vena cava
15 - Left renal vein
16 - Right kidney
17 - Left kidney
18 - Spleen
19 - Lumbar vertebra I
20 - Psoas major muscle
21 - Quadratus lumborum muscle
22 - Erector spinae muscle

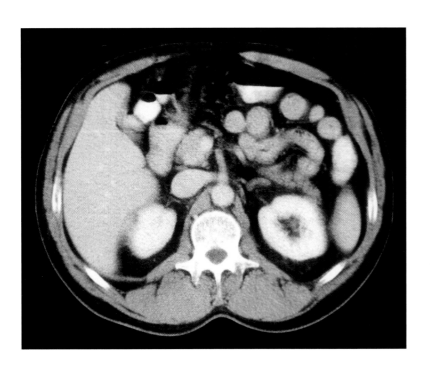

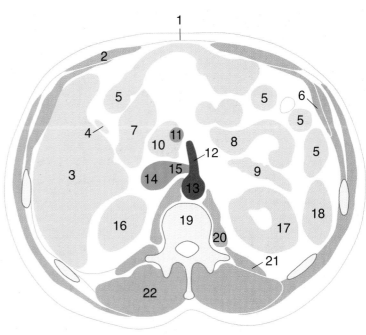

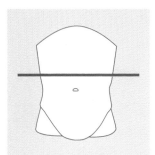

Axial CT of abdomen

1 - Linea alba
2 - Rectus abdominis muscle
3 - Transversus abdominis muscle
4 - Internal oblique muscle
5 - External oblique muscle
6 - Colon
7 - Liver
8 - Duodenum, pars descendens (second part)
9 - Common bile duct
10 - Head of pancreas
11 - Superior mesenteric vein
12 - Superior mesenteric artery
13 - Coils of jejunum
14 - Right renal artery
15 - Inferior vena cava
16 - Left renal vein
17 - Right kidney
18 - Crus of diaphragm
19 - Aorta
20 - Left kidney
21 - Psoas major muscle
22 - Lumbar vertebra I
23 - Quadratus lumborum muscle
24 - Latissimus dorsi muscle
25 - Erector spinae muscle
26 - Renal fascia

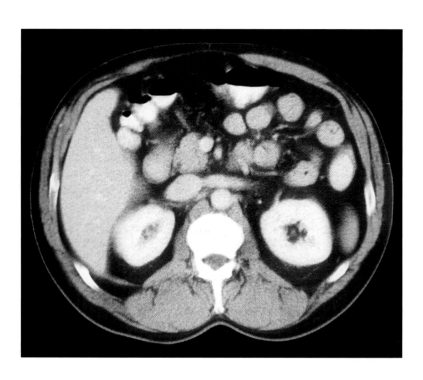

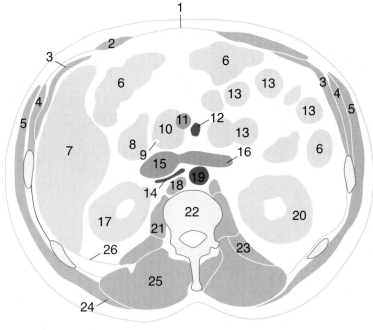

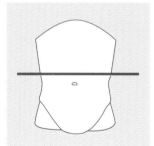

Axial CT of abdomen

1 - Linea alba
2 - Rectus abdominis muscle
3 - Transversus abdominis muscle
4 - Internal oblique muscle
5 - External oblique muscle
6 - Colon
7 - Liver
8 - Duodenum
9 - Head of pancreas
10 - Superior mesenteric vein
11 - Superior mesenteric artery
12 - Coils of jejunum
13 - Right renal vein
14 - Inferior vena cava
15 - Left renal vein
16 - Left renal artery
17 - Left kidney
18 - Right kidney
19 - Crus of diaphragm
20 - Intervertebral disc between lumbar vertebrae I-II
21 - Psoas major muscle
22 - Quadratus lumborum muscle
23 - Latissimus dorsi muscle
24 - Serratus posterior inferior muscle
25 - Erector spinae muscle
26 - Inferior mesenteric vein

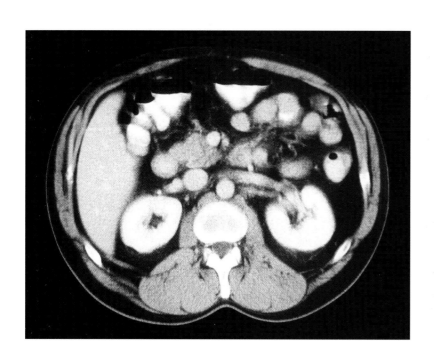

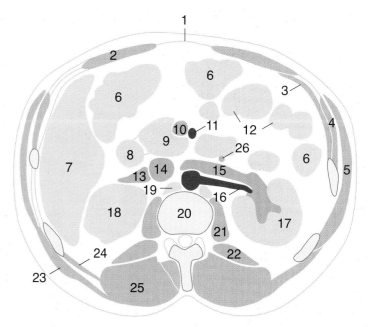

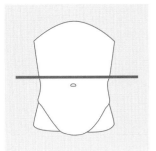

Axial CT of abdomen

1 - Linea alba	13 - Right kidney
2 - Rectus abdominis muscle	14 - Right renal vein
3 - Transversus abdominis muscle	15 - Inferior vena cava
	16 - Aorta
4 - Internal oblique muscle	17 - Left renal vein
5 - External oblique muscle	18 - Left kidney
6 - Colon	19 - Psoas major muscle
7 - Liver	20 - Lumbar vertebra II
8 - Duodenum, pars descendens (second part)	21 - Quadratus lumborum muscle
9 - Head and uncinate process of pancreas	22 - Latissimus dorsi muscle
10 - Superior mesenteric vein	23 - Serratus posterior inferior muscle
11 - Superior mesenteric artery	24 - Erector spinae muscle
12 - Coils of jejunum	25 - Posterior pararenal space II
	26 - Rib

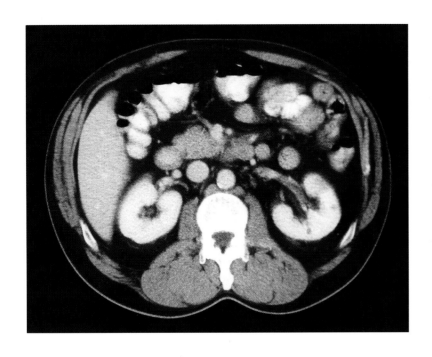

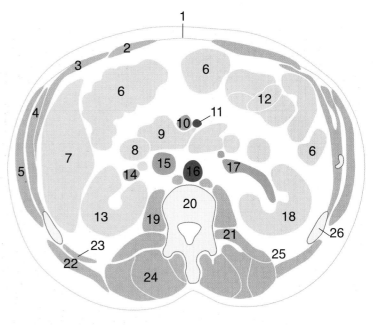

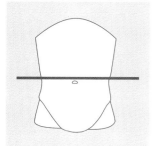

Axial CT of abdomen

1 - Linea alba
2 - Rectus abdominis muscle
3 - Transversus abdominis muscle
4 - Internal oblique muscle
5 - External oblique muscle
6 - Colon
7 - Liver
8 - Duodenum, pars horizontalis inferior (third part)
9 - Superior mesenteric vein
10 - Superior mesenteric artery
11 - Coils of jejunum
12 - Right kidney
13 - Upper ureter
14 - Inferior vena cava
15 - Aorta
16 - Inferior mesenteric vein
17 - Renal pelvis
18 - Renal cyst
19 - Psoas major muscle
20 - Lumbar vertebra II
21 - Quadratus lumborum muscle
22 - Latissimus dorsi muscle
23 - Erector spinae muscle

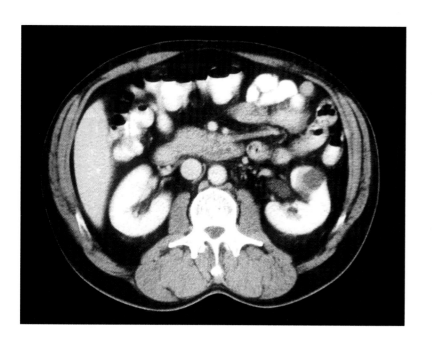

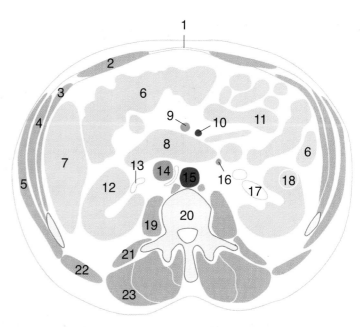

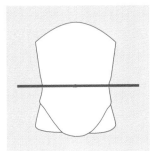

Axial CT of abdomen

1 - Umbilicus
2 - Rectus abdominis muscle
3 - Transversus abdominis and internal oblique muscles
4 - External oblique muscle
5 - Ascending colon
6 - Branches of superior mesenteric artery
7 - Coils of jejunum
8 - Right kidney

9 - Inferior vena cava
10 - Aorta
11 - Inferior mesenteric artery
12 - Inferior mesenteric vein
13 - Gonadal vessels
14 - Left kidney
15 - Psoas major muscle
16 - Quadratus lumborum muscle
17 - Lumbar vertebra III-IV
18 - Erector spinae muscle

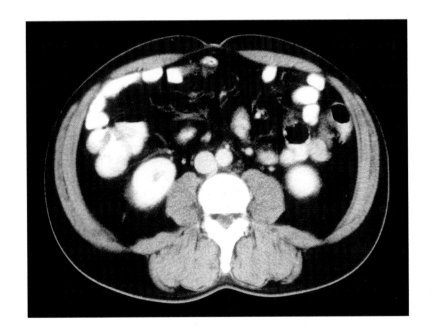

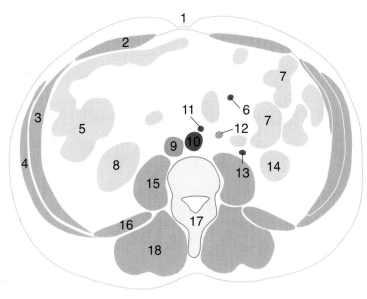

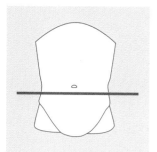

Axial CT of abdomen

1 - Linea alba
2 - Rectus abdominis muscle
3 - Terminal loop of ileum
4 - Ileocaecal valve
5 - Transversus abdominis and internal oblique muscles
6 - External oblique muscle
7 - Caecum
8 - Gonadal vessels
9 - Psoas major muscle
10 - Inferior vena cava
11 - Aorta
12 - Inferior mesenteric vein
13 - Coils of jejunum
14 - Colon
15 - Iliac crest
16 - Erector spinae muscle

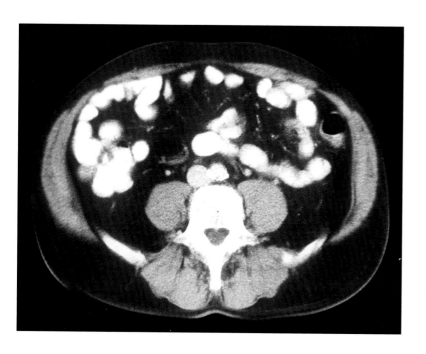

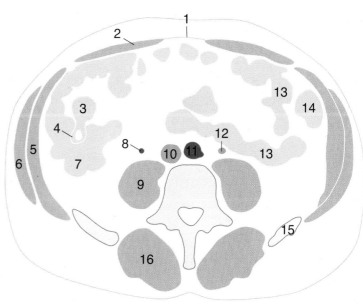

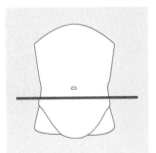

Axial CT of abdomen

1 - Linea alba
2 - Rectus abdominis muscle
3 - Transversus abdominis and internal oblique muscles
4 - External oblique muscle
5 - Terminal ileal loops
6 - Coils of ileum
7 - Descending colon
8 - Caecum

9 - Terminal loop of ileum
10 - Gonadal vessels
11 - Inferior vena cava
12 - Common iliac arteries
13 - Inferior mesenteric vein
14 - Psoas major muscle
15 - Iliac crest
16 - Erector spinae muscle
17 - Lumbar vertebra IV

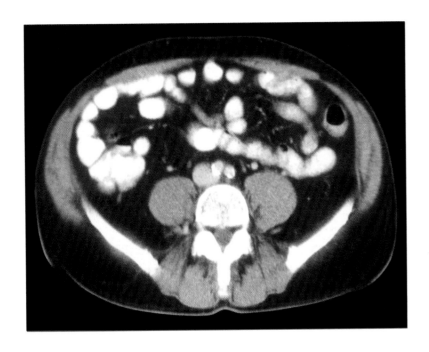

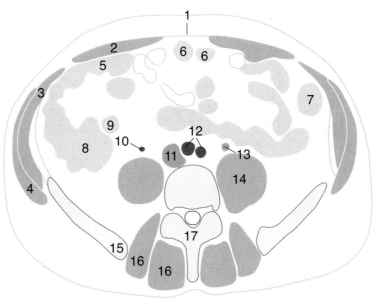

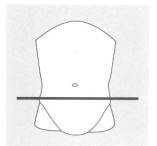

Axial CT of abdomen

1 - Linea alba
2 - Rectus abdominis muscle
3 - Transversus abdominis and internal oblique muscles
4 - External oblique muscle
5 - Coils of ileum
6 - Descending colon
7 - Psoas major muscle
8 - Right common iliac vein
9 - Right common iliac artery
10 - Left common iliac vein
11 - Left common iliac artery
12 - Iliacus muscle
13 - Lumbosacral junction
14 - Gluteus medius muscle
15 - Ilium
16 - Erector spinae muscle
17 - Sacro-iliac joint

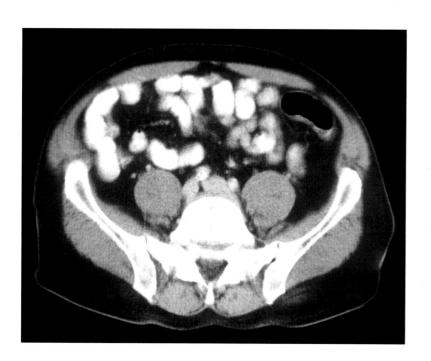

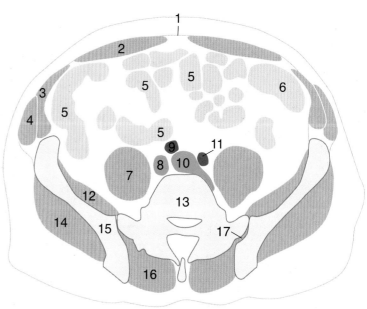

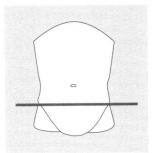

Axial CT of abdomen

1 - Linea alba
2 - Rectus abdominis muscle
3 - Anterolateral abdominal
    muscles
4 - Ileum
5 - Sigmoid colon
6 - Gluteus medius muscle
7 - Ilium
8 - Iliacus muscle
9 - Psoas major muscle
10 - Right common iliac
     artery
11 - Right common iliac vein
12 - Left common iliac vein
13 - Left common iliac artery
14 - Sacrum
15 - Gluteus maximus muscle
16 - Sacro-iliac joint

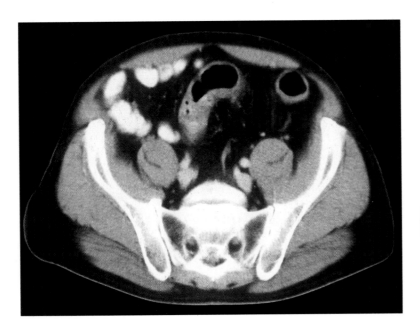

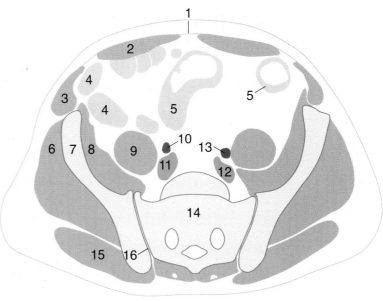

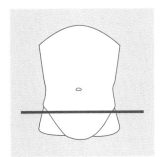

Axial CT of abdomen

1 - Linea alba
2 - Rectus abdominis muscle
3 - Coils of ileum
4 - Sigmoid colon
5 - Iliopsoas muscle
6 - Right external iliac artery
7 - Right external iliac vein
8 - Left external iliac artery

9 - Left external iliac vein
10 - Gluteus medius muscle
11 - Gluteus minimus muscle
12 - Ilium
13 - Right internal iliac artery
14 - Internal iliac veins
15 - Gluteus maximus muscle
16 - Sacrum

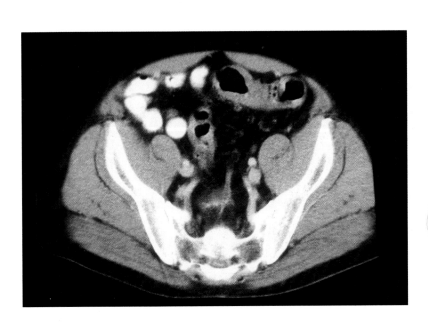

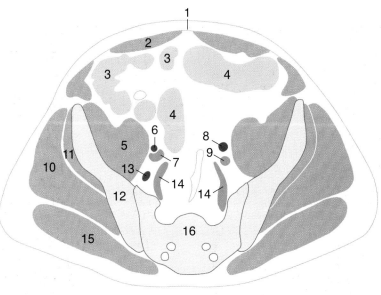

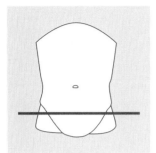

Axial CT of abdomen

1 - Linea alba
2 - Rectus abdominis muscle
3 - Anterolateral abdominal muscles
4 - Coils of ileum
5 - Sigmoid colon
6 - Peritoneum
7 - Iliopsoas muscle
8 - Right external iliac vessels

9 - Left external iliac artery
10 - Left external iliac vein
11 - Ilium
12 - Median sacral vessels
13 - Gluteus minimus muscle
14 - Gluteus medius muscle
15 - Gluteus maximus muscle
16 - Sacrum

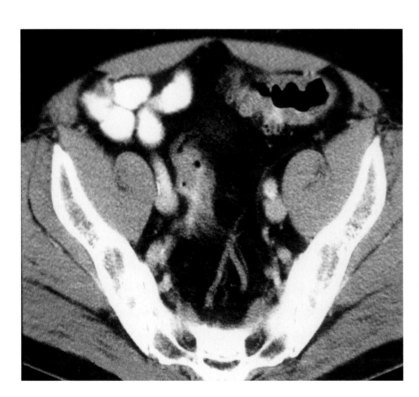

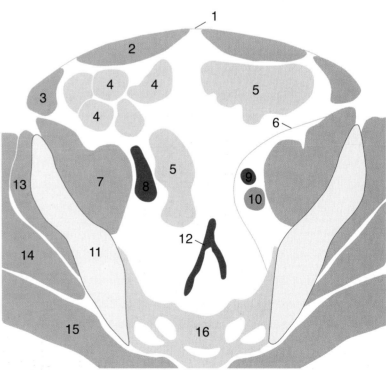

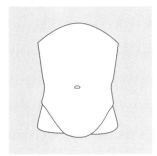

Double contrast barium study of stomach and duodenum

1 - Spine
2 - Fundus
3 - Lesser curvature
4 - Magenstrasse
5 - Greater curvature
6 - First part of duodenum (duodenal cap)
7 - Pylorus
8 - Longitudinal mucosal folds in body of stomach
9 - Superior (first) part of duodenum
10 - Descending (second) part of duodenum
11 - Pyloric canal
12 - Horizontal inferior (third) part of duodenum
13 - Pyloric antrum
14 - Proximal loops of jejunum

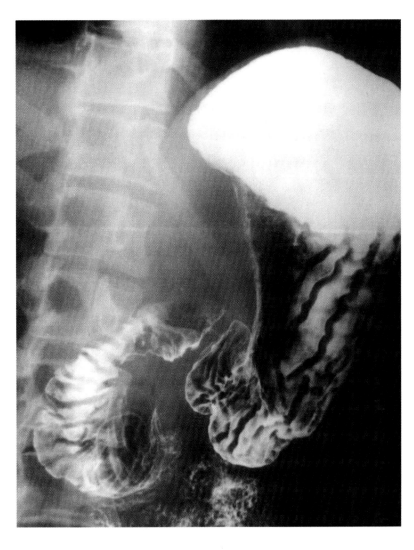

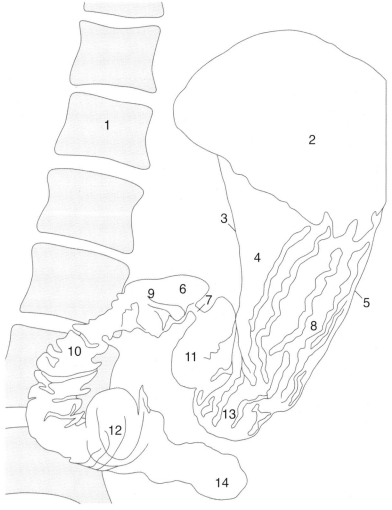

ABDOMEN

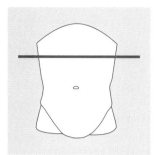

Axial CT of stomach

1 - Liver
2 - Stomach filled with water
3 - Left dome of diaphragm
4 - Wall of stomach
5 - Coeliac trunk
6 - Inferior vena cava
7 - Right adrenal gland
8 - Aorta

9 - Left adrenal gland
10 - Spleen
11 - Right kidney
12 - Right crus of diaphragm
13 - Hemiazygos vein
14 - Left kidney
15 - Vertebra

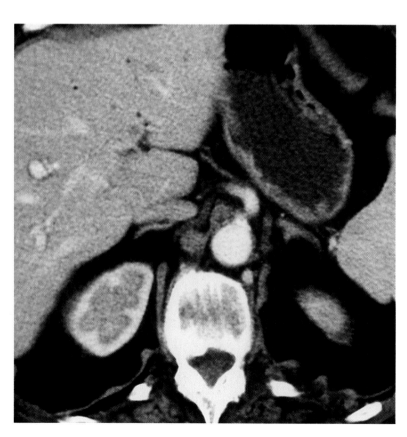

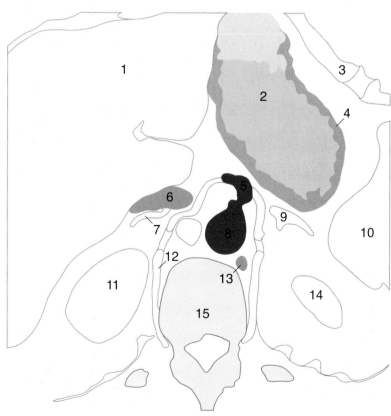

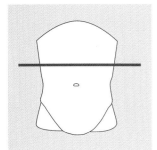

Axial CT of duodenum

1 - Liver
2 - Stomach
3 - Colon
4 - Gall bladder (with lucent gall stone)
5 - Portal vein and confluence
6 - Duodenum, first/second part transition
7 - Pancreas (body)
8 - Splenic artery

9 - Kidney
10 - Renal vein
11 - Inferior vena cava
12 - Superior mesenteric artery
13 - Aorta
14 - Left renal vein
15 - Lumbar vertebra I
16 - Psoas major muscle

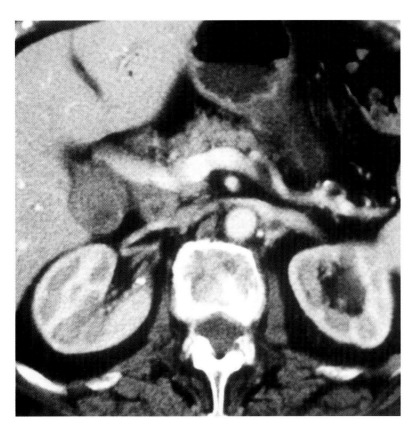

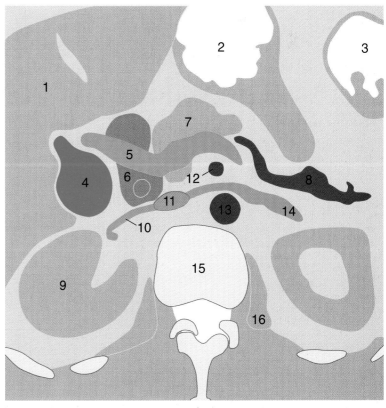

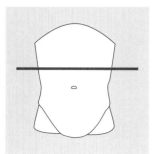

Axial CT of duodenum

1 - Liver
2 - Stomach
3 - Jejunum
4 - Gall bladder
5 - Duodenum, pars superior (first part)
6 - Duodenum, pars descendens (second part)
7 - Pancreas
8 - Superior mesenteric vein
9 - Splenic vein
10 - Superior mesenteric artery
11 - Kidney
12 - Inferior vena cava
13 - Aorta
14 - Renal vein
15 - Disc between lumbar vertebrae I-II
16 - Psoas major muscle

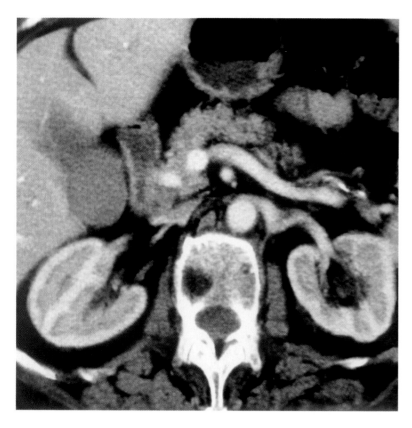

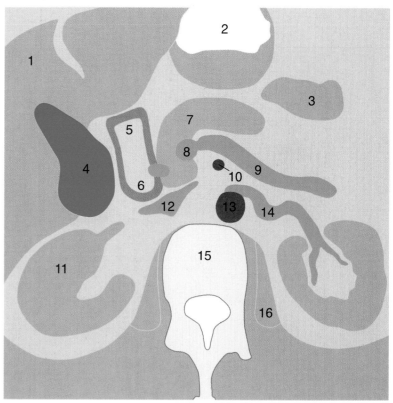

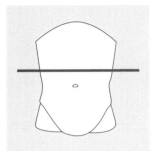

Axial CT of duodenum

1 - Liver
2 - Stomach
3 - Jejunum
4 - Gall bladder
5 - Duodenum, pars superior (first part)
6 - Duodenum, pars descendens (second part)
7 - Pancreas, head
8 - Confluence of superior mesenteric and splenic veins
9 - Pancreas, tail
10 - Superior mesenteric artery
11 - Aorta
12 - Left renal vein
13 - Kidney
14 - Inferior vena cava
15 - Psoas major muscle
16 - Disc between lumbar vertebrae I-II

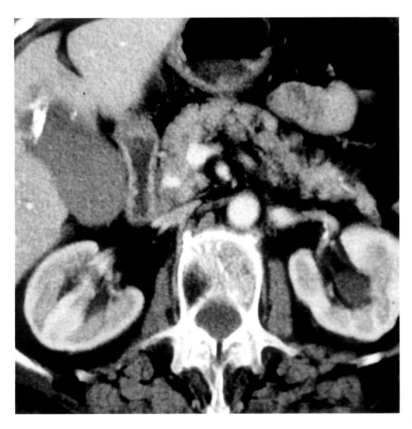

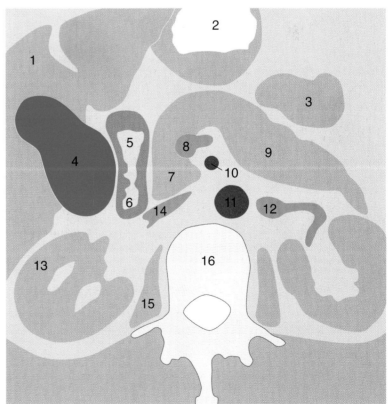

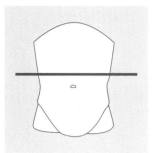

Axial CT of duodenum

1 - Stomach
2 - Falciform fissure and
    ligamentum teres
3 - Gall stone
4 - Liver
5 - Gall bladder
6 - Duodenum, pars
    descendens (second part)
7 - Head of pancreas

8 - Superior mesenteric vein
9 - Superior mesenteric artery
10 - Jejunum
11 - Kidney
12 - Inferior vena cava
13 - Aorta
14 - Psoas major muscle
15 - Lumbar vertebra II
16 - Renal pelvis

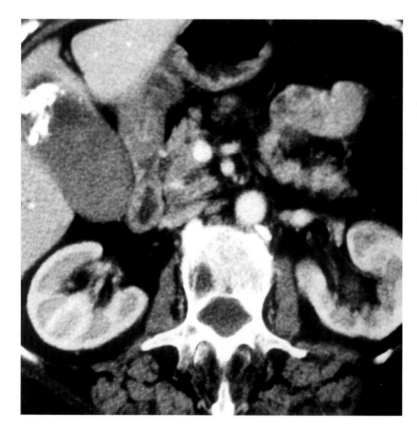

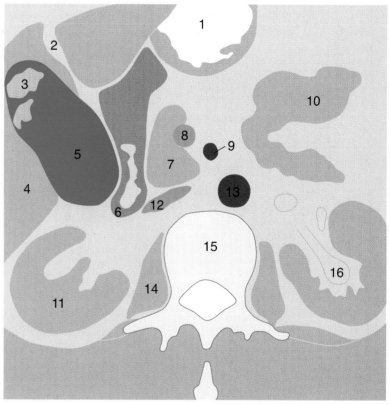

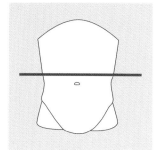

Axial CT of duodenum

1 - Liver
2 - Gall bladder
3 - Gall stone
4 - Groove for ligamentum teres
5 - Stomach (pylorus/antrum)
6 - Duodenum, pars descendens (second part)
7 - Head of pancreas

8 - Superior mesenteric vein
9 - Superior mesenteric artery
10 - Jejunum
11 - Kidney
12 - Inferior vena cava
13 - Aorta
14 - Psoas major muscle
15 - Lumbar vertebra II
16 - Quadratus lumborum muscle

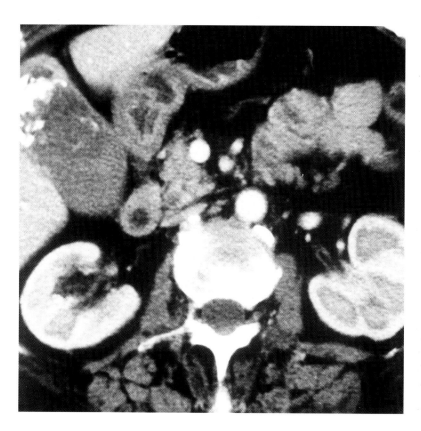

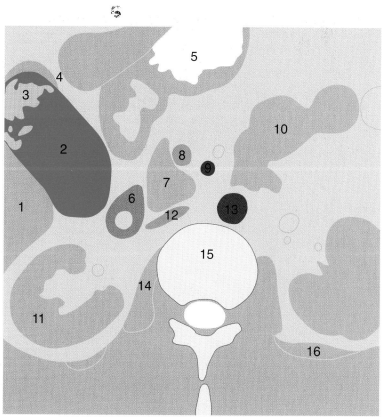

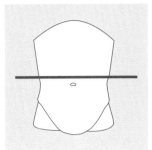

Axial CT of duodenum

1 - Liver
2 - Gall bladder with gall stones
3 - Pyloric stomach
4 - Superior mesenteric vein
5 - Superior mesenteric artery
6 - Jejunum
7 - Duodenum, pars descendens (second part)
8 - Head of pancreas
9 - Inferior vena cava

10 - Aorta
11 - Branch of right renal artery
12 - Kidney (medullary pyramid)
13 - Disc between lumbar vertebrae II-III
14 - Psoas major muscle
15 - Quadratus lumborum muscle

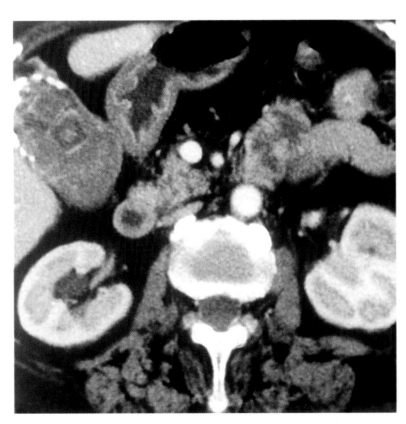

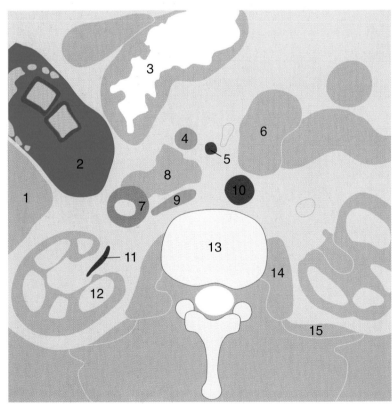

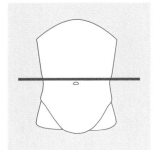

Axial CT of duodenum

1 - Gall bladder
2 - Colon, hepatic flexure
3 - Transverse colon
4 - Duodenum pars
    horizontalis (third part)
5 - Superior mesenteric vein
6 - Superior mesenteric artery
7 - Kidney

8 - Inferior vena cava
9 - Aorta
10 - Psoas major muscle
11 - Lumbar vertebra III
12 - Quadratus lumborum
     muscle
13 - Erector spinae muscle

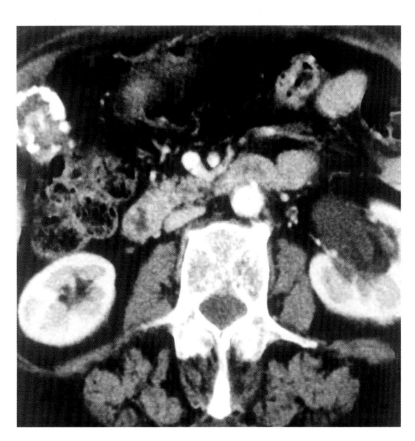

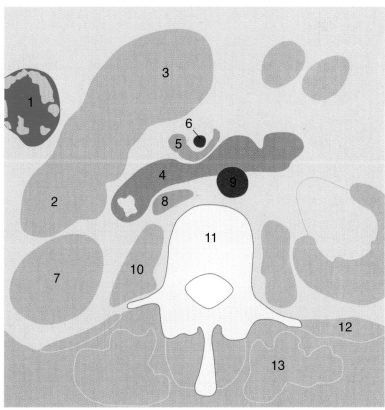

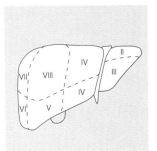

Segmental anatomy of liver, axial CT

Left lobe:
- I. Caudate lobe
- II. Lateral superior segment
- III. Lateral inferior segment
- IV. Medial superior and medial inferior segments

Right lobe:
- V. Anterior inferior segment
- VI. Posterior inferior segment
- VII. Posterior superior segment
- VIII. Anterior superior segment

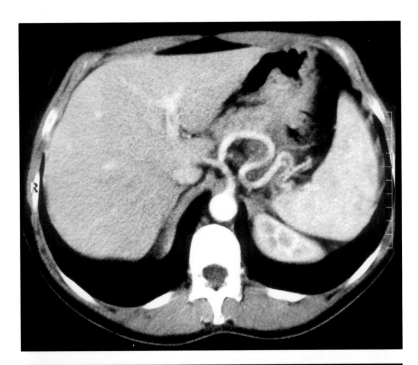

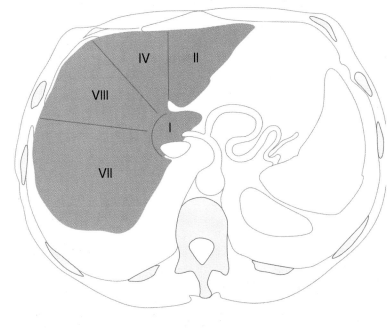

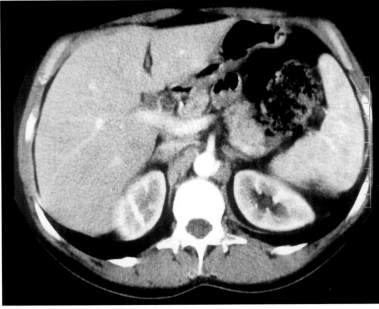

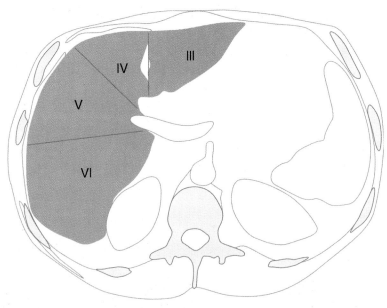

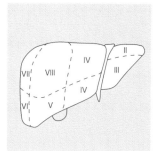

Segmental anatomy of liver, axial CT

Left lobe:
- I. Caudate lobe
- II. Lateral superior segment
- III. Lateral inferior segment
- IV. Medial superior and medial inferior segments

Right lobe:
- V. Anterior inferior segment
- VI. Posterior inferior segment
- VII. Posterior superior segment
- VIII. Anterior superior segment

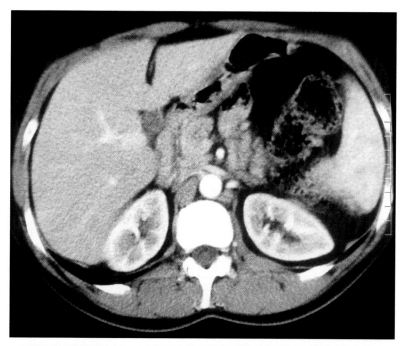

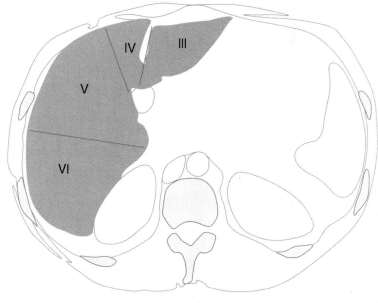

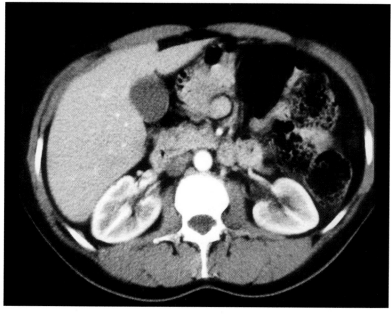

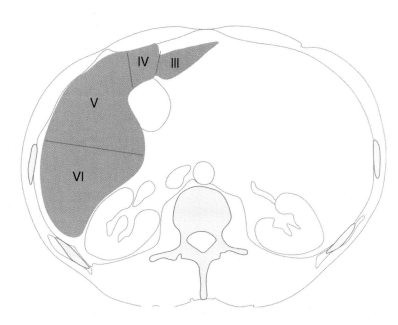

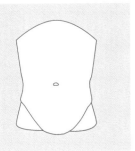

Ultrasonogram of porta hepatis, transverse oblique view

1 - Left lobe of liver   4 - Right lobe of liver
2 - Common bile duct   5 - Portal vein
3 - Hepatic artery   6 - Inferior vena cava

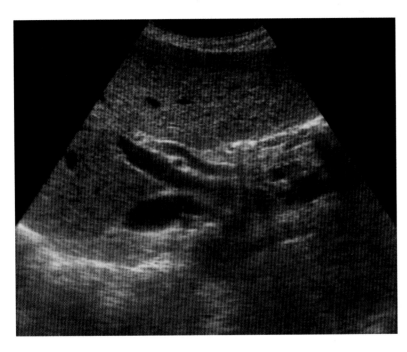

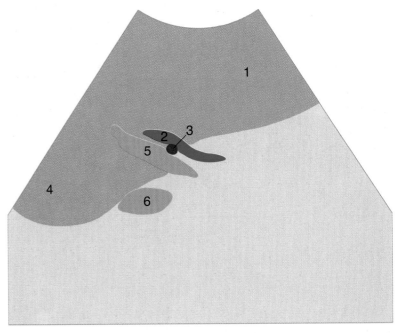

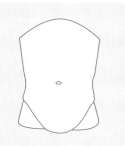

Hepatic arteriogram, anteroposterior view

1 - Terminal intrahepatic branches
2 - Phrenic branch
3 - Right branch of hepatic artery
4 - Left branch of hepatic artery

5 - Hepatic artery proper
6 - Common hepatic artery
7 - Gastroduodenal artery
8 - Right gastric artery

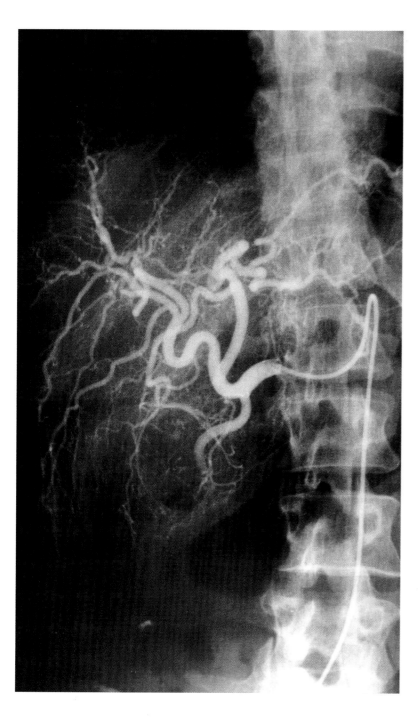

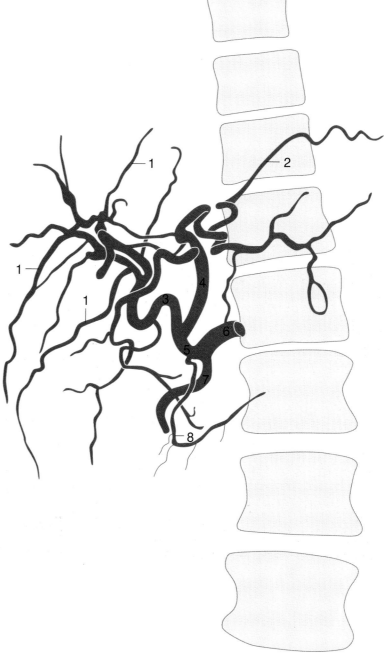

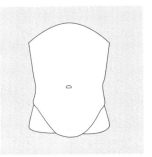

Colour Doppler ultrasonogram of hepatic veins, axial view

1 - Hepatic parenchyma   3 - Inferior vena cava
2 - Middle hepatic vein   4 - Right hepatic vein

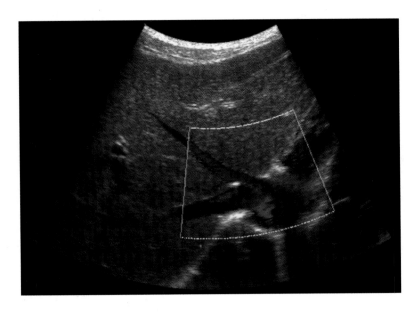

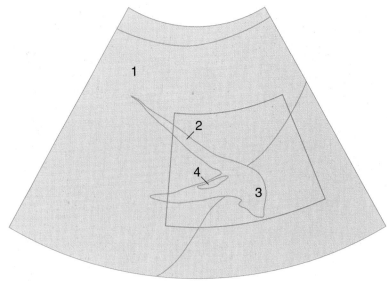

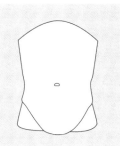

Endoscopic retrograde cholangiography (ERC) of bile passages

1 - Intrahepatic bile ducts
2 - Left hepatic duct
3 - Right hepatic duct
4 - Common bile duct
5 - Cystic duct

6 - Gall bladder
7 - Endoscope
8 - Lumbar vertebra
9 - Major duodenal papilla
10 - Endoscopic cannula

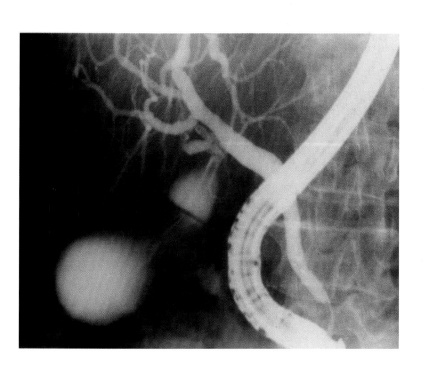

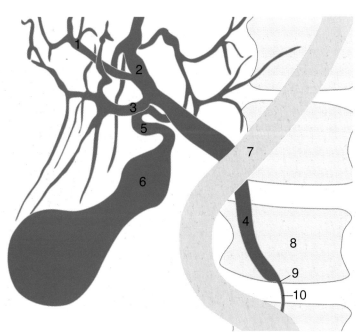

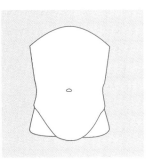

3D ultrasonogram of gall bladder

A – sagittal section, B – reconstruction image in the transverse plane, C – reconstruction image in the coronal plane, D – reconstructed 3D image.

1 - Wall of gall bladder   3 - Bile fluid in gall bladder
2 - Stone in gall bladder

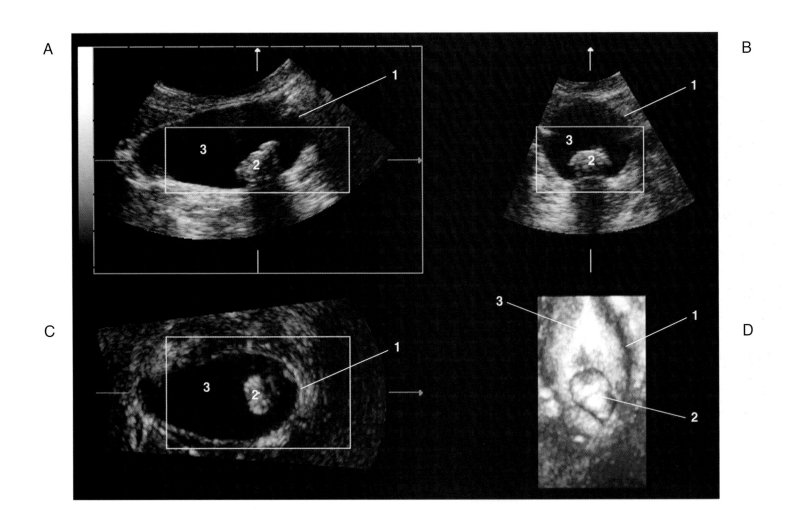

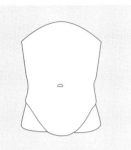

Helical CT cholangiography, SSD reconstruction

1 - Intrahepatic bile ducts of
    the left lobe

2 - Intrahepatic bile ducts of
    the right lobe

3 - Left hepatic duct

4 - Right hepatic duct

5 - Common bile duct

6 - Calculus in the distal part
    of the bile duct

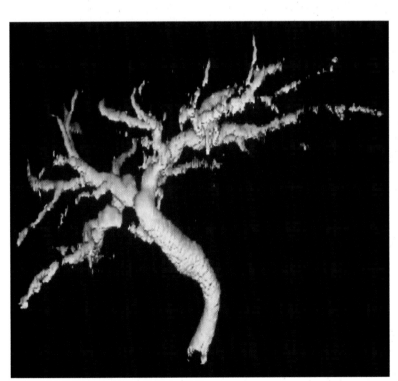

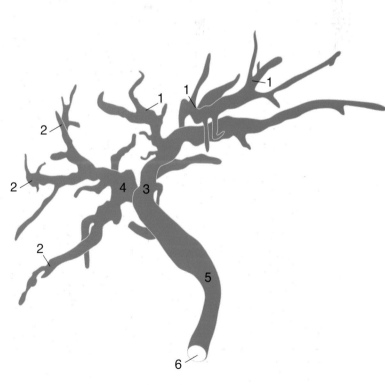

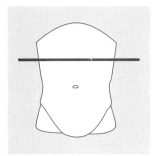

Axial CT of pancreas

1 - Fissure for ligamentum teres
2 - Left lobe of liver (segment III)
3 - Stomach (air bubble)
4 - Right lobe of liver
5 - Porta hepatis
6 - Body of pancreas
7 - Confluence of superior mesenteric and splenic veins
8 - Superior mesenteric artery
9 - Splenic vein
10 - Splenic artery
11 - Left colic (splenic) flexure
12 - Spleen
13 - Inferior vena cava
14 - Left renal vein
15 - Aorta
16 - Tail of pancreas
17 - Adrenal gland
18 - Psoas major muscle
19 - Vertebra
20 - Left kidney

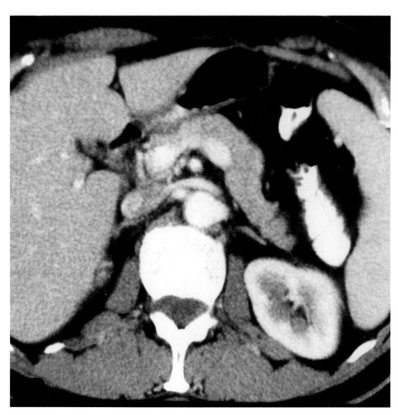

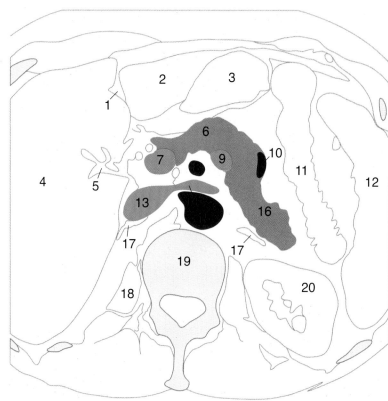

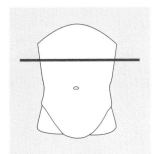

Axial CT of pancreas

1 - Liver	10 - Left renal vein
2 - Pyloric stomach	11 - Aorta
3 - Body of stomach	12 - Tail of pancreas
4 - Left colic (splenic) flexure	13 - Adrenal gland
5 - Body of pancreas	14 - Right kidney
6 - Splenic vein	15 - Psoas major muscle
7 - Superior mesenteric artery	16 - Vertebra
8 - Spleen	17 - Left kidney
9 - Inferior vena cava	

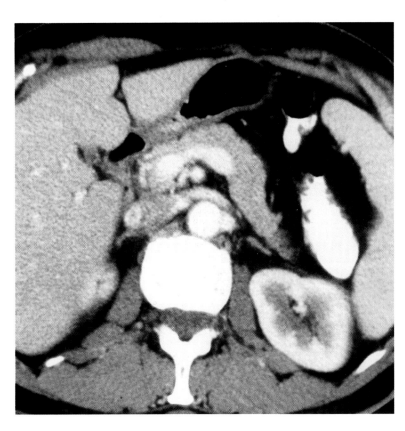

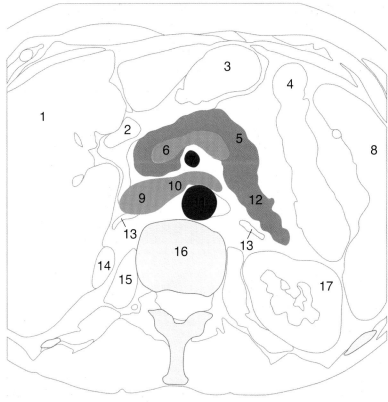

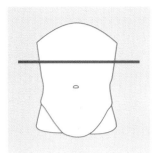

Axial CT of pancreas

1 - Stomach
2 - Left colic (splenic) flexure
3 - Liver
4 - Duodenum
5 - Head of pancreas
6 - Confluence of superior
    mesenteric and splenic
    veins
7 - Uncinate process of
    pancreas
8 - Superior mesenteric artery
9 - Tail of pancreas
10 - Small intestine
11 - Spleen
12 - Inferior vena cava
13 - Aorta
14 - Left renal vein
15 - Right kidney
16 - Vertebra
17 - Psoas major muscle
18 - Left renal artery
19 - Quadratus lumborum
     muscle

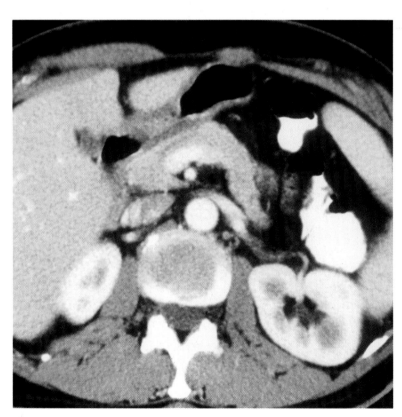

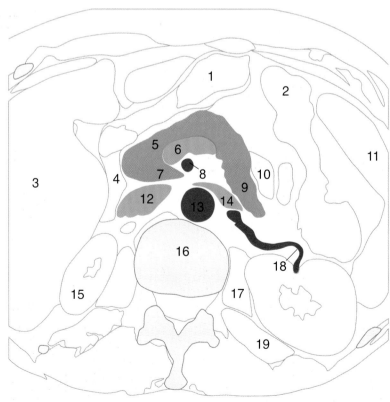

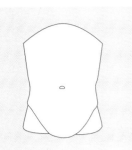

Endoscopic retrograde pancreatography (ERP) of pancreatic ducts

1 - Nasoduodenal tube
2 - Main pancreatic duct (Wirsung)
3 - Spine
4 - Duodenum
5 - Accessory pancreatic duct (of Santorini)
6 - Major duodenal papilla (of Vater) and opening of

major pancreatic duct
7 - Excretory ducts of the pancreatic body
8 - Excretory ducts of the pancreatic head
9 - Cannula of endoscope

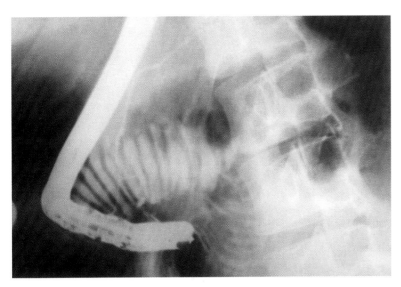
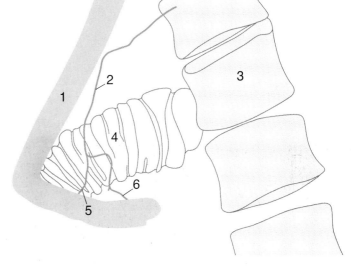

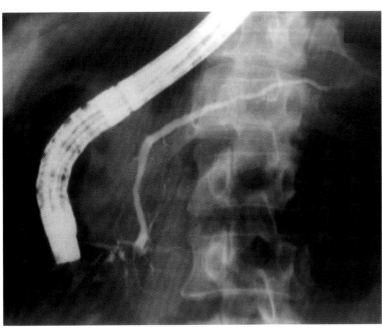
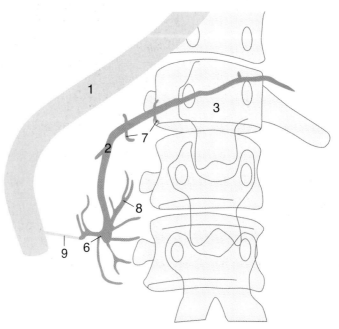

ABDOMEN

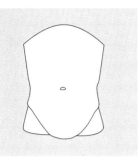

Ultrasonogram of pancreas, transverse view

1 - Pancreas
2 - Splenic vein
3 - Superior mesenteric artery

4 - Inferior vena cava
5 - Aorta
6 - Vertebra

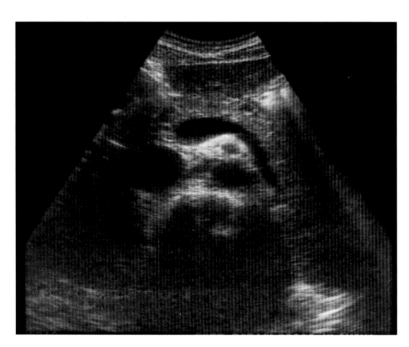

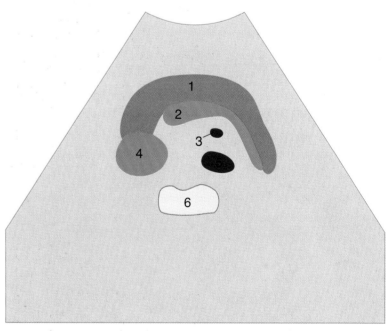

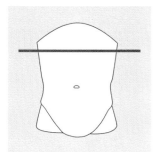

Axial CT of spleen

1 - Liver
2 - Air bubble of stomach
3 - Rib
4 - Inferior vena cava
5 - Aorta
6 - Splenic artery
7 - Fundus of stomach
    adjacent to gastric facet of
    spleen
8 - Spleen
9 - Vertebra
10 - Diaphragm
11 - Costodiaphragmatic
     recess with inferior lobe
     of left lung within

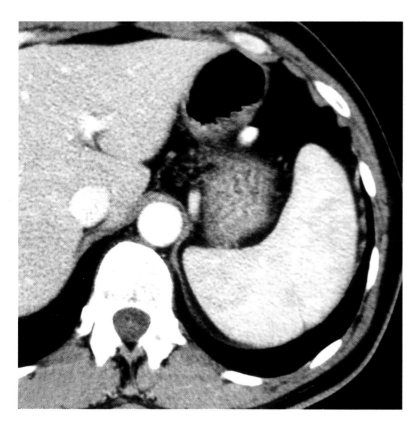

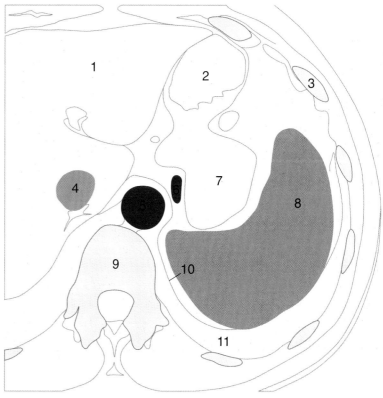

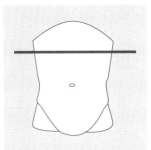

Axial CT of spleen

1 - Left lobe of liver
2 - Stomach
3 - Rib
4 - Portal vein
5 - Caudate lobe of liver
6 - Splenic artery
7 - Left colic flexure
8 - Inferior vena cava
9 - Aorta

10 - Hilum of spleen (visceral surface)
11 - Right lobe of liver
12 - Right adrenal gland
13 - Right crus of diaphragm
14 - Vertebra
15 - Diaphragmatic surface of spleen

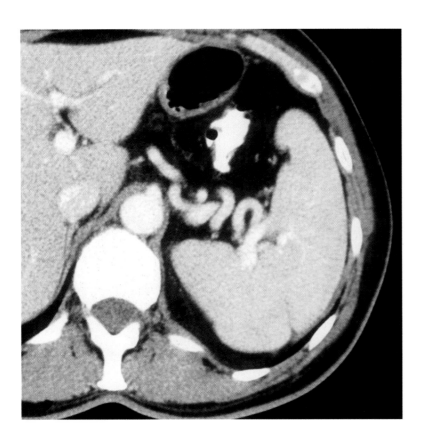
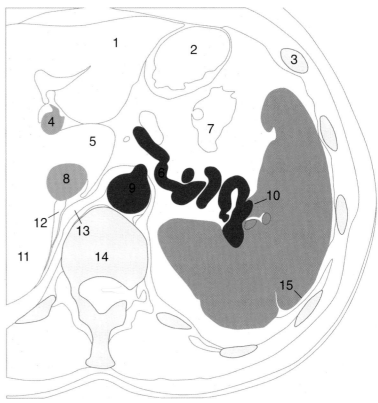

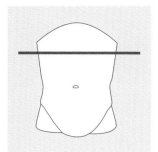

Axial CT of spleen

1 - Left lobe of liver
2 - Stomach
3 - Colic facet of spleen adjacent to left colic flexure
4 - Portal vein
5 - Coeliac trunk
6 - Splenic artery
7 - Inferior vena cava

8 - Aorta
9 - Splenic vein
10 - Tail of pancreas
11 - Right adrenal gland
12 - Right crus of diaphragm
13 - Vertebra
14 - Left adrenal gland
15 - Renal facet of spleen adjacent to left kidney

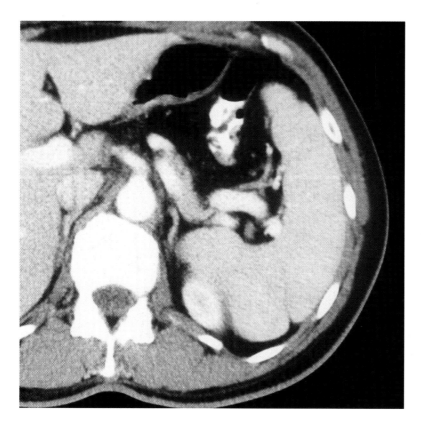

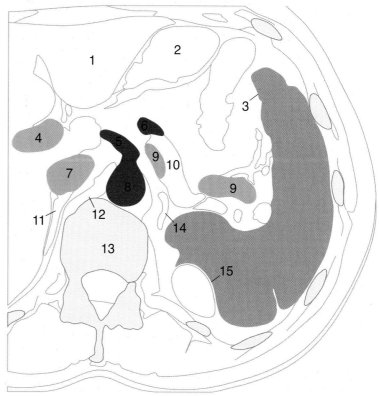

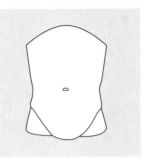

Small intestine, enteroclysis

1 - Nasojejunal tube
2 - Jejunal loops
3 - Ileal loops

4 - Ascending colon
5 - Descending colon

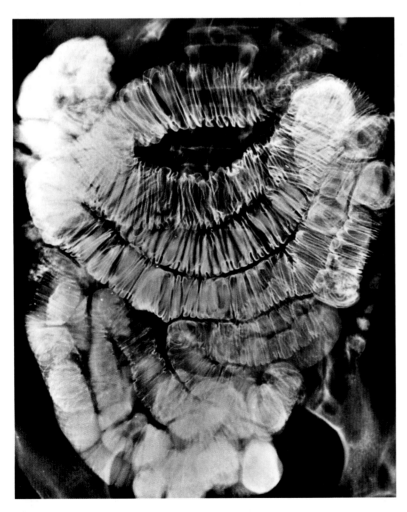

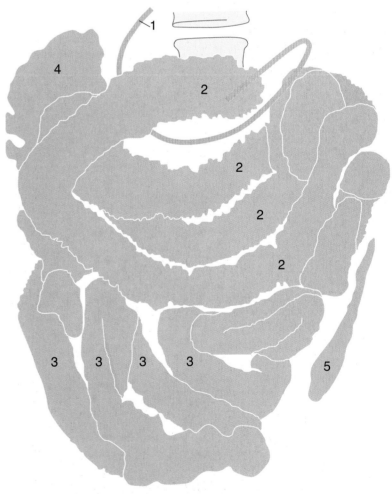

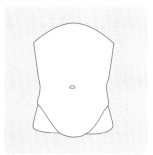

Barium enema study of caecum and vermiform appendix

1 - Haustra of transverse
    colon
2 - Ascending colon
3 - Caecum
4 - Sigmoid colon

5 - Sacro-iliac joint
6 - Lateral part of sacrum
7 - Vermiform appendix
8 - Ilium

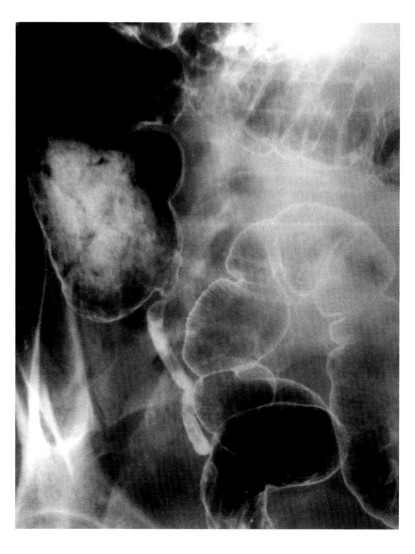

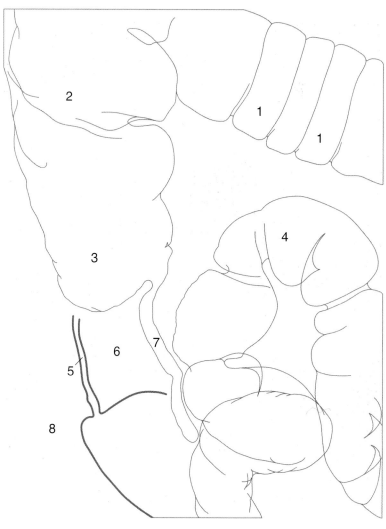

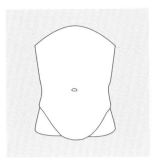

Double contrast barium enema study of large intestine

1 - Caecum
2 - Ascending colon
3 - Right colic (hepatic) flexure
4 - Transverse colon

5 - Left colic (splenic) flexure
6 - Descending colon
7 - Sigmoid colon
8 - Rectum, upper part

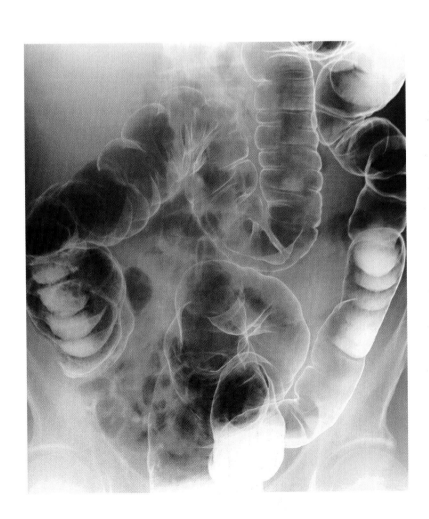

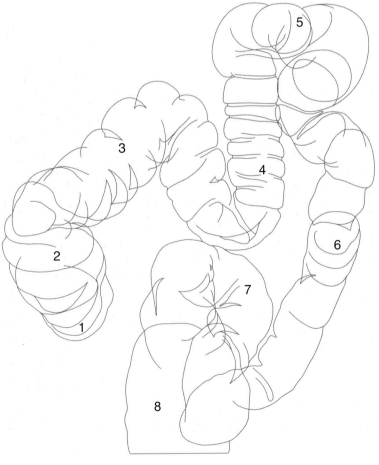

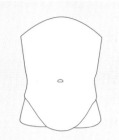

Arteriogram of abdominal aorta, anteroposterior view

1 - Aorta
2 - Superior mesenteric artery
3 - Right renal artery
4 - Accessory renal artery
5 - Right colic artery
6 - Ileocolic artery
7 - Ileal branches
8 - Jejunal branches
9 - Median sacral artery from bifurcation of aorta

10 - Lumbar artery
11 - Right common iliac artery
12 - Lateral sacral artery (variation)
13 - Iliolumbar artery
14 - Origin of left internal iliac artery
15 - External iliac artery

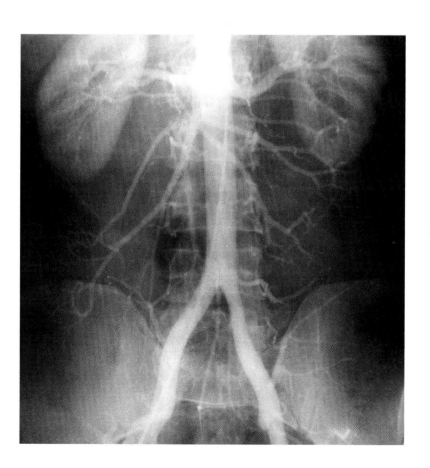

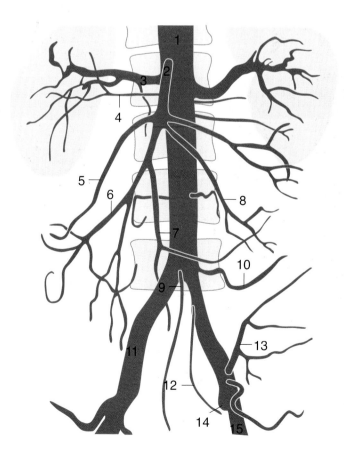

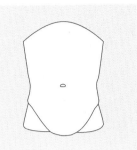

Arteriogram of coeliac trunk, anteroposterior view

1 - Phrenic branch of left hepatic artery
2 - Left hepatic artery
3 - Left gastric artery
4 - Intrahepatic terminal branches
5 - Cystic artery
6 - Hepatic artery proper
7 - Common hepatic artery
8 - Coeliac trunk
9 - Splenic artery
10 - Gastroduodenal artery
11 - Posterior superior pancreaticoduodenal artery
12 - Anterior superior pancreaticoduodenal artery
13 - Right gastro-epiploic artery
14 - Left gastro-epiploic artery

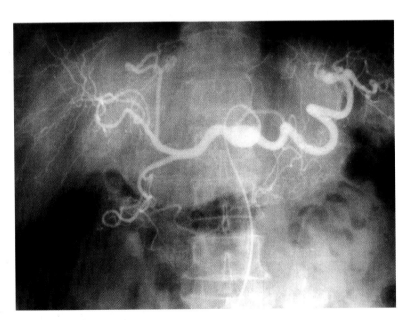

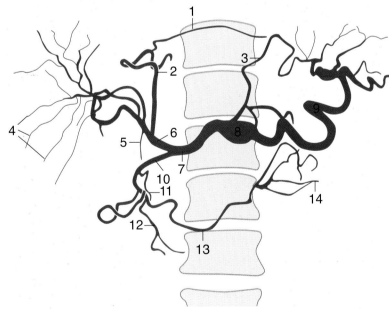

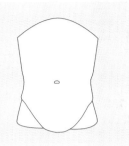

Arteriogram of coeliac trunk, anteroposterior view

1 - Intrahepatic branches
2 - Right hepatic artery
3 - Left hepatic artery
4 - Hepatic artery proper
5 - Common hepatic artery

6 - Splenic artery
7 - Gastroduodenal artery
8 - Left gastro-epiploic artery
9 - Right gastro-epiploic artery

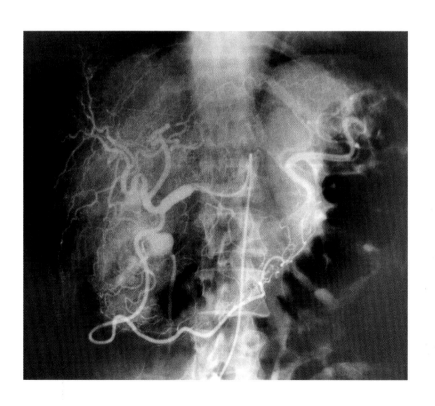

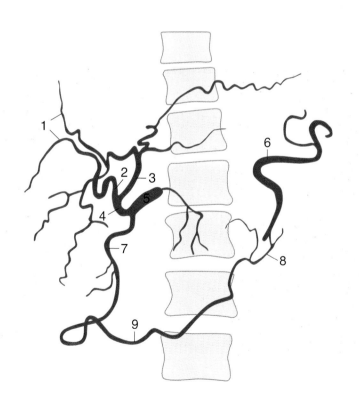

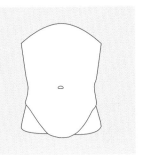

Arteriogram of superior mesenteric artery, anteroposterior view

1 - Superior mesenteric artery
2 - Middle colic artery
3 - Right colic artery

4 - Jejunal arteries
5 - Ileocolic artery
6 - Ileal arteries

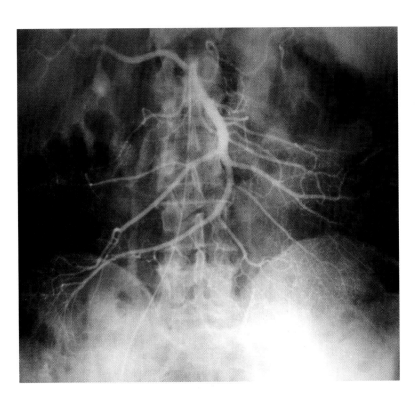

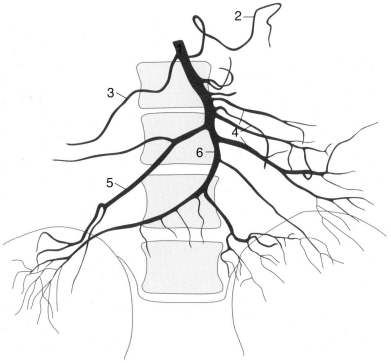

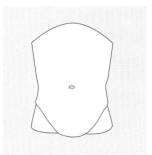

Arteriogram of superior mesenteric artery, anteroposterior view

1 - Middle colic artery
2 - Inferior pancreatico-
    duodenal artery
3 - Superior mesenteric artery
4 - Ileal arteries
5 - Jejunal arteries

6 - Arcade of jejunal artery
7 - First arcade of ileal artery
8 - Second arcade of ileal
    artery
9 - Third arcade of ileal
    artery

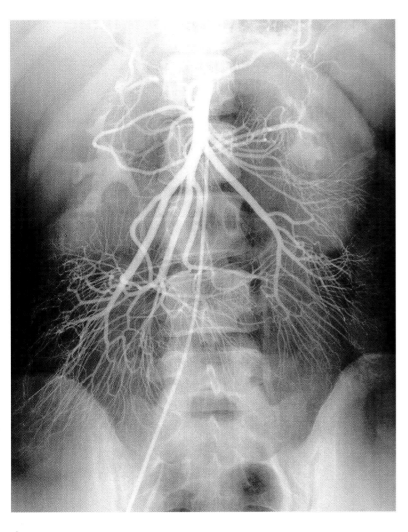

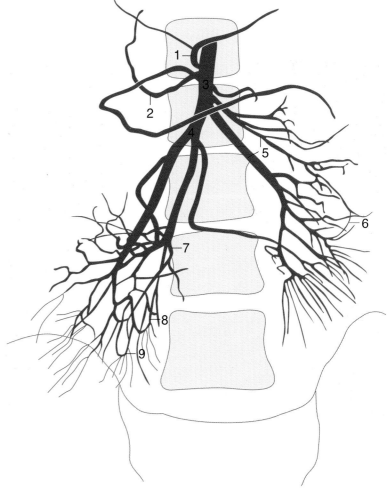

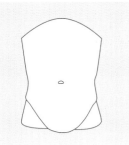

Arteriogram of inferior mesenteric artery, anteroposterior view

1 - Inferior mesenteric artery
2 - Left colic artery
3 - Left colic artery,
    ascending branch

4 - Sigmoid arteries
5 - Sigmoidea ima (lowest
    sigmoid) artery
6 - Superior rectal artery

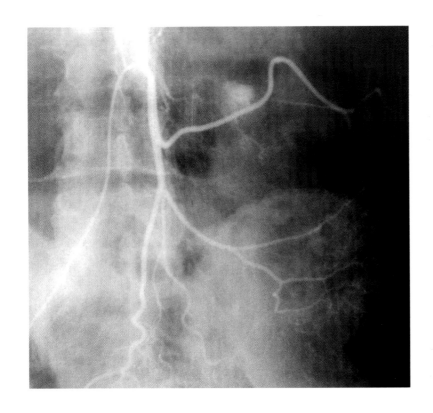

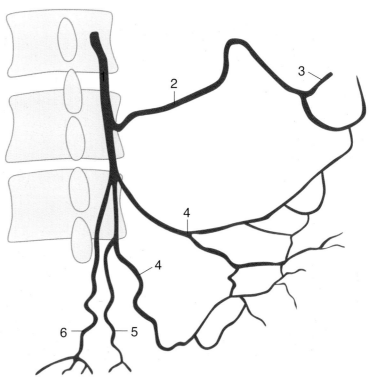

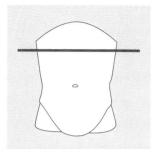

Axial CT image of peritoneal spaces, supramesocolic compartment

The pathological accumulation of abdominal fluid (ascites) highlights the peritoneal spaces and ligaments. However, some abdominal organs appear displaced or distorted.

1 - Falciform ligament
2 - Liver
3 - Aorta
4 - Cardia, oesophagogastric junction

5 - Gastrosplenic ligament
6 - Spleen
7 - Retroperitoneum

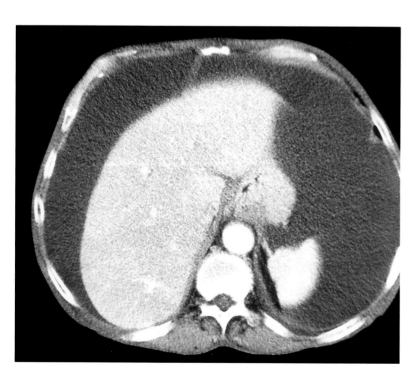

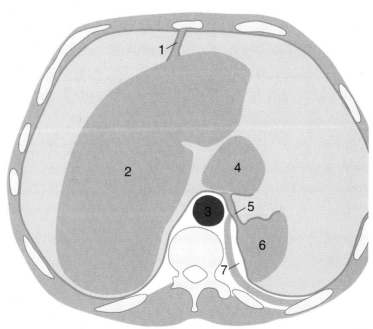

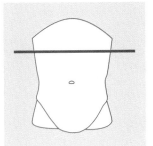

Axial CT image of peritoneal spaces, supramesocolic compartment

The pathological accumulation of abdominal fluid (ascites) highlights the peritoneal spaces and ligaments. However, some abdominal organs appear displaced or distorted.

1 - Liver
2 - Portal vein
3 - Free edge of lesser omentum
4 - Caudate lobe of liver
5 - Stomach
6 - Gastrosplenic ligament
7 - Crus of diaphragm
8 - Aorta
9 - Lienorenal (splenorenal) ligament
10 - Omental bursa (lesser sac)
11 - Left kidney
12 - Spleen
13 - Peritoneal cavity
14 - Parietal peritoneum

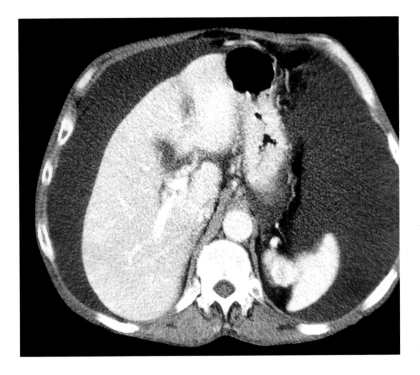

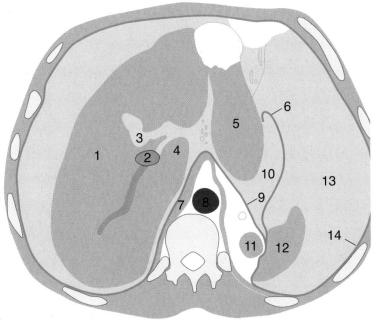

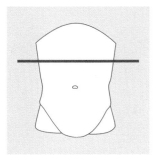

Axial CT image of peritoneal spaces, supramesocolic compartment

The pathological accumulation of abdominal fluid (ascites) highlights the peritoneal spaces and ligaments. However, some abdominal organs appear displaced or distorted.

1 - Liver
2 - Gall bladder
3 - Hepatogastric ligament
4 - Stomach
5 - Transverse colon
6 - Portal vein
7 - Hepatic artery
8 - Left gastric artery
9 - Splenic artery
10 - Omental bursa (lesser sac)
11 - Epiploic foramen
12 - Inferior vena cava
13 - Aorta
14 - Splenic vein
15 - Lienorenal (splenorenal) ligament
16 - Left gastro-epiploic artery in gastrosplenic ligament
17 - Right kidney
18 - Left kidney
19 - Retroperitoneum (perirenal fat)
20 - Spleen

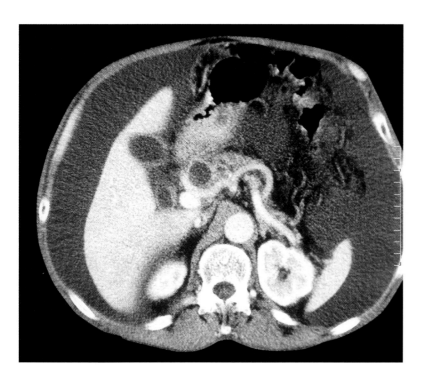

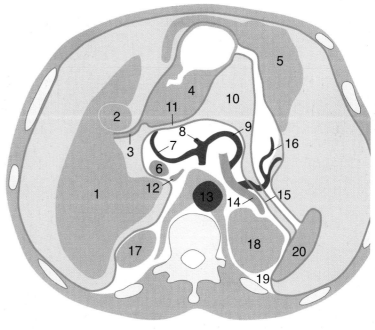

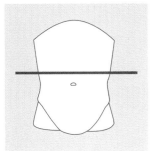

Axial CT image of peritoneal spaces, supramesocolic compartment

The pathological accumulation of abdominal fluid (ascites) highlights the peritoneal spaces and ligaments. However, some abdominal organs appear displaced or distorted.

1 - Transverse mesocolon
2 - Transverse colon
3 - Jejunum
4 - Mesentery
5 - Root of mesentery
6 - Superior mesenteric vessels
7 - Duodenum
8 - Duodenojejunal flexure
9 - Aorta
10 - Inferior vena cava
11 - Right kidney
12 - Psoas major muscle
13 - Descending colon
14 - Retroperitoneum (perirenal fat)

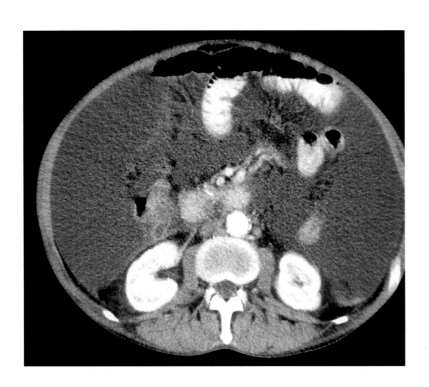

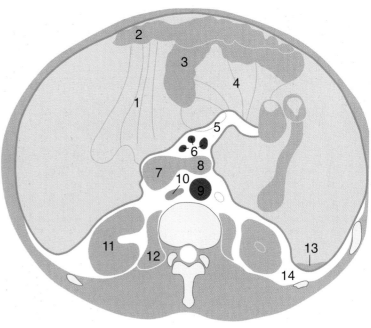

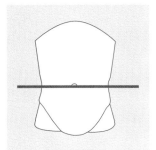

Axial CT image of peritoneal spaces, inframesocolic compartment

The pathological accumulation of abdominal fluid (ascites) highlights the peritoneal spaces and ligaments. However, some abdominal organs appear displaced or distorted.

1 - Ileum
2 - Mesentery
3 - Jejunum
4 - Ascending colon
5 - Root of mesentery
6 - Inferior vena cava

7 - Aorta
8 - Paracolic recess
9 - Right kidney
10 - Psoas major muscle
11 - Retroperitoneum
12 - Descending colon

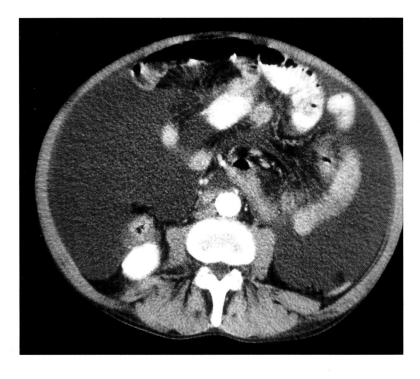

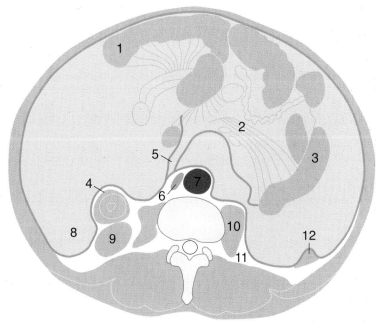

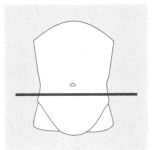

Axial CT image of peritoneal spaces, inframesocolic compartment

The pathological accumulation of abdominal fluid (ascites) highlights the peritoneal spaces and ligaments. However, some abdominal organs appear displaced or distorted.

1 - Ileum
2 - Mesentery
3 - Jejunum
4 - Caecum
5 - Root of mesentery
6 - Inferior vena cava

7 - Aorta
8 - Psoas major muscle
9 - Descending colon
    (compressed)
10 - Ilium

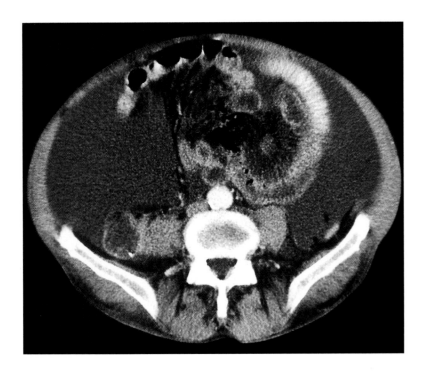

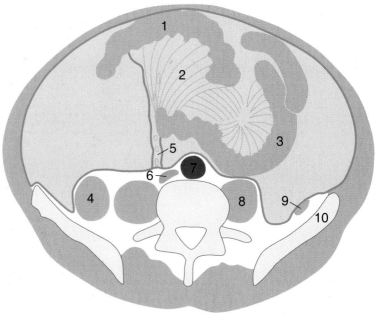

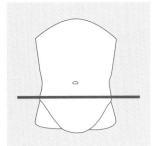

Axial CT image of peritoneal spaces, inframesocolic compartment

The pathological accumulation of abdominal fluid (ascites) highlights the peritoneal spaces and ligaments. However, some abdominal organs appear displaced or distorted.

1 - Ileum
2 - Jejunum
3 - Ilium
4 - Caecum
5 - Terminal ileum
6 - Root of mesentery

7 - Common iliac arteries
8 - Psoas major muscle
9 - Descending colon
10 - Sacrum
11 - Retroperitoneum

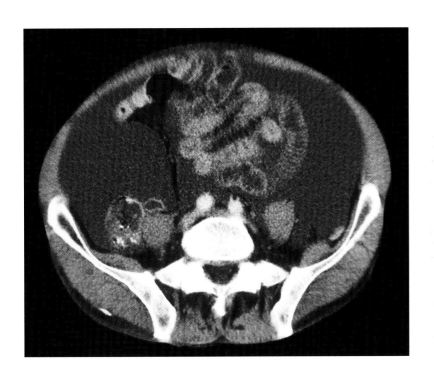

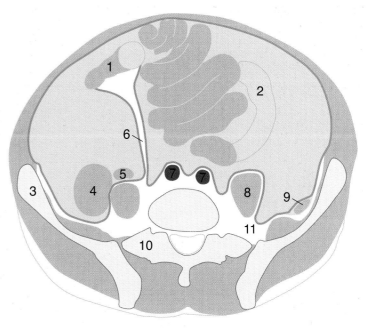

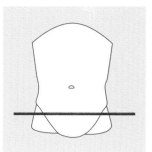

Axial CT image of peritoneal spaces, inframesocolic compartment

The pathological accumulation of abdominal fluid (ascites) highlights the peritoneal spaces and ligaments. However, some abdominal organs appear displaced or distorted.

1 - Rectus abdominis muscle
2 - Parietal peritoneum, pelvic peritoneum
3 - Pouch of Douglas
4 - Sigmoid mesocolon
5 - Sigmoid colon
6 - Rectum, infraperitoneal part

7 - Sacrum
8 - Branches of internal iliac artery
9 - Piriformis muscle
10 - Gluteus maximus muscle
11 - External iliac artery

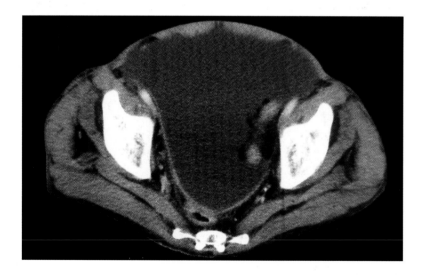

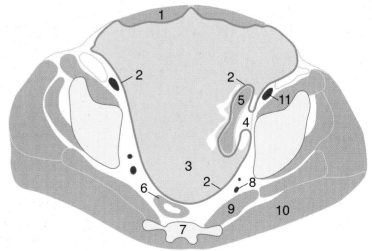

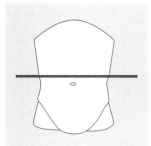

Axial CT of the capsules of kidney

1 - Aorta
2 - Jejunum
3 - Descending colon
4 - Inferior mesenteric vein
5 - Lumbar vertebra II
6 - Psoas major muscle
7 - Renal artery
8 - Kidney
9 - Adipose capsule (anterior perirenal fat)
10 - Anterior lamella of renal fascia (Gerota's fascia)
11 - Lateroconal fascia
12 - Posterior lamella of renal fascia (Zuckerkandl's fascia)
13 - Rib X
14 - Spinal canal
15 - Spinous process
16 - Erector spinae muscle
17 - Quadratus lumborum muscle
18 - Rib XII
19 - Serratus posterior inferior muscle
20 - Latissimus dorsi muscle
21 - Posterior pararenal fat
22 - Rib XI

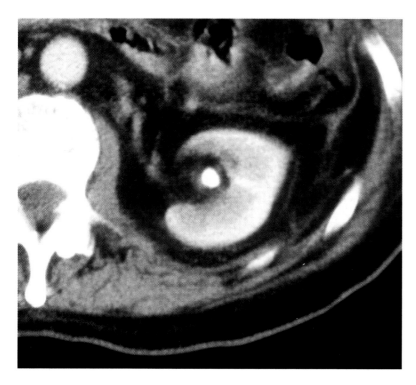

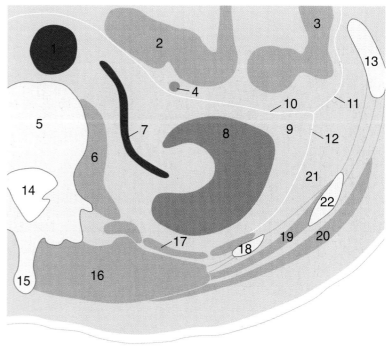

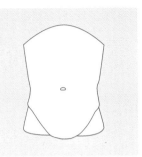

Ultrasonogram of kidney, parasagittal view

1 - Liver
2 - Cortex of kidney
3 - Pyramid of medulla

4 - Renal column
5 - Renal sinus and pelvis

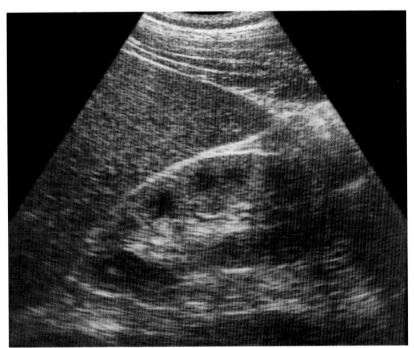

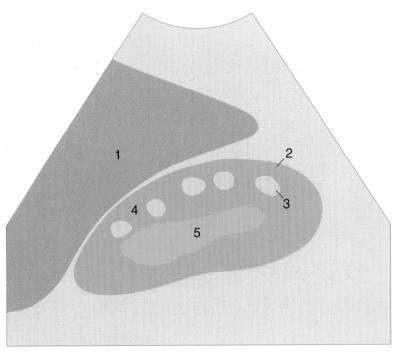

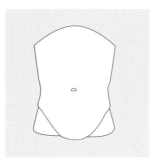

Ultrasonograms of kidney of newborn infant
A – in sagittal and B – transverse planes.

1 - Liver
2 - Right kidney
3 - Renal pelvis

4 - Renal pyramid
5 - Adrenal gland

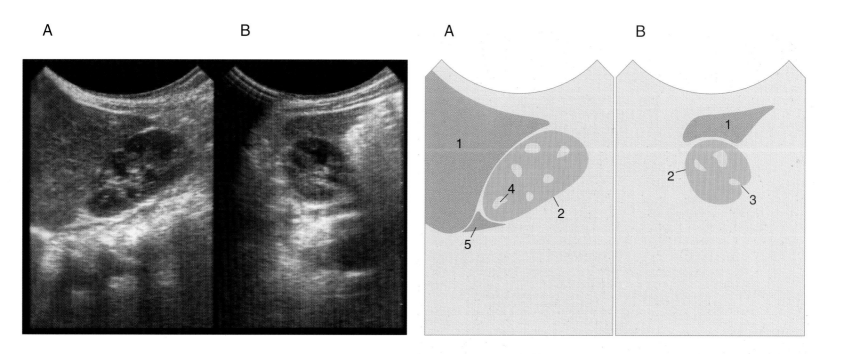

A   B   A   B

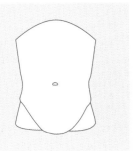

Renal arteriogram, anteroposterior view

1 - Spine
2 - Main renal artery
3 - Posterior division of renal artery
4 - Anterior division of renal artery

5 - Lobar artery
6 - Interlobar artery
7 - Arcuate artery

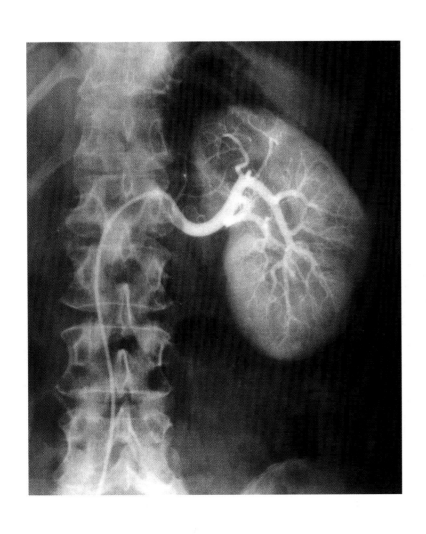

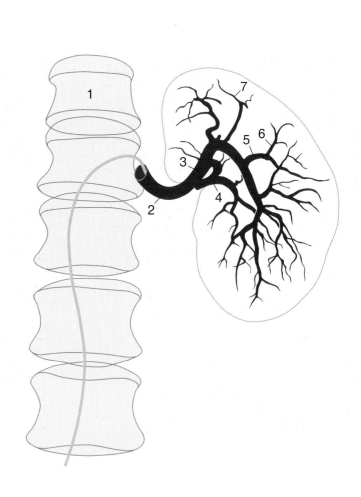

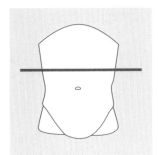

Axial CT of renal vessels

1 - Costal arch	10 - Renal artery
2 - Liver	11 - Aorta
3 - Duodenum, second part	12 - Medulla of kidney
4 - Pancreas, uncinate process	13 - Body of lumbar vertebra I
5 - Superior mesenteric vein	14 - Diaphragm, lumbar part
6 - Superior mesenteric artery	15 - Renal sinus
7 - Small intestine	16 - Spinous process
8 - Inferior vena cava	17 - Rib XII
9 - Renal vein	18 - Cortex of kidney
	19 - Rib XI

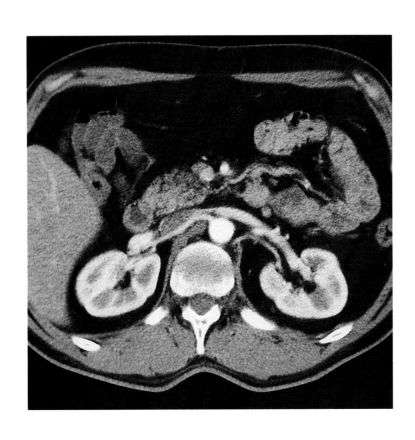

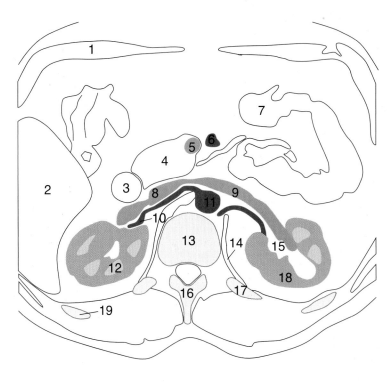

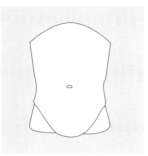

Intravenous urography of renal pelvis and ureter

1 - Rib XI
2 - Calyx minor
3 - Calyx major
4 - Vertebral column
5 - Renal pelvis

6 - Ureter
7 - Psoas major muscle
8 - Sacrum
9 - Ilium
10 - Sacro-iliac joint

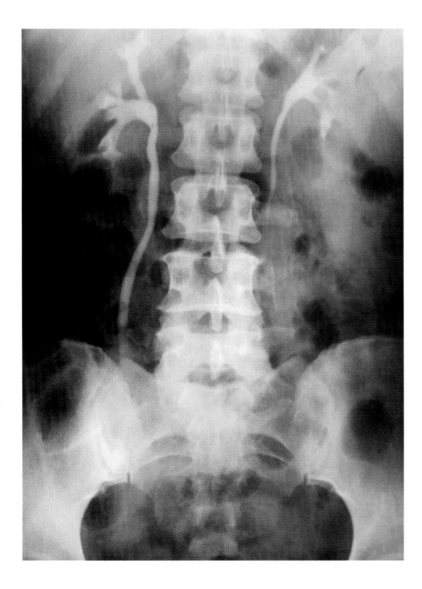

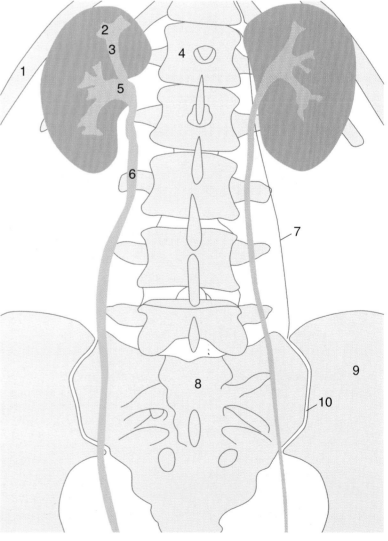

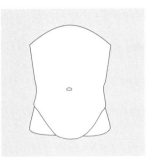

3D CT SSD reconstruction of renal pelvis and ureter

1 - Thoracic vertebra XII
2 - Lumbar vertebra I
3 - Lumbar vertebra II
4 - Lumbar vertebra III
5 - Lumbar vertebra IV
6 - Rib XII
7 - Transverse process (costal process)
8 - Calyx minor
9 - Calyx major

10 - Ureter
11 - Iliac crest
12 - Anterior superior iliac spine
13 - Sacro-iliac joint
14 - Urinary bladder
15 - Pubic symphysis
16 - Superior ramus of pubis
17 - Sacral promontory
18 - Terminal line

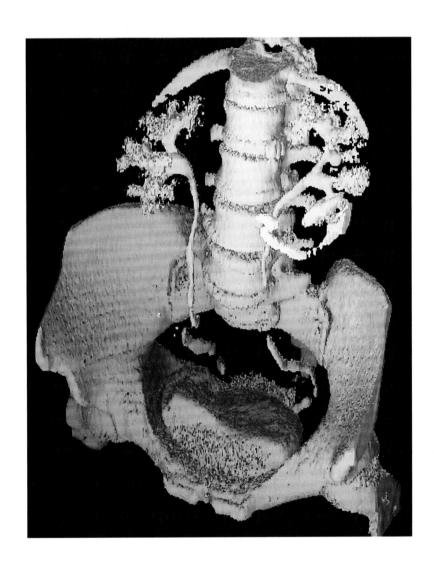

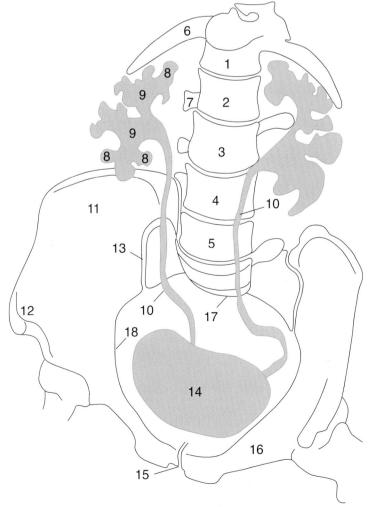

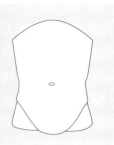

Ultrasonogram of adrenal gland of newborn infant, transverse view

1 - Liver
2 - Right kidney
3 - Lateral crus of adrenal
    gland

4 - Cortex of adrenal gland
5 - Medulla of adrenal gland
6 - Medial crus of adrenal
    gland

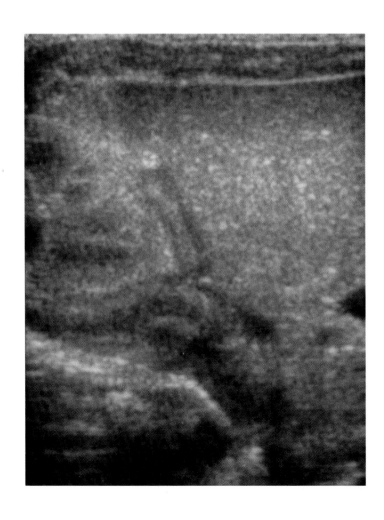

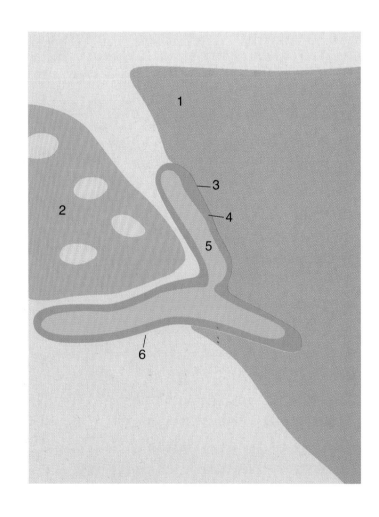

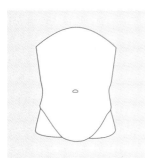

Ultrasonogram of adrenal gland of newborn infant, parasagittal view

1 - Liver
2 - Lateral crus of adrenal
    gland
3 - Right kidney (superior
    pole)

4 - Medial crus of adrenal
    gland

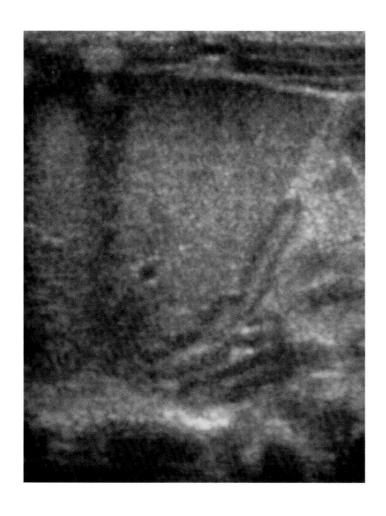

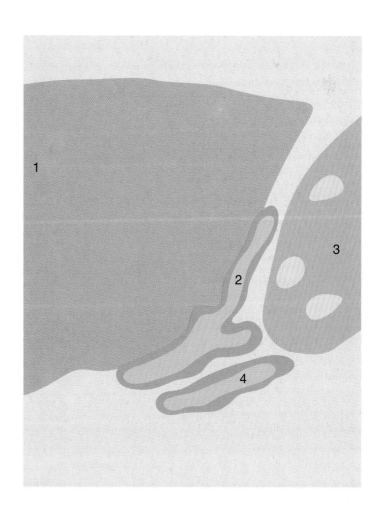

PELVIS

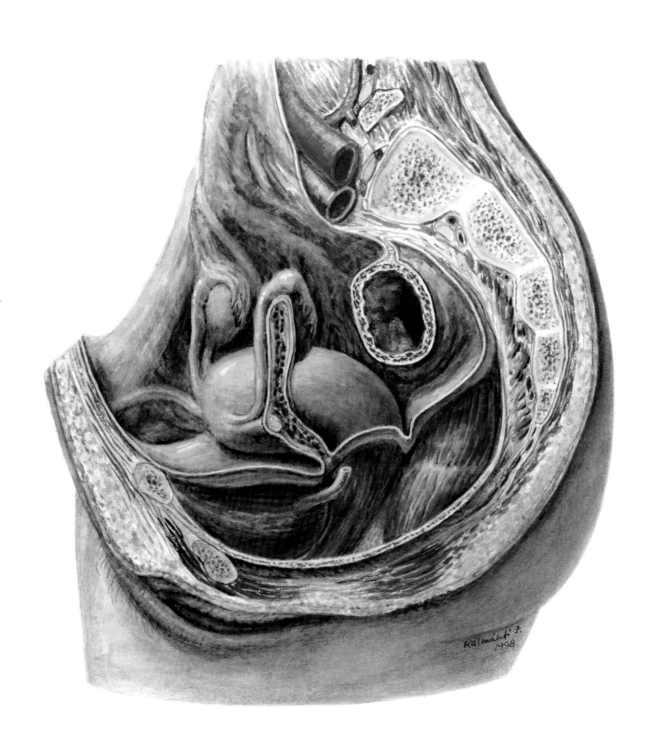

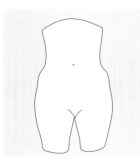

X-ray of osseous pelvis (female), anteroposterior view

1 - Iliac crest
2 - Lumbar vertebra V
3 - Ilium
4 - Sacro-iliac joint
5 - Lateral mass (ala) of sacrum
6 - Spinous process of sacral vertebra I (median sacral crest)
7 - Anterior (pelvic) sacral foramina
8 - Anterior superior iliac spine
9 - Pelvic brim
10 - Coccyx
11 - Anterior inferior iliac spine
12 - Acetabulum
13 - Head of femur
14 - Superior ramus of pubis
15 - Pubic symphysis
16 - Ramus of ischium
17 - Pubic tubercle
18 - Obturator foramen
19 - Inferior ramus of pubis
20 - Neck of femur
21 - Greater trochanter
22 - Intertrochanteric line
23 - Lesser trochanter

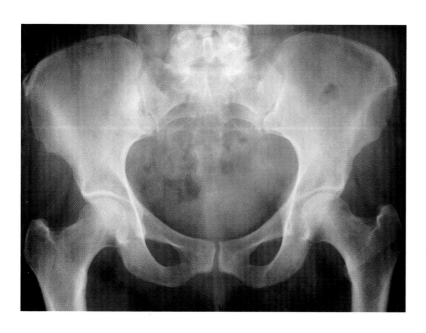

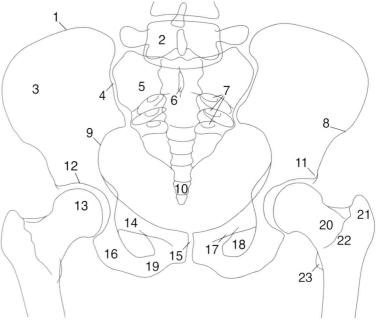

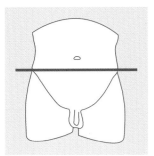

Axial CT of male pelvis

1 - Rectus abdominis muscle
2 - Inferior epigastric vessels
3 - Internal oblique muscle
4 - Iliopsoas muscle
5 - External iliac artery
6 - External iliac vein
7 - Vas deferens
8 - Urinary bladder
9 - Gluteus medius muscle

10 - Gluteus minimus muscle
11 - Ilium
12 - Rectum
13 - Internal iliac artery
14 - Internal iliac vein
15 - Gluteus maximus muscle
16 - Piriformis muscle
17 - Superior rectal artery
18 - Sacrum

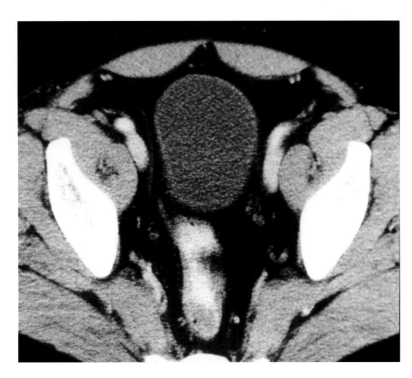

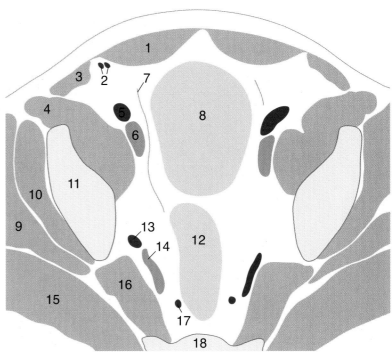

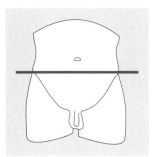

Axial CT of male pelvis

1 - Rectus abdominis muscle
2 - Inguinal canal (deep inguinal ring)
3 - Inferior epigastric vessels
4 - Vas deferens
5 - Iliopsoas muscle
6 - Urinary bladder
7 - External iliac vein
8 - External iliac artery
9 - Gluteus medius and minimus muscles
10 - Ilium
11 - Obturator artery
12 - Gluteal arterial branch
13 - Perirectal fibrous sling
14 - Obturator internus muscle
15 - Piriformis muscle
16 - Gluteus maximus muscle
17 - Sacrum
18 - Rectum

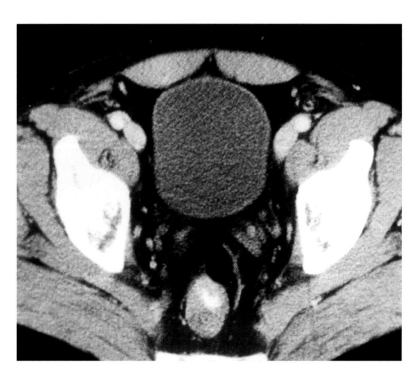

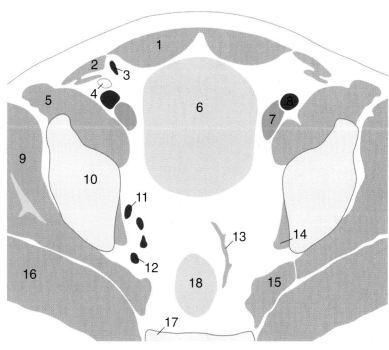

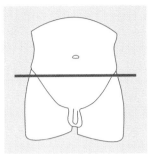

Axial CT of male pelvis

1 - Rectus abdominis muscle	13 - Ureteric orifice
2 - Inguinal canal and spermatic cord	14 - Seminal vesicle
3 - Sartorius muscle	15 - Obturator internus muscle
4 - Gluteus minimus muscle	16 - Gluteus maximus muscle
5 - Iliopsoas muscle	17 - Inferior gluteal artery
6 - Urinary bladder	18 - Levator ani muscle
7 - Femoral vein	19 - Perirectal fibrous sling
8 - Femoral artery	20 - Rectum
9 - Prevesical space of Retzius	21 - Retrorectal space
10 - Gluteus medius muscle	22 - Sacrum
11 - Acetabulum	23 - Perirectal fat
12 - Internal iliac artery	24 - Pararectal fat

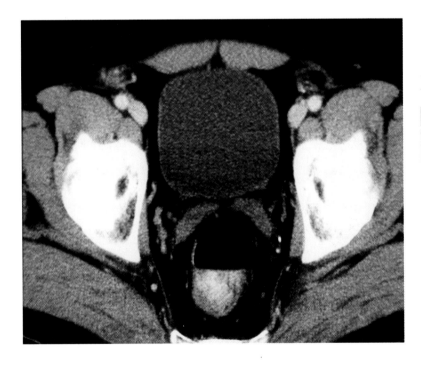

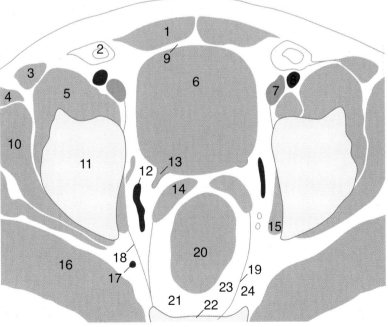

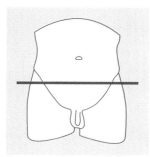

Axial CT of male pelvis

1 - Rectus abdominis muscle
2 - Inguinal canal and spermatic cord
3 - Sartorius muscle
4 - Iliopsoas muscle
5 - Urinary bladder
6 - Femoral canal (femoral septum, lacuna lymphatica)
7 - Femoral vein
8 - Femoral artery

9 - Femoral nerve
10 - Gluteus medius muscle
11 - Head of femur
12 - Acetabulum (pubic part)
13 - Obturator internus muscle
14 - Seminal vesicle
15 - Gluteus maximus muscle
16 - Perirectal fibrous sling
17 - Rectum
18 - Sacrum

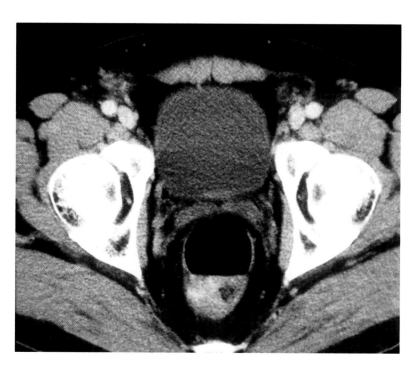

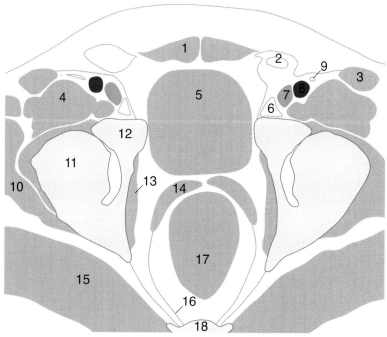

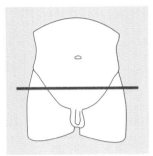

Axial CT of male pelvis

1 - Sartorius muscle
2 - Femoral artery
3 - Femoral vein
4 - Spermatic cord and testicular vessels
5 - Rectus abdominis and pyramidalis muscles
6 - Rectus femoris muscle
7 - Iliopsoas muscle
8 - Pectineus muscle
9 - Urinary bladder
10 - Head of femur
11 - Acetabulum, pubic part
12 - Obturator internus muscle
13 - Prostate
14 - Rectum
15 - Gluteus maximus muscle
16 - Ischio-anal (ischiorectal) fossa
17 - Levator ani muscle
18 - Sacrum
19 - Acetabulum, ischial part

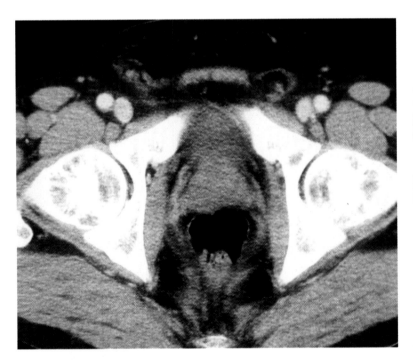

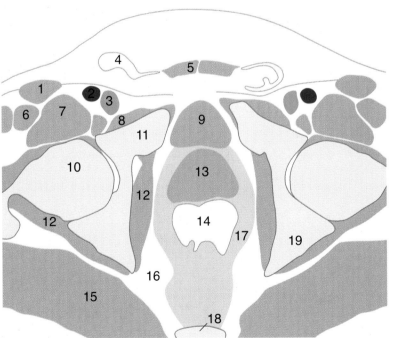

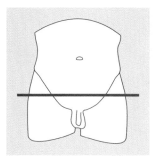

Axial CT of male pelvis

1 - Tensor fasciae latae muscle
2 - Rectus femoris muscle
3 - Sartorius muscle
4 - Spermatic cord and testicular vessels
5 - Rectus abdominis and pyramidalis muscles
6 - Pubis
7 - Pectineus muscle
8 - Femoral vein
9 - Femoral artery
10 - Iliopsoas muscle
11 - Femur
12 - Obturator internus muscle
13 - Prostate
14 - Obturator artery
15 - Rectum
16 - Ischio-anal fossa
17 - Retrorectal space
18 - Levator ani muscle
19 - Gluteus maximus muscle
20 - Coccyx
21 - Coccygeus muscle
22 - Ischial spine

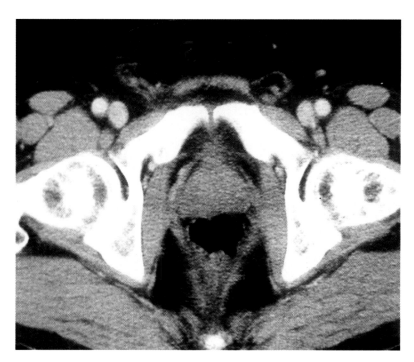

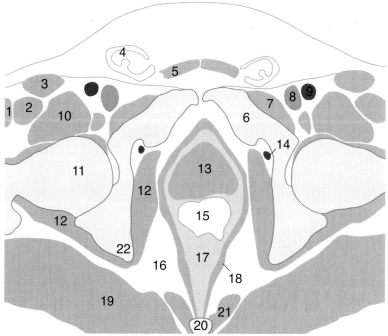

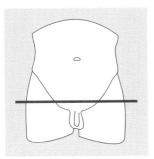

Axial CT of male pelvis

1 - Rectus femoris muscle
2 - Sartorius muscle
3 - Femoral artery
4 - Femoral vein
5 - Pectineus muscle
6 - Insertion of rectus abdominis muscle and pyramidalis muscle
7 - Spermatic cord and testicular vessels
8 - Iliopsoas muscle
9 - Pubis
10 - Femur
11 - Obturator internus muscle
12 - Prostate
13 - Ischio-anal fossa
14 - Rectum
15 - Anococcygeal ligament and coccygeus muscle
16 - Gluteus maximus muscle
17 - Coccyx
18 - Levator ani muscle
19 - Ischial tuberosity

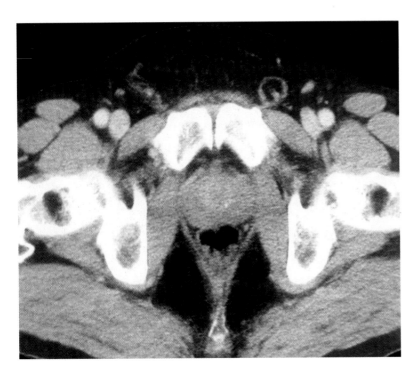

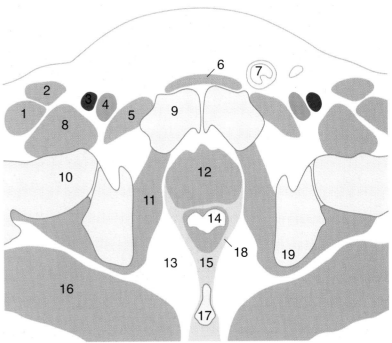

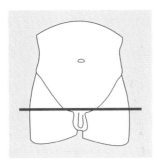

Axial CT of male pelvis

1 - Rectus femoris muscle
2 - Sartorius muscle
3 - Femoral artery
4 - Femoral vein
5 - Pectineus muscle
6 - Insertion of rectus abdominis muscle and pyramidalis muscle
7 - Iliopsoas muscle
8 - Obturator externus muscle
9 - Obturator membrane
10 - Pubis
11 - Obturator internus muscle
12 - Anus
13 - Ischial tuberosity
14 - Gluteus maximus muscle
15 - Anococcygeal ligament
16 - Levator ani muscle

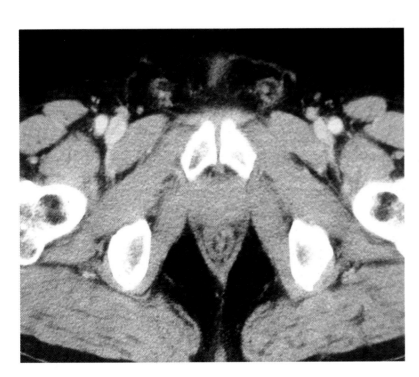

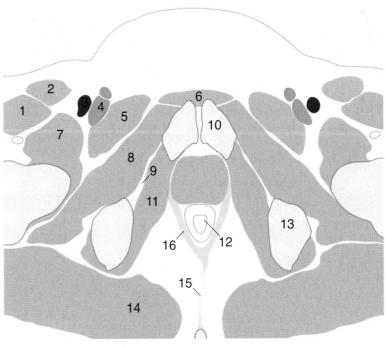

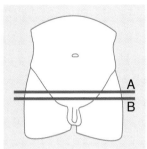

Axial MR of male pelvis and perineum

1 - Sartorius muscle
2 - Tensor fasciae latae muscle
3 - Rectus femoris muscle
4 - Iliopsoas muscle
5 - Femoral artery
6 - Femoral vein
7 - Pectineus muscle
8 - Pyramidalis muscle
9 - Gluteus medius muscle
10 - Head of femur
11 - Obturator externus muscle
12 - Pubic symphysis
13 - Prostate and prostatic urethra

14 - Obturator internus muscle
15 - Greater trochanter
16 - Gemellus superior and gemellus inferior muscles
17 - Ischio-anal fossa
18 - Levator ani muscle
19 - Gluteus maximus muscle
20 - Superior pubic ligament
21 - Adductor brevis muscle
22 - Urogenital triangle (urogenital diaphragm)
23 - Ischial tuberosity
24 - Urethra (membranous part)
25 - Rectum

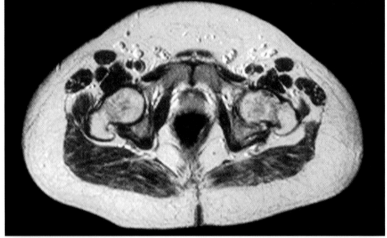

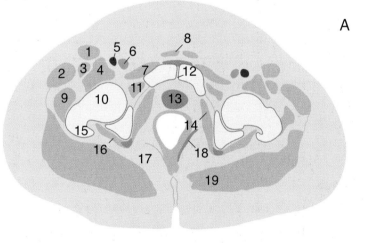

A

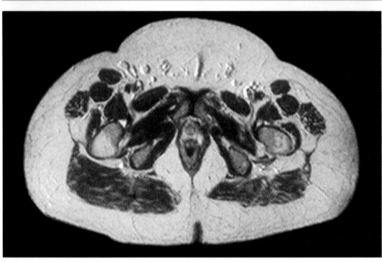

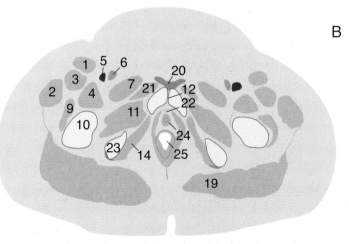

B

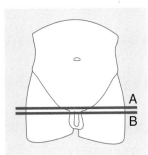

Axial MR of male pelvis and perineum

1 - Sartorius muscle
2 - Femoral vessels
3 - Inguinal lymph node
4 - Corpus cavernosum of penis
5 - Rectus femoris muscle
6 - Tensor fasciae latae muscle
7 - Vastus lateralis muscle
8 - Vastus intermedius muscle
9 - Pectineus muscle
10 - Adductor brevis muscle
11 - Adductor minimus muscle
12 - Femur
13 - Obturator externus muscle
14 - Ramus of ischium

15 - Urethra (bulb of urethra)
16 - Quadratus femoris muscle
17 - Rectum
18 - Ischio-anal fossa
19 - Gluteus maximus muscle
20 - Adductor longus muscle
21 - Corpus spongiosum of penis
22 - Adductor minimus and obturator externus muscle
23 - Ischiocavernosus muscle and crus of penis
24 - Anal canal
25 - Sciatic nerve
26 - Natal cleft

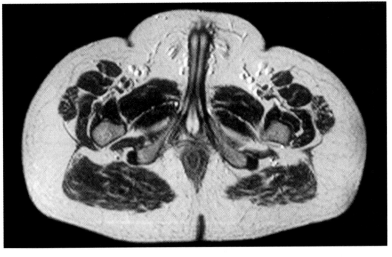
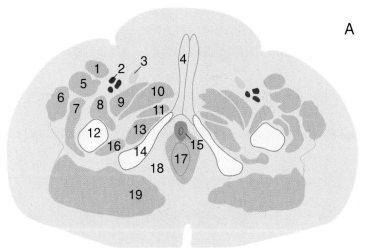

A

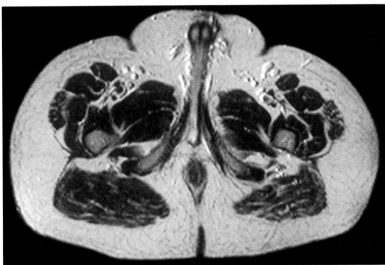
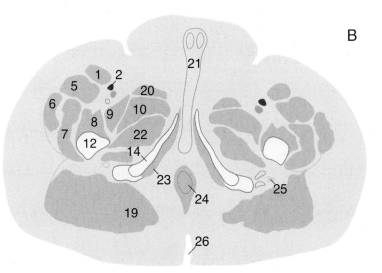

B

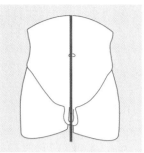

Sagittal MR of male pelvis and perineum

1 - Rectus abdominis muscle	10 - Glans of penis
2 - Sacrum	11 - Corpus cavernosum
3 - Urinary bladder	12 - Corpus spongiosum
4 - Pubis	13 - Bulb of penis
5 - Prevesical space of Retzius	14 - External anal sphincter
6 - Prostate	15 - Anal canal
7 - Urethra, prostatic part	16 - Coccyx
8 - Rectovesical pouch	17 - Testis
9 - Rectum	

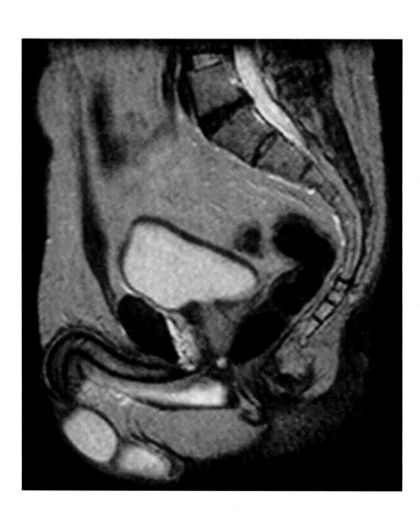

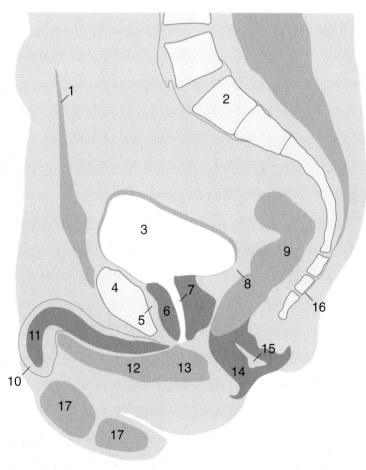

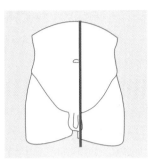

Sagittal MR of male pelvis and perineum

1 - Rectus abdominis muscle
2 - Urinary bladder
3 - Pubis
4 - Prevesical space of Retzius
5 - Prostate
6 - Seminal vesicle
7 - Rectum
8 - Sacrum

9 - Anococcygeal ligament
10 - Glans of penis
11 - Corpus cavernosum
12 - Urogenital diaphragm and levator prostatae muscle (part of levator ani muscle)
13 - Testis

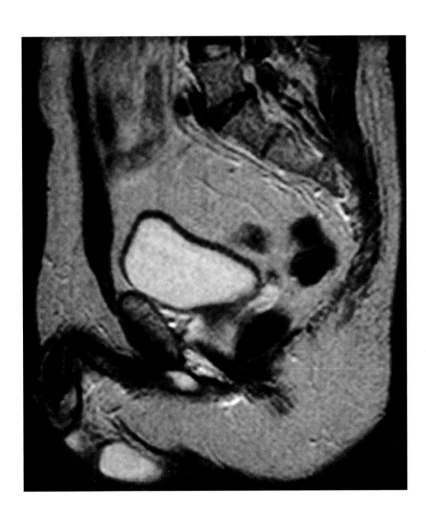

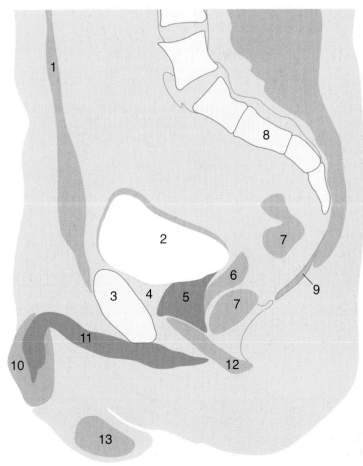

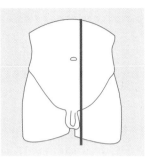

Sagittal MR of male pelvis and perineum

1 - Rectus abdominis muscle
2 - Urinary bladder
3 - Pubis
4 - Seminal vesicle
5 - Rectum
6 - Glans of penis
7 - Testicular vessels,
    spermatic cord and
    epididymis

8 - Levator prostatae and
    puborectalis muscles
    (parts of levator ani
    muscle)
9 - Anococcygeal ligament
10 - Scrotal sac

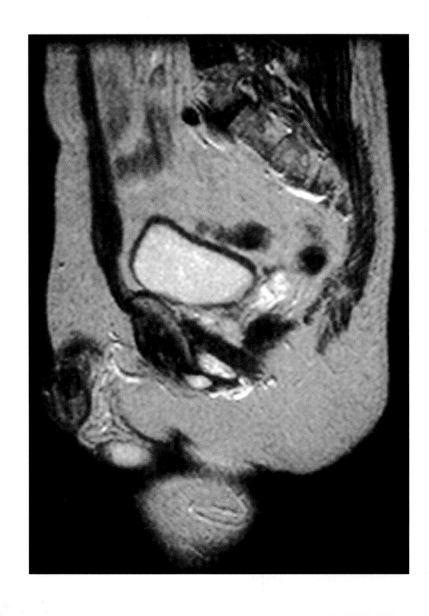

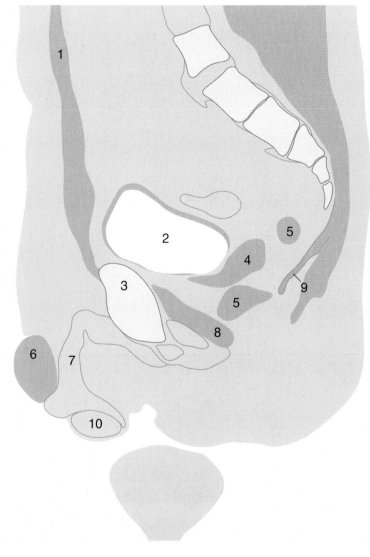

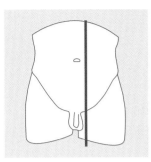

Sagittal MR of male pelvis and perineum

1 - Rectus abdominis muscle
2 - Sacrum
3 - Sigmoid colon
4 - Urinary bladder
5 - Pubis
6 - Seminal vesicle
7 - Glans of penis
8 - Spermatic cord and testicular vessels
9 - Levator prostatae and puborectalis muscles (parts of levator ani muscle)

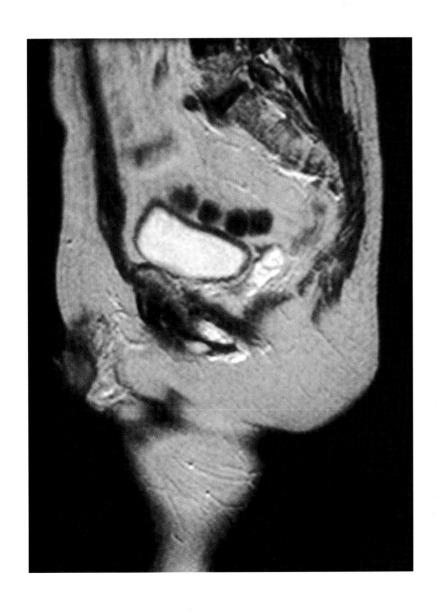

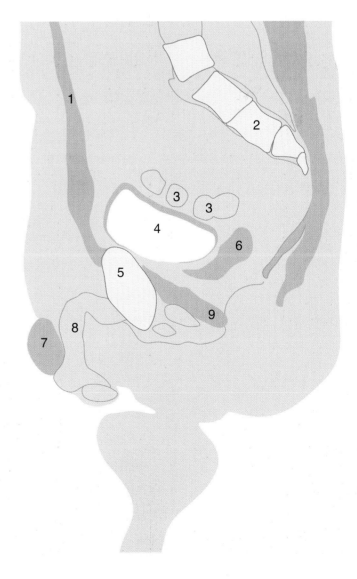

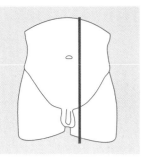

Sagittal MR of male pelvis and perineum

1 - Rectus abdominis muscle
2 - Sacrum
3 - Sigmoid colon
4 - Urinary bladder
5 - Pubis
6 - Seminal vesicle
7 - Gracilis muscle
8 - Levator prostatae and puborectalis muscles (parts of levator ani muscle)

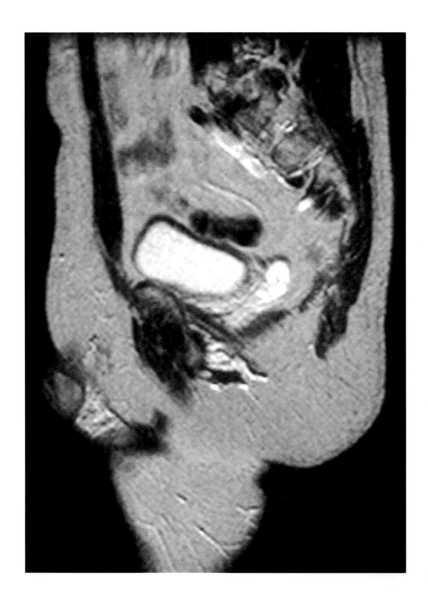

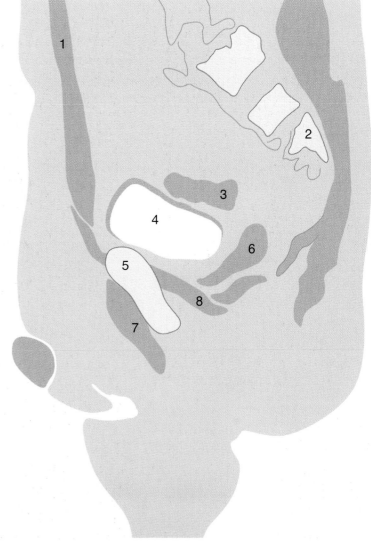

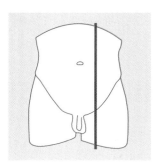

Sagittal MR of male pelvis and perineum

1 - Rectus abdominis muscle
2 - Pubis
3 - Urinary bladder
4 - Sigmoid colon

5 - Seminal vesicle
6 - Gluteus maximus muscle
7 - Gracilis muscle

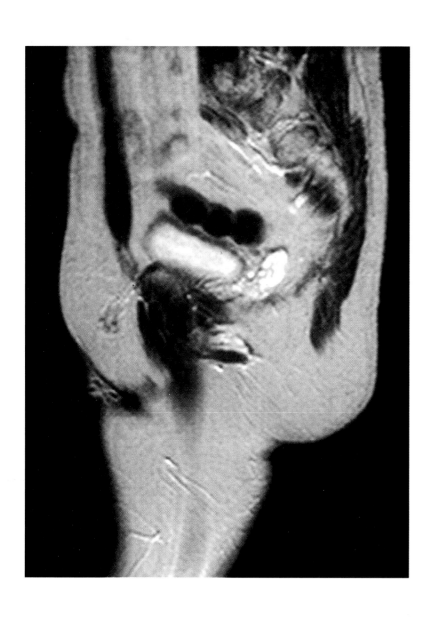

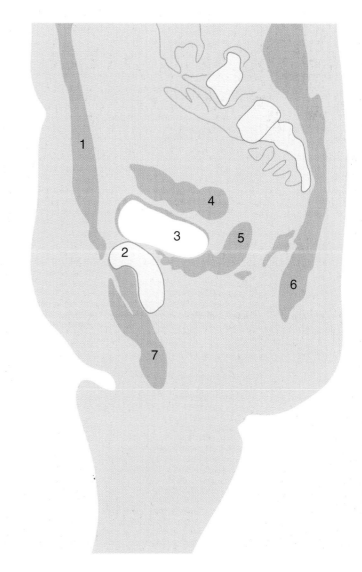

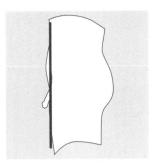

Coronal MR of male pelvis and perineum

1 - Inferior epigastric artery
2 - Rectus abdominis muscle
3 - Pyramidalis muscle
4 - Inguinal ligament
5 - Penis

6 - Corpus cavernosum
7 - Corpus spongiosum
8 - Testicular vessels and
    spermatic cord
9 - Testis

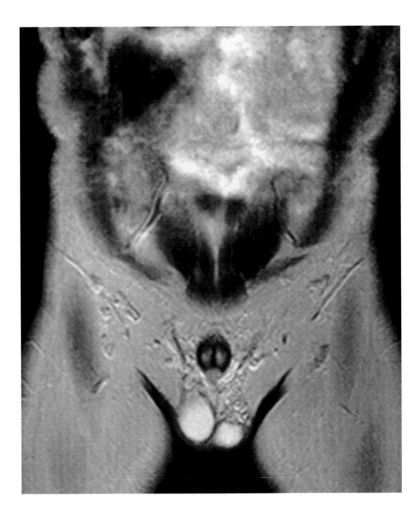

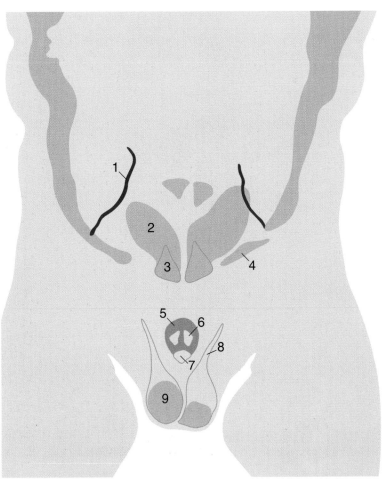

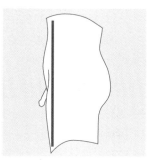

Coronal MR of male pelvis and perineum

1 - Anterolateral abdominal
    muscles
2 - Rectus abdominis muscle
3 - Inguinal ligament
4 - Sartorius muscle
5 - Penis

6 - Corpus cavernosum
7 - Corpus spongiosum
8 - Scrotal sac
9 - Testis
10 - Vastus lateralis muscle

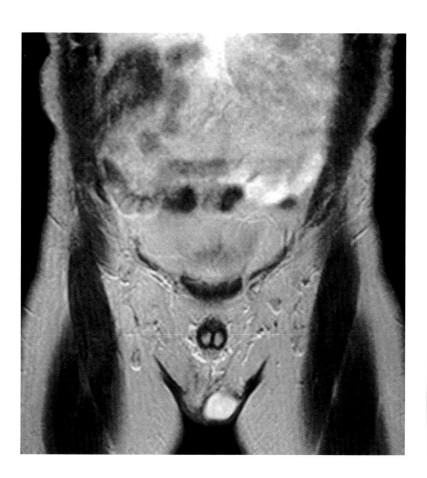

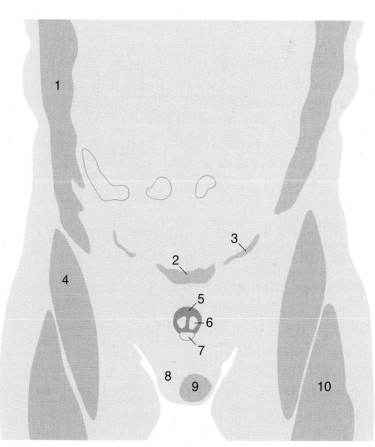

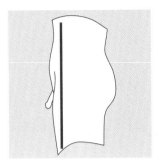

Coronal MR of male pelvis and perineum

1 - Anterolateral abdominal muscles
2 - Terminal ileum
3 - Descending colon
4 - Urinary bladder
5 - Tensor fasciae latae muscle
6 - Iliopsoas muscle
7 - Pubis

8 - Inguinal ligament
9 - Subinguinal hiatus
10 - Quadriceps femoris muscle
11 - Pubic symphysis
12 - Dorsal penile vein
13 - Corpus cavernosum
14 - Corpus spongiosum
15 - Testis

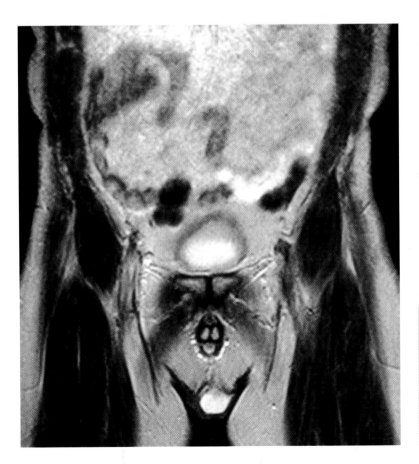

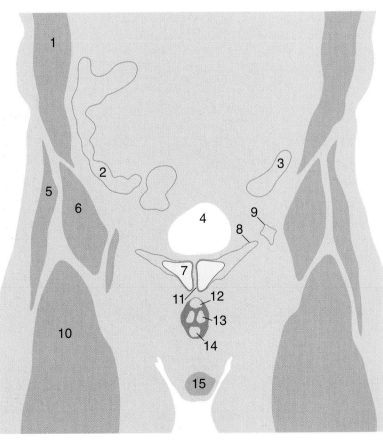

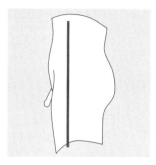

Coronal MR of male pelvis and perineum

1 - Anterolateral abdominal muscles
2 - Terminal ileum
3 - Sigmoid colon
4 - Urinary bladder
5 - Tensor fasciae latae muscle
6 - Ilipsoas muscle
7 - Subinguinal hiatus and femoral vessels (lacuna vasorum)
8 - Pectineus muscle

9 - Pubic symphysis
10 - Pecten of pubis
11 - Vastus lateralis muscle
12 - Rectus femoris muscle
13 - Corpus cavernosum
14 - Corpus spongiosum
15 - Scrotal sac
16 - Femoral vein (superficial branch)
17 - Femoral artery (deep branch)

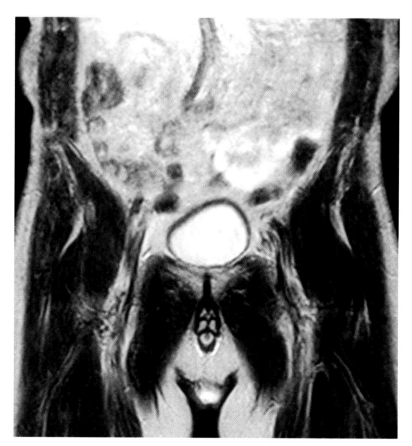

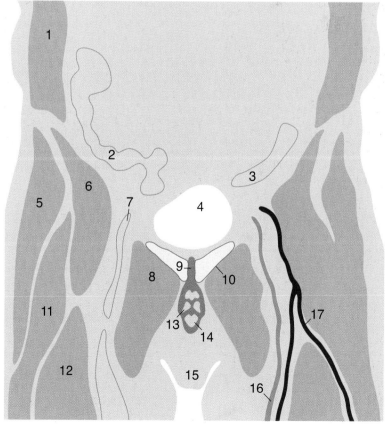

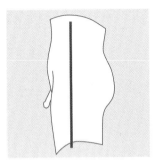

Coronal MR of male pelvis and perineum

1 - Anterolateral abdominal
    muscle
2 - Abdominal cavity
3 - Tensor fasciae latae and
    gluteus medius muscles
4 - Iliopsoas muscle
5 - Urinary bladder
6 - Sigmoid colon

7 - Descending colon
8 - Pubis
9 - Pubic symphysis
10 - Quadriceps femoris
    muscle
11 - Femoral adductors
12 - Corpus cavernosum
13 - Corpus spongiosum

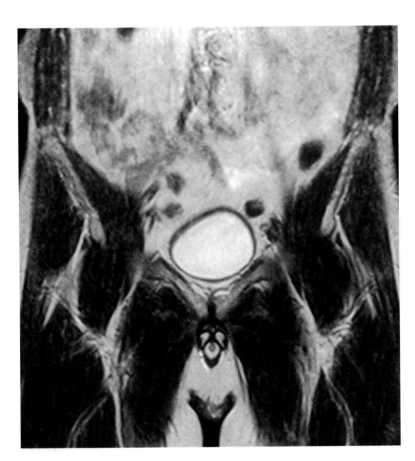

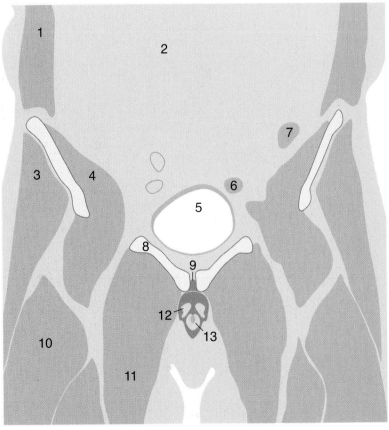

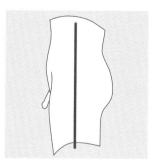

Coronal MR of male pelvis and perineum

1 - Caecum and ascending colon
2 - Terminal ileum
3 - Psoas major muscle
4 - Lumbar vertebra
5 - Descending colon
6 - Gluteus medius and minimus muscles
7 - Ilium
8 - Iliacus muscle
9 - Urinary bladder
10 - Sigmoid colon
11 - Tensor fasciae latae muscle
12 - Femoral extensors
13 - Femoral adductors
14 - Obturator internus muscle
15 - Prostate
16 - Urogenital diaphragm
17 - Crus of penis (corpus cavernosum)
18 - Bulb of penis (corpus spongiosum)

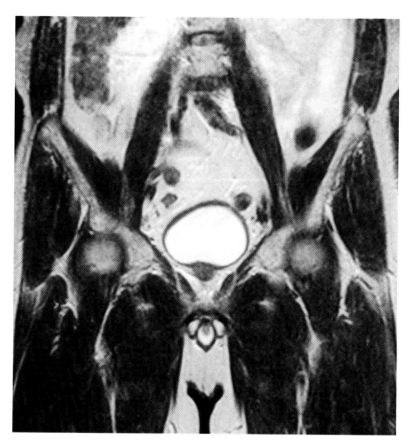

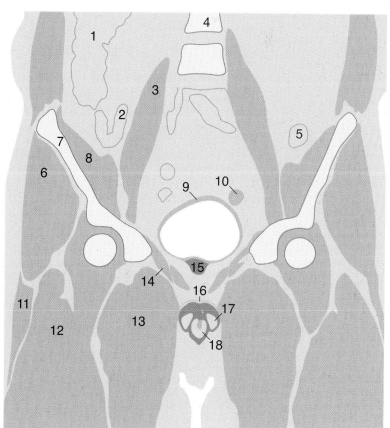

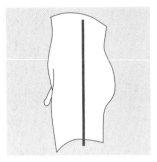

Coronal MR of male pelvis and perineum

1 - Anterolateral abdominal muscles
2 - Psoas major muscle
3 - Lumbar vertebra
4 - Descending colon
5 - Gluteus medius muscle
6 - Gluteus minimus muscle
7 - Acetabulum
8 - Urinary bladder
9 - Sigmoid colon
10 - Head of femur
11 - Obturator internus muscle
12 - Prostate
13 - Obturator externus muscle
14 - Femoral extensors
15 - Femoral adductors
16 - Crus of penis (corpus cavernosum)
17 - Bulb of penis (corpus spongiosum)
18 - Gracilis muscle

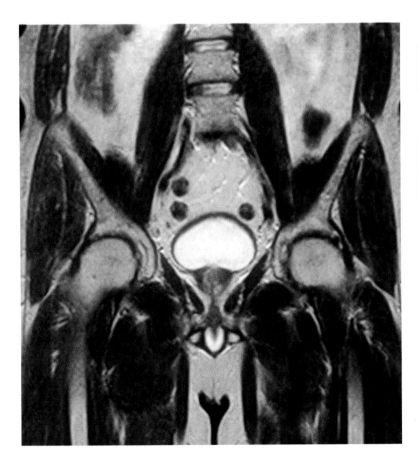

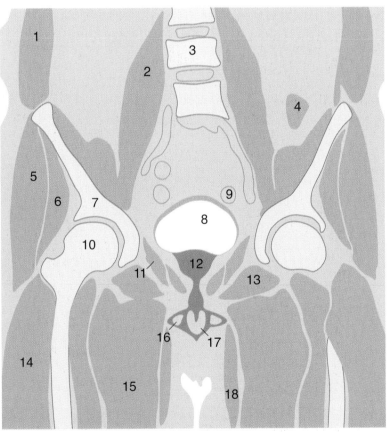

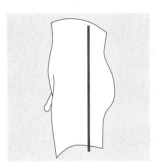

Coronal MR of male pelvis and perineum

1 - Sacral promontory
2 - Gluteus medius and gluteus maximus muscles
3 - Acetabulum
4 - Obturator internus muscle
5 - Seminal vesicle
6 - Sigmoid colon
7 - Greater trochanter
8 - Obturator externus muscle
9 - Rectum
10 - Levator ani muscle
11 - Anus
12 - Femoral extensors
13 - Femoral adductors

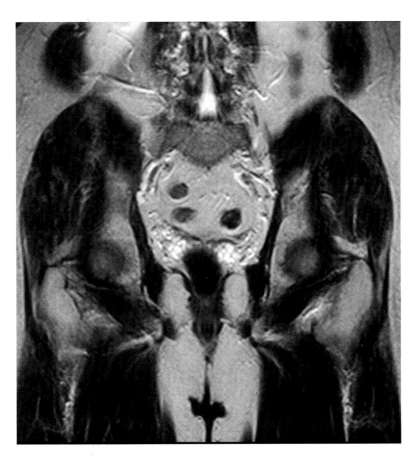

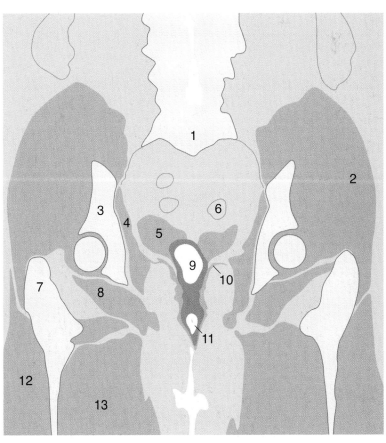

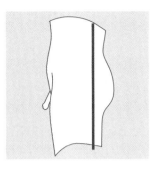

Coronal MR of male pelvis and perineum

1 - Ilium
2 - Sacrum
3 - Sacro-iliac joint
4 - Gluteus maximus muscle
5 - Obturator internus muscle

6 - Seminal vesicle
7 - Rectum
8 - Levator ani muscle
9 - Ischio-anal fossa
10 - Femoral adductors
11 - Anus

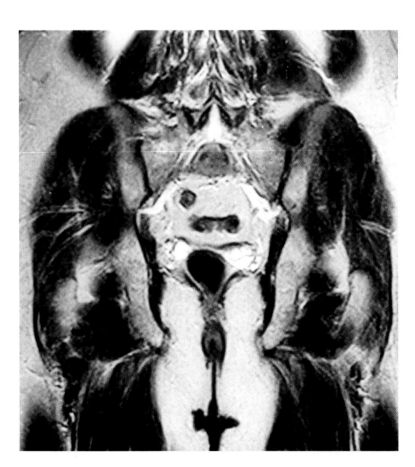

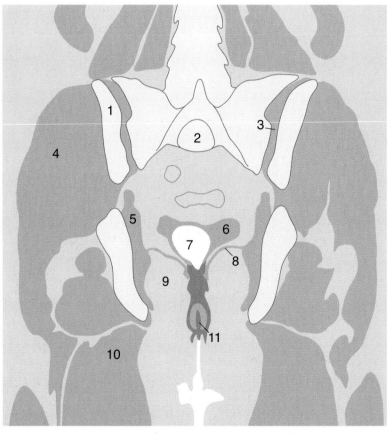

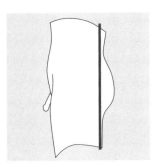

Coronal MR of male pelvis and perineum

1 - Erector spinae muscle
2 - Gluteus maximus muscle
3 - Ilium
4 - Sacrum
5 - Sacro-iliac joint

6 - Piriformis muscle
7 - Coccyx
8 - Coccygeus muscle
9 - Natal cleft

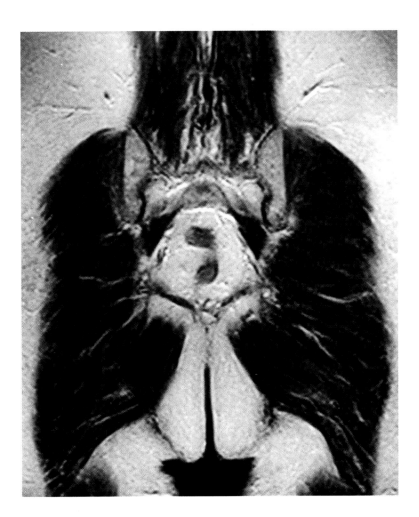

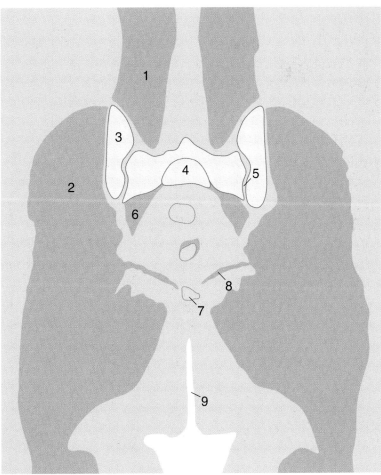

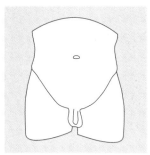

Pelvis and urinary bladder, intravenous urography, anteroposterior view

1 - Iliac crest
2 - Ilium
3 - Sacro-iliac joint
4 - Sacral foramina
5 - Median sacral crest
6 - Hip joint
7 - Ischial spine
8 - Pelvic brim (terminal line)
9 - Contrast medium in urinary bladder
10 - Prostatic indentation
11 - Pubic symphysis

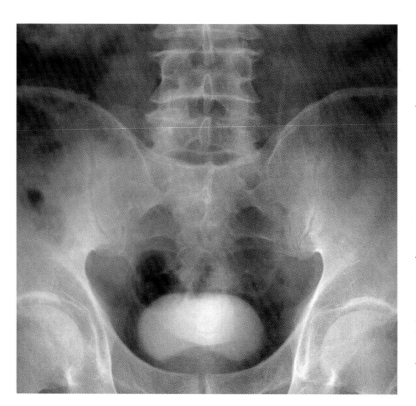

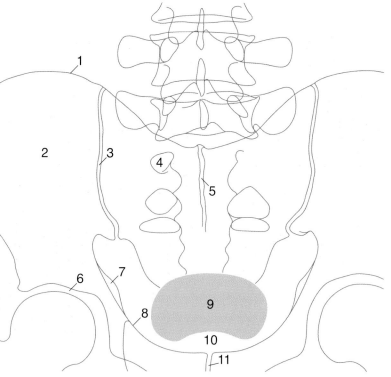

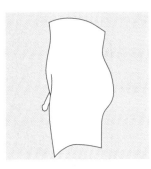

Retrograde urethrogram of male urethra, oblique view

1 - Head of femur
2 - Pubic symphysis
3 - Neck of urinary bladder
4 - Prostatic urethra

5 - Membranous urethra
6 - Bulbar urethra
7 - Penile urethra
8 - Navicular fossa

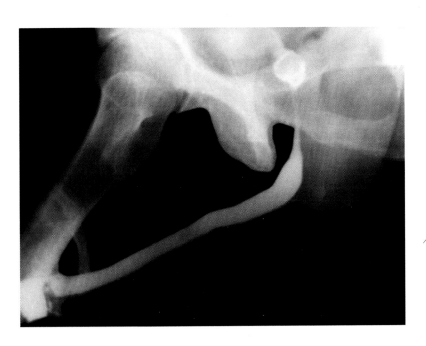

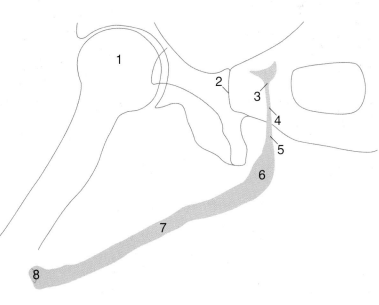

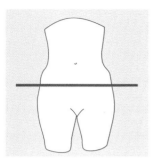

Axial CT of female pelvis

1 - Ileal loops	6 - Sigmoid colon
2 - Iliopsoas muscle	7 - Ilium
3 - External iliac artery	8 - Rectum
4 - External iliac vein	9 - Piriformis muscle
5 - Uterus	10 - Sacrum

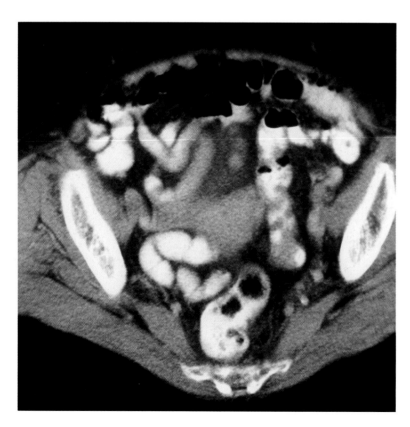

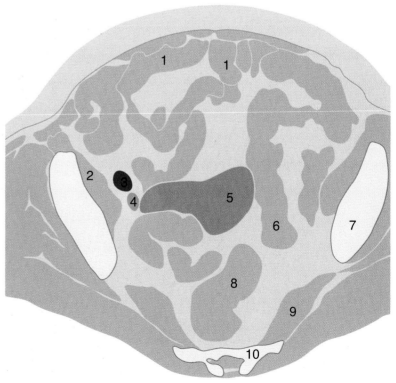

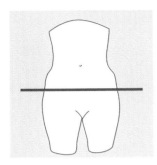

Axial CT of female pelvis

1 - Rectus abdominis muscle
2 - Iliopsoas muscle
3 - Ileal loops
4 - External iliac artery
5 - External iliac vein
6 - Urinary bladder
7 - Body of uterus
8 - Ovary and uterine tube
9 - Acetabulum
10 - Piriformis muscle
11 - Rectum
12 - Sacrum

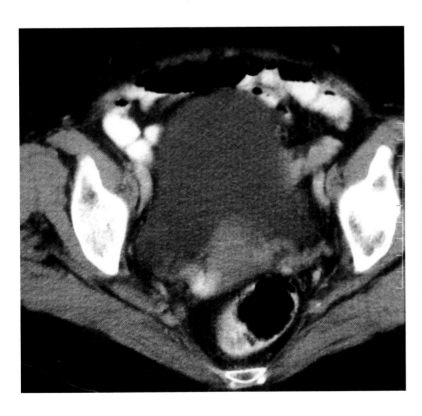

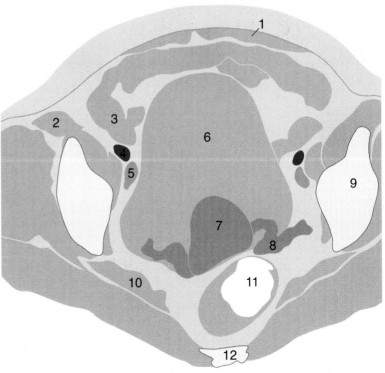

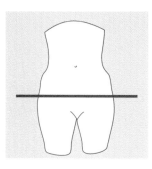

Axial CT of female pelvis

1 - Ileal loop	7 - Urinary bladder
2 - External iliac artery	8 - Vagina
3 - External iliac vein	9 - Internal iliac vessels
4 - Iliopsoas muscle	10 - Rectum
5 - Acetabulum	11 - Coccyx
6 - Head of femur	

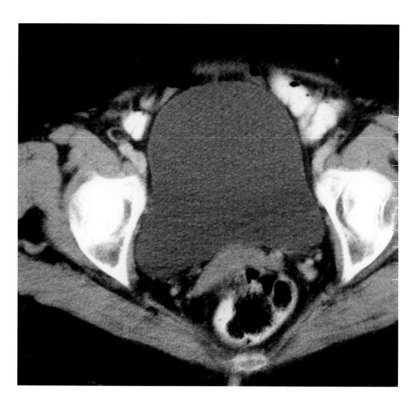

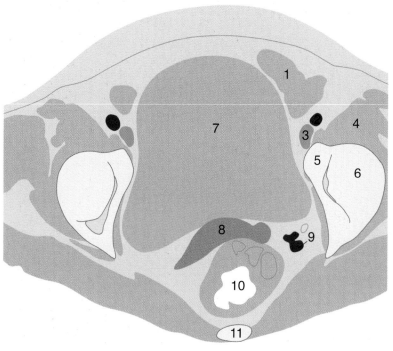

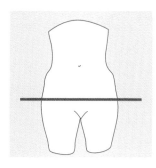

Axial CT of female pelvis

1 - Femoral artery
2 - Femoral vein
3 - Urinary bladder (heavily distended)
4 - Iliopsoas muscle
5 - Head of femur
6 - Acetabulum (pubic part)
7 - Obturator internus muscle
8 - Vagina
9 - Rectum
10 - Coccyx

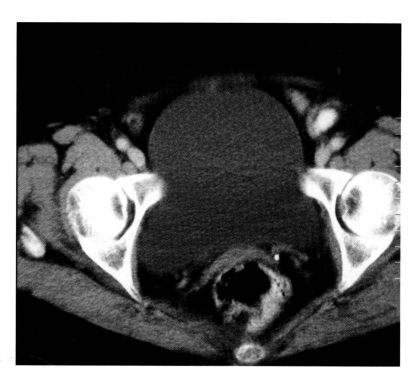

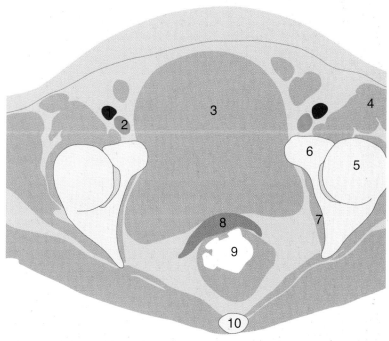

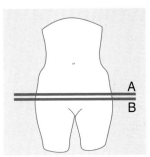

Axial MR of female pelvis and perineum

1 - Tensor fasciae latae muscle
2 - Rectus femoris muscle
3 - Sartorius muscle
4 - Femoral vessels
5 - Pectineus muscle
6 - Gluteus medius muscle
7 - Iliopsoas muscle
8 - Femur
9 - Acetabulum (pubic part)
10 - Urinary bladder
11 - Greater trochanter
12 - Superior and inferior gemellus muscles
13 - Tendon of obturator internus muscle
14 - Obturator internus muscle
15 - Vagina
16 - Rectum
17 - Ischio-anal fossa
18 - Pudendal canal
19 - Gluteus maximus muscle
20 - Natal cleft
21 - Superior pubic ligament
22 - Obturator externus muscle
23 - Pubic symphysis and arcuate ligament
24 - Urethra
25 - Quadratus femoris muscle
26 - Ischial tuberosity

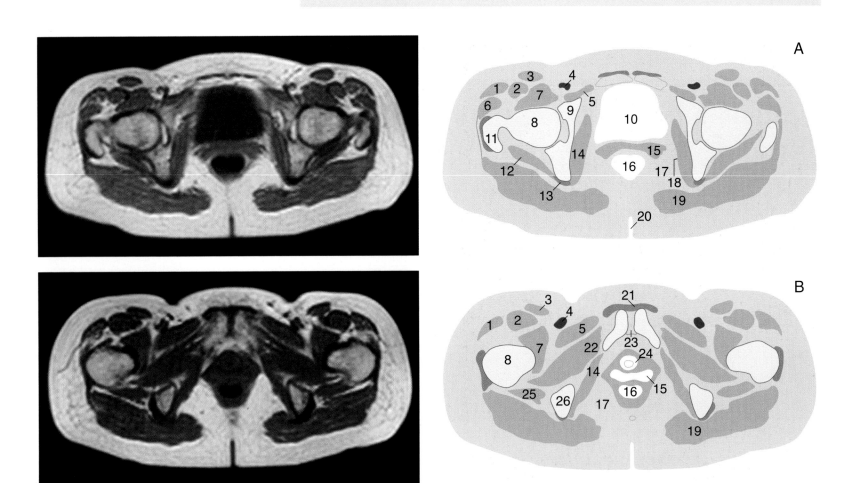

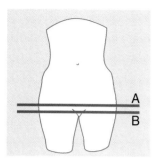

Axial MR of female pelvis and perineum

1 - Tensor fasciae latae muscle
2 - Rectus femoris muscle
3 - Sartorius muscle
4 - Femoral vessels
5 - Adductor brevis muscle
6 - Pubic symphysis
7 - Vastus lateralis muscle
8 - Vastus intermedius muscle
9 - Femur
10 - Pectineus muscle
11 - Adductor longus muscle
12 - Obturator externus muscle
13 - Urogenital triangle (urogenital diaphragm)
14 - Urethra
15 - Quadratus femoris muscle
16 - Vagina
17 - Ischio-anal fossa
18 - Gluteus maximus muscle
19 - Rectum
20 - Labia majora
21 - Adductor magnus muscle
22 - Vestibule of vagina

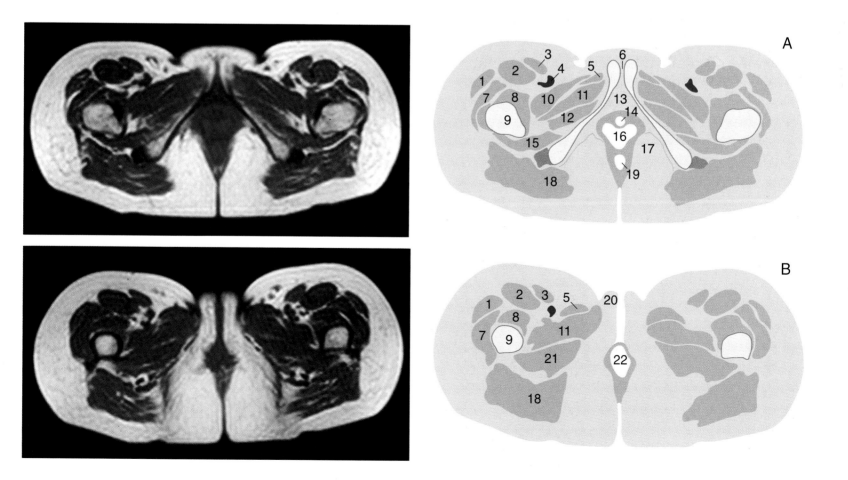

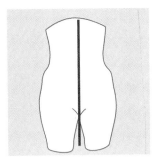

Sagittal MR of female pelvis and perineum

1 - Lumbar vertebrae
2 - Sacrum
3 - Rectus abdominis muscle
4 - Coccyx
5 - Ileum
6 - Rectum
7 - Recto-uterine pouch
  (pouch of Douglas)
8 - Uterus
9 - Vesico-uterine pouch
10 - Urinary bladder
11 - Prevesical space of Retzius
12 - Pubis
13 - Urethra
14 - Urethrovaginal septum
15 - Vagina
16 - Rectovaginal septum
  (peritoneo-perineal
  aponeurosis)
17 - Rectum, anal canal
18 - External anal sphincter
19 - Anococcygeal ligament

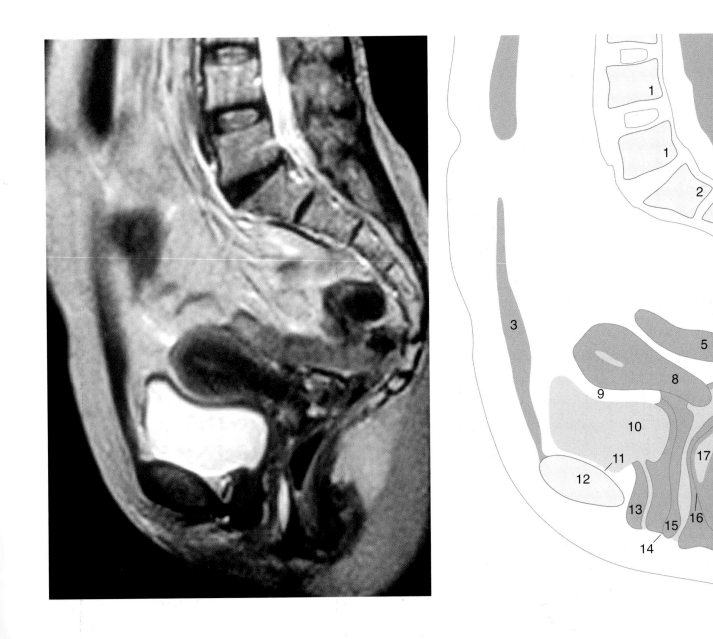

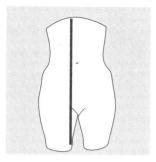

Sagittal MR of female pelvis and perineum

1 - Lumbar vertebrae
2 - Aorta
3 - Rectus abdominis muscle
4 - Rectum
5 - Uterus
6 - Uterine cavity and cervical canal
7 - Cervix of uterus, vaginal part
8 - Posterior fornix of vagina

9 - Anococcygeal ligament
10 - Anterior fornix of vagina
11 - Vesico-uterine pouch
12 - Urinary bladder
13 - Pubic symphysis
14 - Prevesical space of Retzius
15 - Vagina
16 - Perineal body, urogenital diaphragm
17 - Sacrum

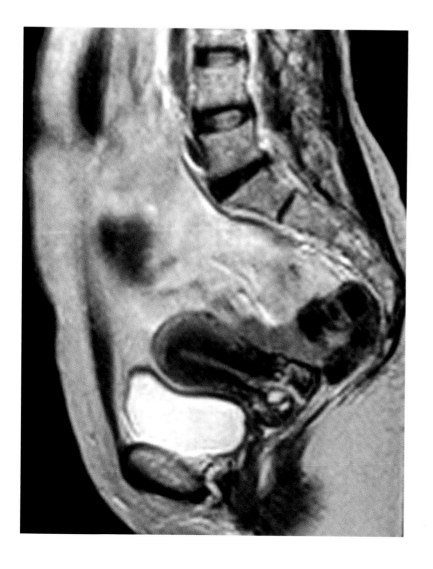

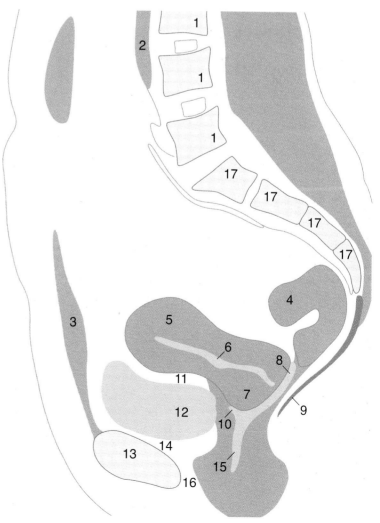

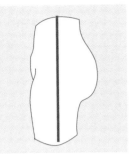

Coronal MR of female pelvis and perineum

1 - Inferior vena cava
2 - Abdominal aorta
3 - Common iliac artery
4 - Coils of ileum
5 - Gluteus medius and
    minimus muscles
6 - Ilium
7 - Iliacus muscle
8 - Psoas major muscle
9 - External iliac/femoral
    artery

10 - Suspensory ligament of
     ovary
11 - Ovary
12 - Uterus
13 - External iliac vein
14 - Pubis
15 - Urinary bladder
16 - Extensors of thigh
17 - Adductors of thigh
18 - Labia majora

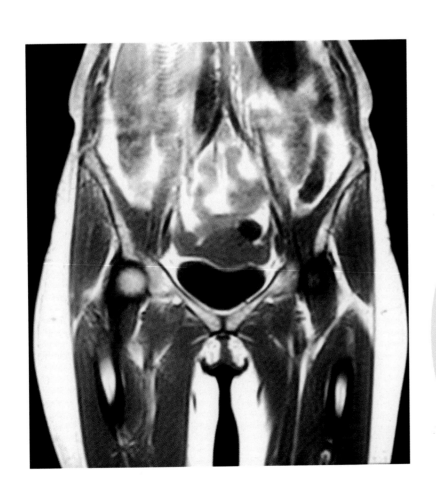

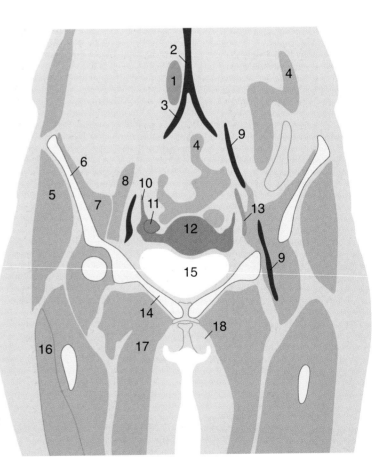

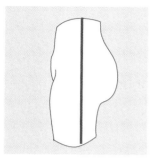

Coronal MR of female pelvis and perineum

1 - Anterolateral abdominal muscles
2 - Lumbar vertebra
3 - Psoas major muscle
4 - Common iliac vein
5 - Gluteus medius muscle
6 - Gluteus minimus muscle
7 - Ilium
8 - Iliacus muscle
9 - Uterine (Fallopian) tube

10 - Uterus
11 - Sigmoid colon
12 - Head of femur
13 - Pubis
14 - Vestibule of vagina
15 - Labia majora
16 - Extensors of thigh and tensor fasciae latae muscle
17 - Adductors of thigh
18 - Urinary bladder

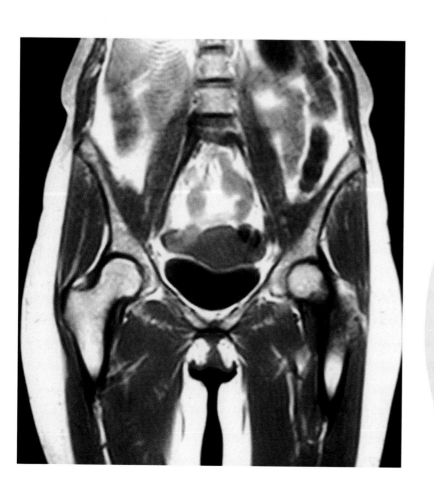

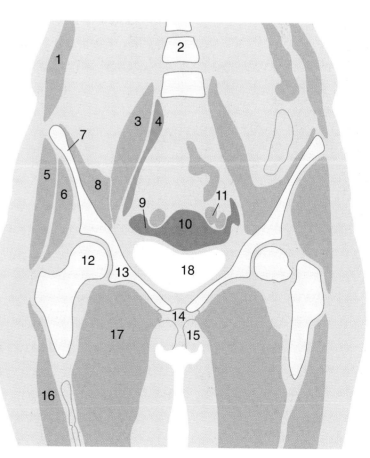

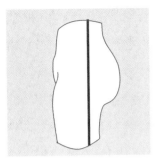

Coronal MR of female pelvis and perineum

1 - Anterolateral abdominal muscles
2 - Psoas major muscle
3 - Lumbar vertebra
4 - Ilium
5 - Iliacus muscle
6 - Gluteus medius muscle
7 - Gluteus minimus muscle
8 - Ileal loop
9 - Acetabulum (iliac portion)
10 - Uterus
11 - Tubovarian complex
12 - Greater trochanter
13 - Obturator internus muscle
14 - Urinary bladder
15 - Obturator externus muscle
16 - Pectineus muscle
17 - Pelvic floor including vagina
18 - Vastus lateralis muscle
19 - Vastus medialis muscle
20 - Adductor magnus muscle
21 - Labia majora

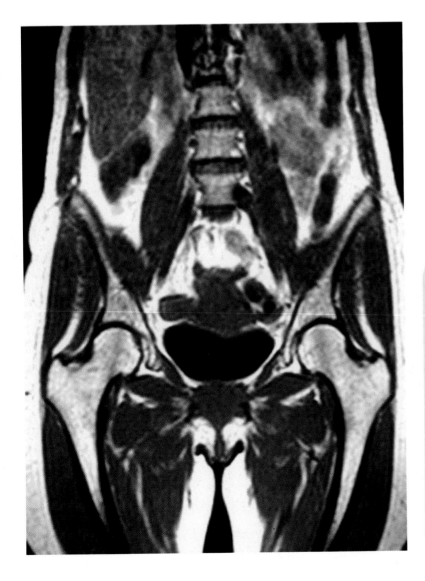

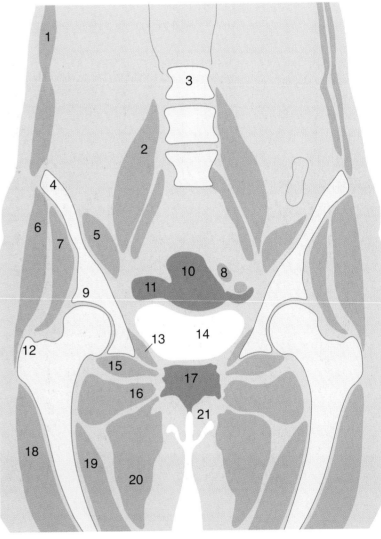

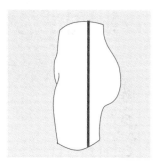

Coronal MR of female pelvis and perineum

1 - Anterolateral abdominal muscles
2 - Psoas major muscle
3 - Lumbar vertebra
4 - Ilium
5 - Iliacus muscle
6 - Ileum
7 - Gluteus medius and gluteus maximus muscles
8 - Gluteus minimus muscle
9 - Acetabulum
10 - Uterus
11 - Sigmoid colon
12 - Head of femur
13 - Obturator internus muscle
14 - Urinary bladder
15 - Tensor fasciae latae muscle
16 - Obturator externus muscle
17 - Pectineus muscle
18 - Pelvic floor including vagina
19 - Adductors of thigh

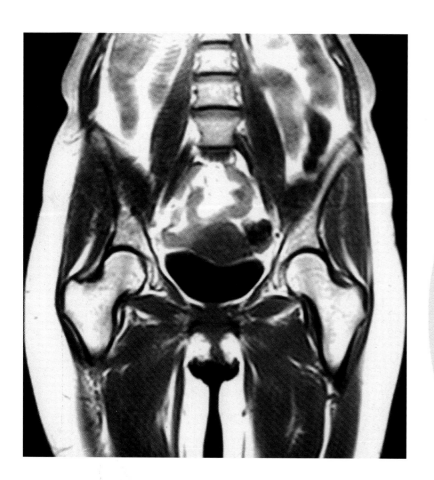

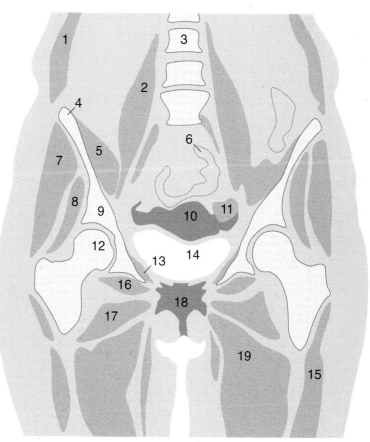

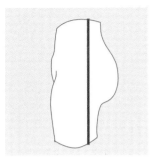

Coronal MR of female pelvis and perineum

1 - Anterolateral abdominal muscles
2 - Psoas major muscle
3 - Lumbar vertebra
4 - Gluteus medius and gluteus maximus muscles
5 - Iliacus muscle
6 - Ileum
7 - Gluteus minimus muscle
8 - Uterus
9 - Sigmoid colon
10 - Acetabulum
11 - Head of femur
12 - Obturator internus muscle
13 - Urinary bladder
14 - Greater trochanter of femur
15 - Gluteus maximus muscle
16 - Pelvic floor including vagina
17 - Obturator externus muscle
18 - Pectineus muscle
19 - Adductors of thigh
20 - Gracilis muscle

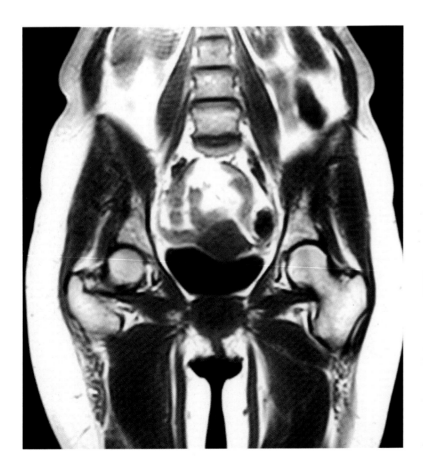

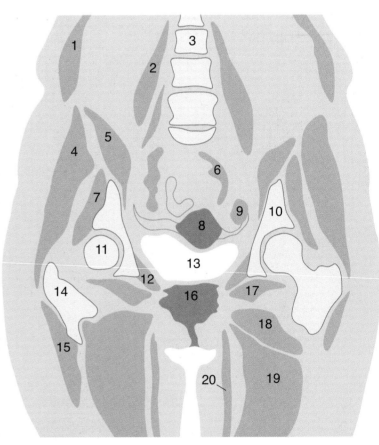

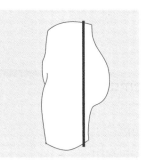

Coronal MR of female pelvis and perineum

1 - Iliacus muscle
2 - Psoas major muscle
3 - Gluteus maximus muscle
4 - Uterus
5 - Obturator internus muscle
6 - Obturator externus muscle

7 - Urinary bladder
8 - Vagina
9 - Pectineus muscle
10 - Adductors of thigh
11 - Gracilis muscle

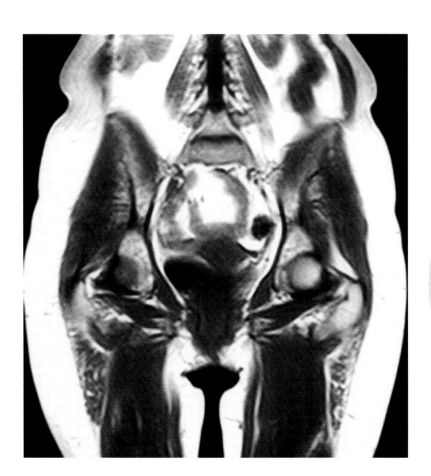

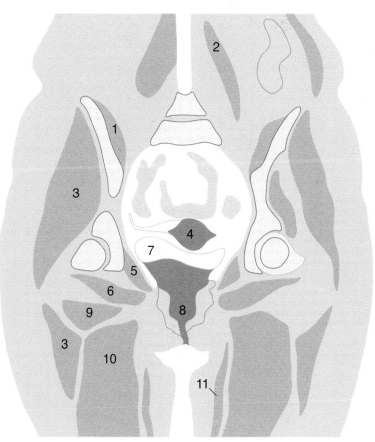

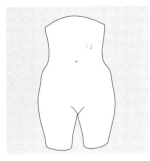

Hystero-salpingogram of uterus and uterine (Fallopian) tubes

1 - Ampulla of Fallopian tube
2 - Isthmus of Fallopian tube
3 - Uterine cornu
4 - Fundus of uterus with inflated catheter inside
5 - Peritoneal spill of contrast material

6 - Pelvic brim (superior pubic ramus)
7 - Pubic symphysis
8 - Obturator foramen

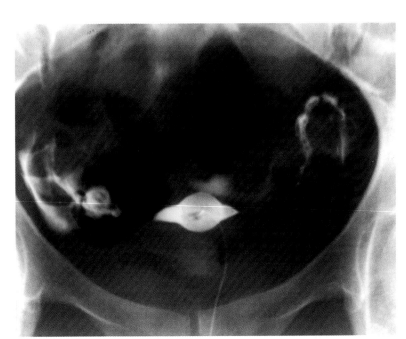
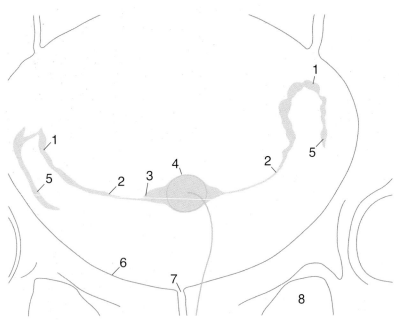

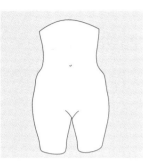

Ultrasonogram of 12-week-old foetus in pregnant uterus

1 - Amniotic cavity
2 - Hand
3 - Head

4 - Forearm
5 - Chest
6 - Placenta

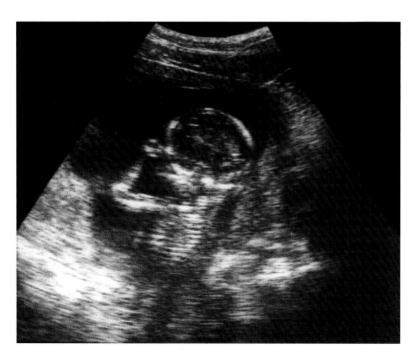

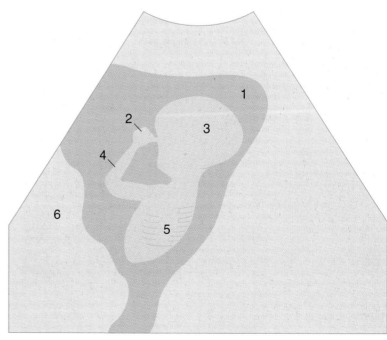

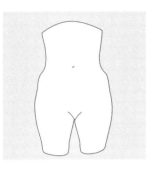

Ultrasonogram of head of foetus in pregnant uterus

1 - Thoracic vertebrae
2 - Neck

3 - Cerebellum
4 - Cerebral hemispheres

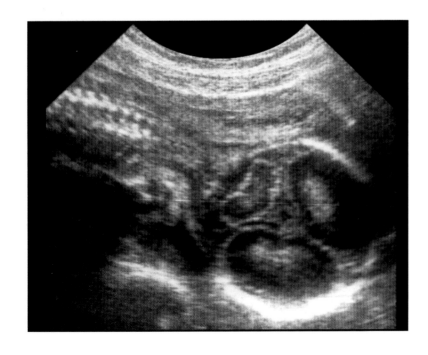

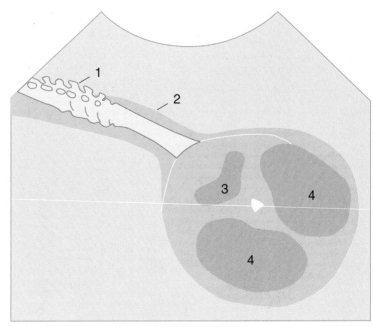

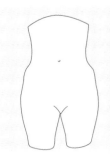

Internal iliac arteriogram, anteroposterior view

1 - Iliolumbar artery
2 - Internal iliac artery
3 - Posterior trunk of internal iliac artery
4 - Anterior trunk of internal iliac artery
5 - Lateral sacral artery

6 - Superior gluteal artery
7 - Internal pudendal artery
8 - Uterine artery
9 - Superior vesical artery
10 - Inferior gluteal artery
11 - Obturator artery

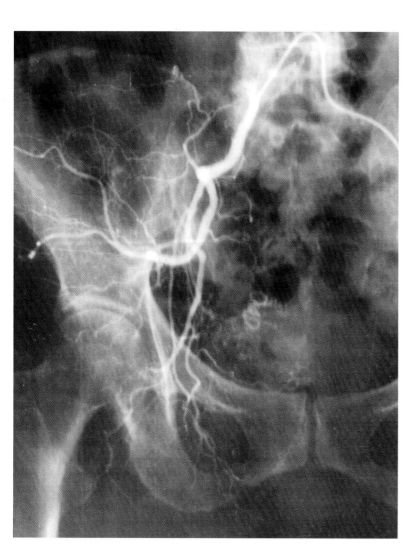

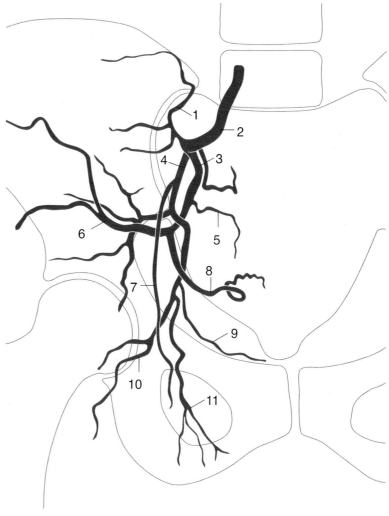

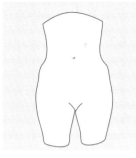

Uterine artery, common iliac arteriogram, anteroposterior view. The uterus is marked blue

1 - External iliac artery
2 - Internal iliac artery
3 - Superior gluteal artery
4 - Posterior trunk of internal iliac artery
5 - Anterior trunk of internal iliac artery
6 - Lateral sacral artery
7 - Inferior gluteal artery
8 - Uterine artery

9 - Femoral artery
10 - Obturator artery
11 - Superior vesical artery
12 - Lateral circumflex femoral artery
13 - Deep branch of femoral artery
14 - Superficial branch of femoral artery

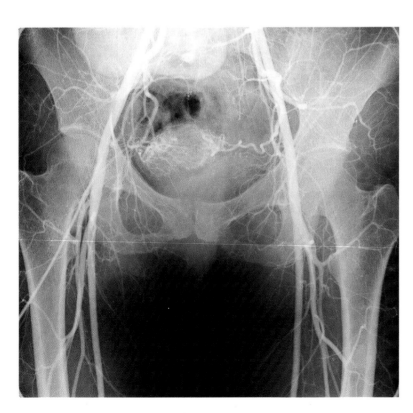

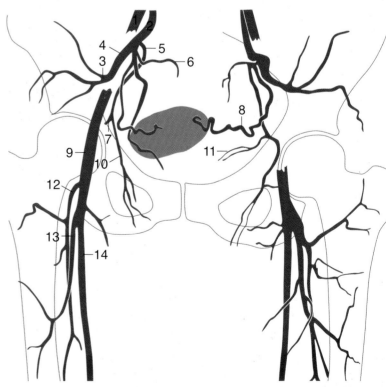

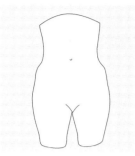

Iliopelvic lymphatic structures, lymphangiography, front view. Note filling defect in right paracaval system

1 - Lumbar spine
2 - Para-aortic lymphatic tract
3 - Ilium
4 - Sacro-iliac joint
5 - Sacrum
6 - Left common iliac nodes and vessels
7 - Enlarged metastatic lymph node with filling defect in the upper pole

8 - External iliac nodes and vessels
9 - Head of femur
10 - Pelvic brim
11 - Pubic symphysis
12 - Obturator foramen
13 - Inguinal lymph nodes and vessels

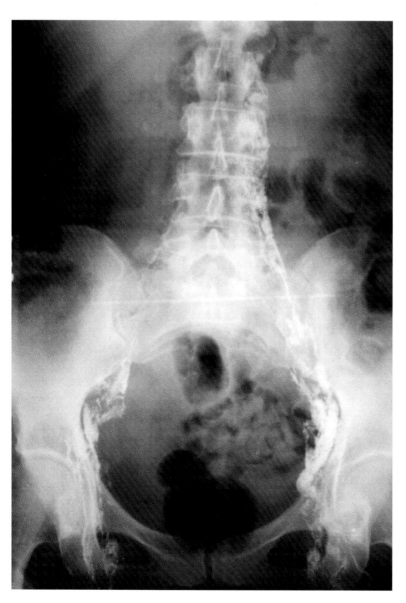

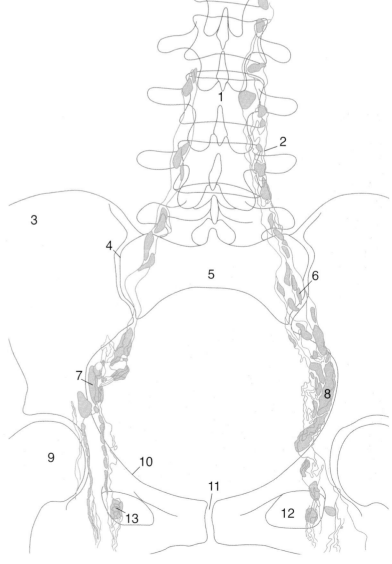

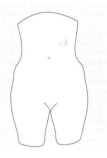

Lymphangiography of pelvic lymphatic tracts, oblique view
External iliac group.

E – External lymphatic chain
M – Middle lymphatic chain
I – Internal lymphatic chain

C – Common iliac lymphatic
    bundle

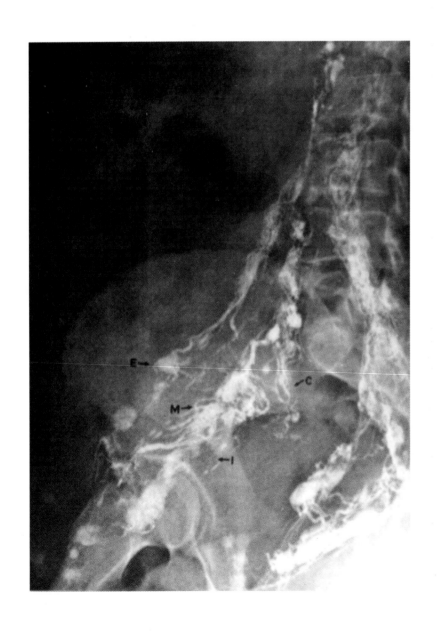

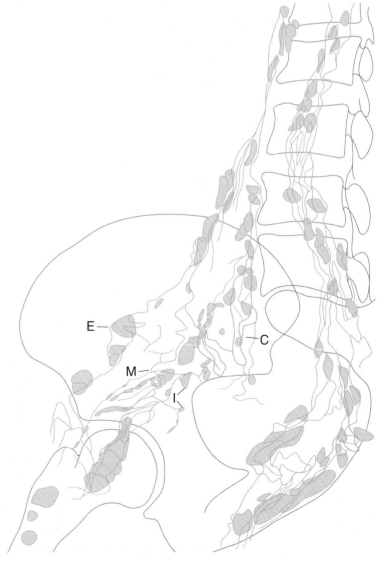

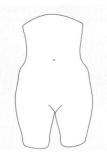

Lymphadenography of lumbosacral (abdomino-aortic) lymphatic system, front view

1 - Lumbar spine
2 - Paracaval nodes
3 - Pre-aortic nodes
4 - Para-aortic nodes

5 - Sacro-iliac joint
6 - Common iliac group
7 - Sacrum
8 - External iliac group

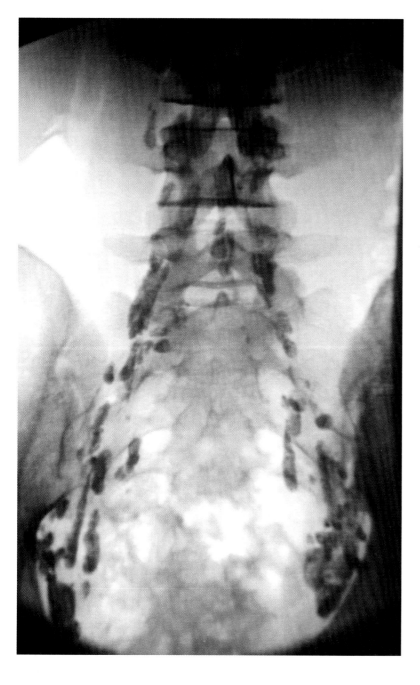

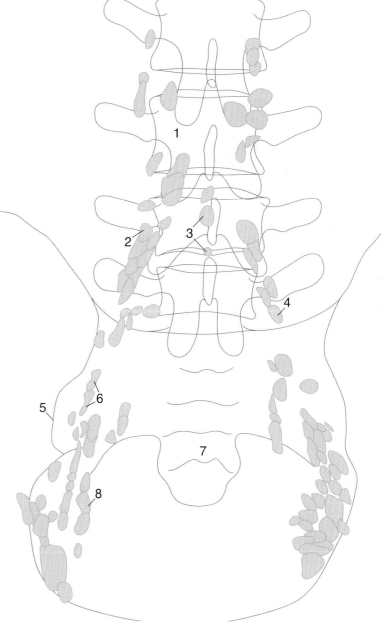

SPINE AND BACK

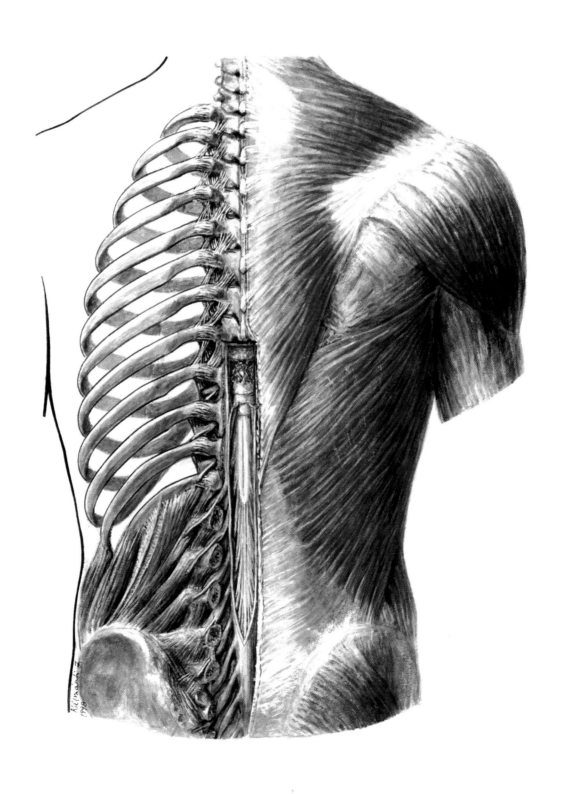

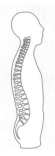

SPECT image of skeletal system

1 - Skull
2 - Nasal cavity
3 - Mandible
4 - Acromion
5 - Humerus
6 - Ribs
7 - Lumbar vertebrae
8 - Forearm
9 - Hand
10 - Ilium
11 - Head of femur
12 - Ischium

13 - Bladder containing
     radioactive isotope
14 - Shaft of femur
15 - Tibia
16 - Fibula
17 - Cervical vertebrae
18 - Scapula
19 - Thoracic vertebrae
20 - Sacrum
21 - Acetabulum
22 - Coccyx

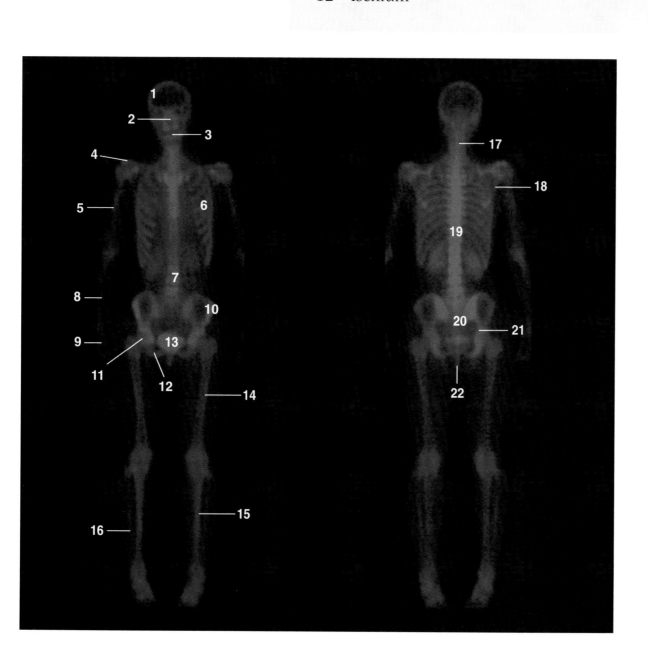

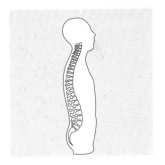

Anteroposterior radiograph of cervical spine

1 - Axis
2 - Transverse process
3 - Vertebral body
4 - Intervertebral foramen
5 - Raised lip of upper
    surface of vertebral body
    (uncovertebral process)

6 - Intervertebral disc
7 - Thoracic vertebra I
8 - Rib III

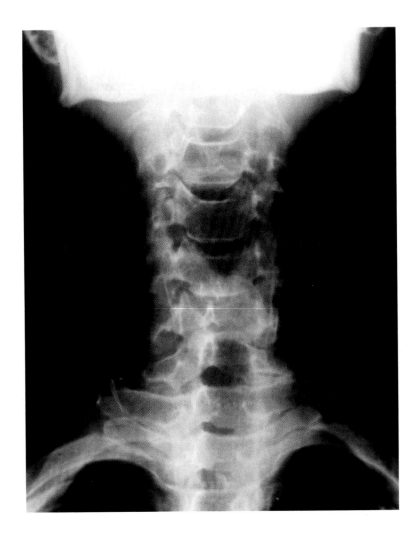

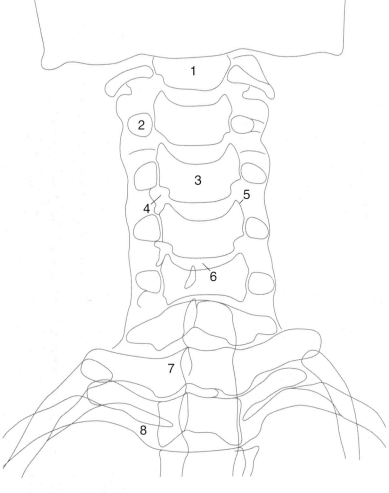

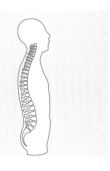

Lateral radiograph of cervical spine

1 - Dens of axis
2 - Anterior arch of atlas
3 - Spinous process of axis
4 - Zygapophyseal joint

5 - Body of vertebra
6 - Intervertebral disc
7 - Spinous process of
   vertebra prominens (VII)

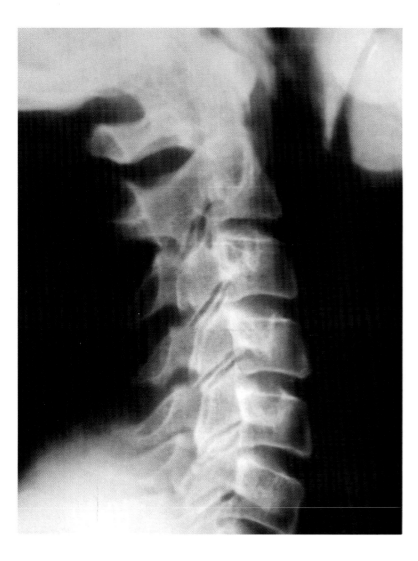

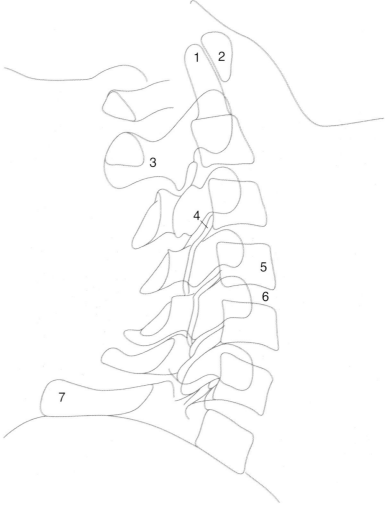

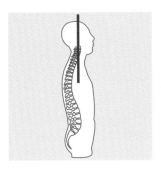

Coronal CT of craniocervical region

1 - Mastoid antrum
2 - Petro-occipital fissure
3 - Aeration of petrous apex
4 - Petrous temporal
5 - Tympanic cavity
6 - External acoustic meatus
7 - Clivus
8 - Jugular bulb
9 - Styloid process (origin of ossified stylohyoid ligament)
10 - Transverse process of atlas
11 - Lateral mass of atlas
12 - Odontoid process (dens) of axis
13 - Occipital condyle
14 - Atlanto-occipital joint
15 - Superior facet of axis
16 - Atlanto-axial joint
17 - Body of axis
18 - Transverse process of axis
19 - Cervical vertebra III

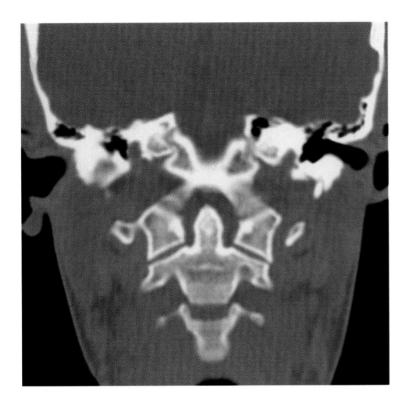

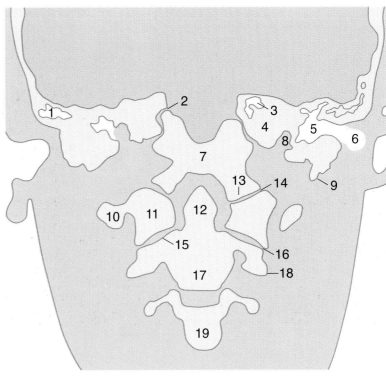

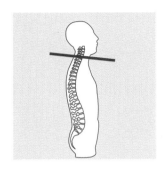

Axial CT of cervical vertebra, superior aspect

1 - Body of vertebra
2 - Foramen transversarium
3 - Anterior tubercle of
    transverse process
4 - Intertubercular lamella
5 - Posterior tubercle of
    transverse process

6 - Superior articular facet
7 - Vertebral canal
8 - Pedicle
9 - Lamina
10 - Spinous process

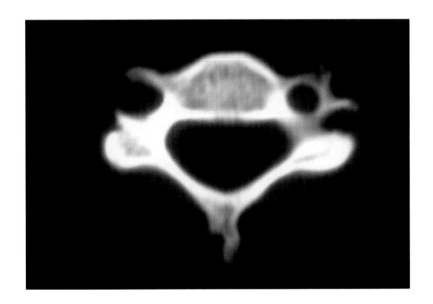

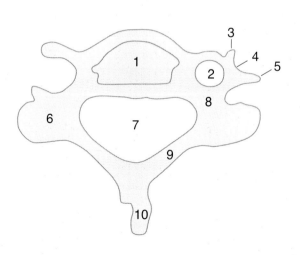

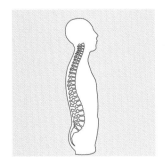

3D CT SSD reconstruction of cervical vertebra, superior aspect

1 - Sulcus for spinal nerve
2 - Body of vertebra
3 - Anterior tubercle of transverse process
4 - Intertubercular lamella
5 - Posterior tubercle of transverse process
6 - Foramen transversarium
7 - Pedicle
8 - Superior articular facet
9 - Vertebral foramen
10 - Lamina
11 - Spinous process

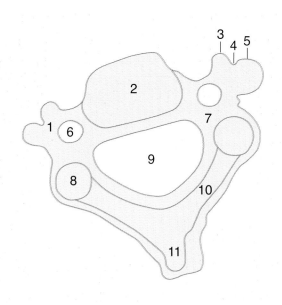

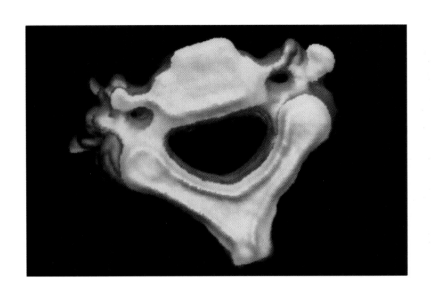

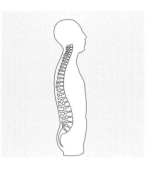

3D CT SSD reconstruction of cervical vertebrae, inferior oblique aspect

1 - Foramen transversarium
2 - Transverse process
3 - Body of vertebra
4 - Inferior articular facet
5 - Lamina
6 - Vertebral canal
7 - Bifid spinous process

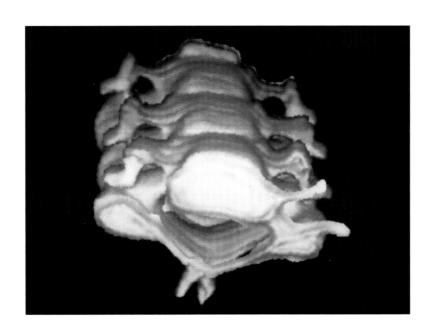

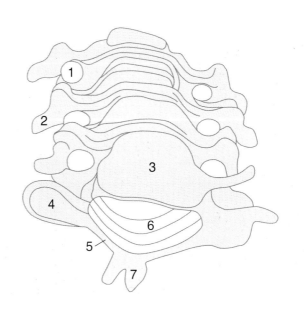

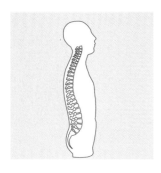

Anteroposterior radiograph of thoracic spine

1 - Rib I
2 - Clavicle
3 - Body of thoracic vertebra VI
4 - Transverse process of
    thoracic vertebra VIII

5 - Intervertebral disc
6 - Spinous process
7 - Pedicle

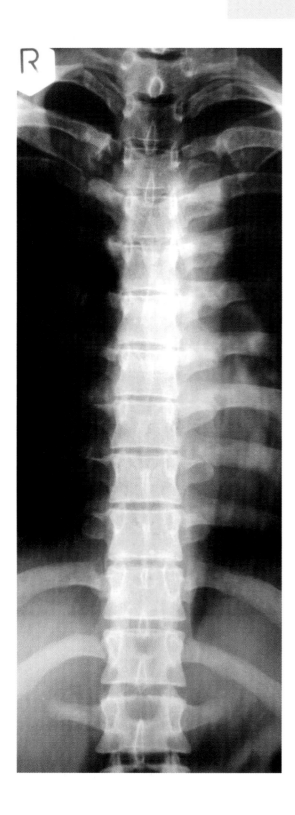

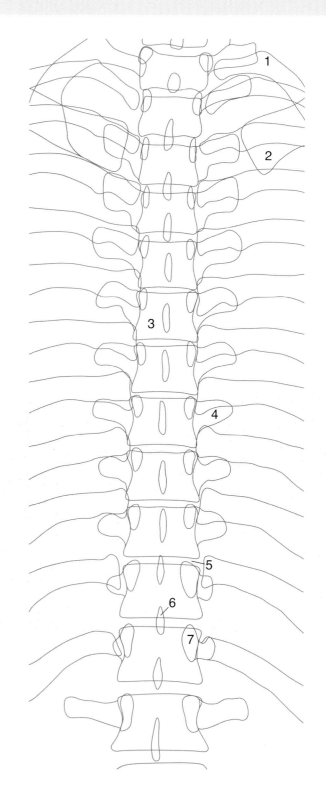

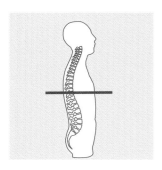

Axial CT of thoracic vertebra

1 - Body of vertebra
2 - Semilunar facet
3 - Rib
4 - Pedicle
5 - Vertebral foramen
6 - Superior articular process
7 - Lamina
8 - Costal tubercle
9 - Spinous process
10 - Costal facet of transverse process

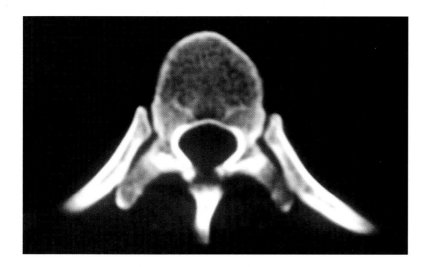

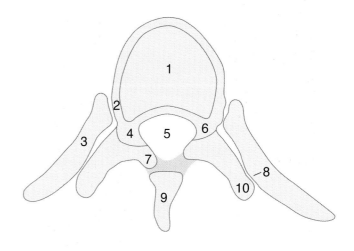

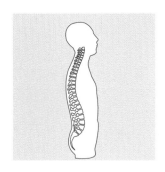

3D CT SSD reconstruction of thoracic vertebra and rib, superior aspect

1 - Body of vertebra
2 - Costovertebral joint
3 - Rib
4 - Vertebral foramen

5 - Lamina
6 - Transverse process
7 - Spinous process

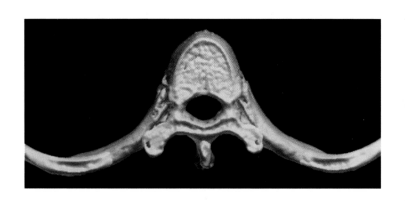

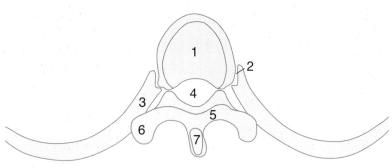

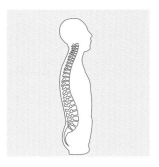

3D CT SSD reconstruction of thoracic vertebrae and ribs, anterosuperior oblique aspect

1 - Spinous process
2 - Transverse process
3 - Lamina
4 - Vertebral canal

5 - Body of vertebra
6 - Costotransverse joint
7 - Rib
8 - Costovertebral joint

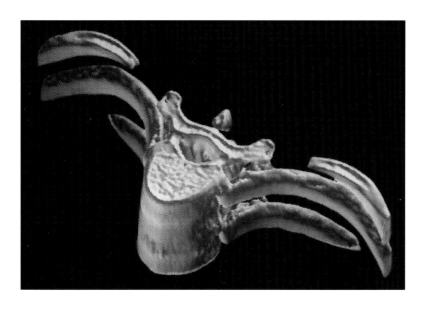

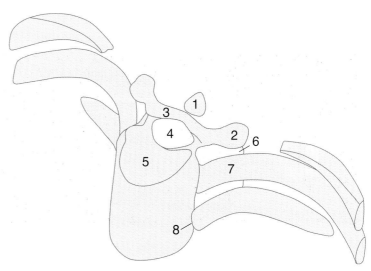

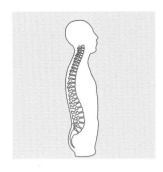

3D CT SSD reconstruction of thoracic vertebrae and ribs, posterior aspect

1 - Spinous process
2 - Costal tubercle
3 - Rib
4 - Costotransverse joint

5 - Transverse process
6 - Inferior articular process
    (zygapophyseal joint)

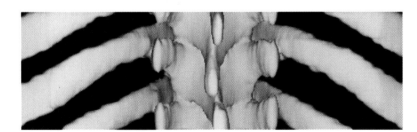

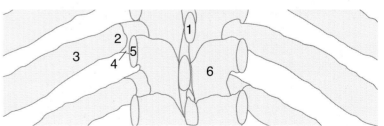

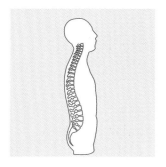

Anteroposterior radiograph of lumbar spine
(note lumbarization of first sacral vertebra)

1 - Rib XII (floating rib)
2 - Transverse (costal) process
3 - Pedicle
4 - Spinous process
5 - Body of vertebra

6 - Superior articular process
7 - Inferior articular process
8 - Sacro-iliac joint
9 - Lateral part of sacrum
10 - Ilium

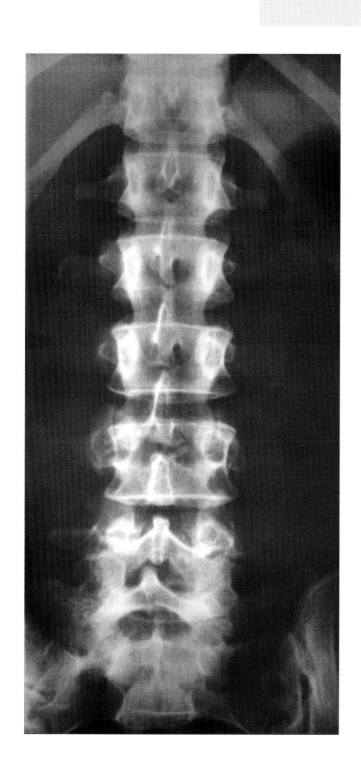

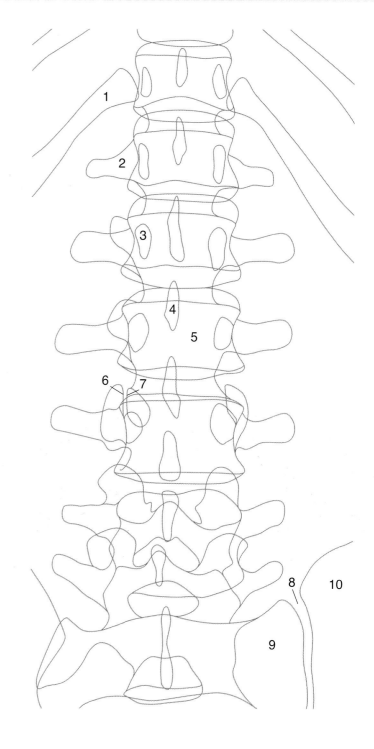

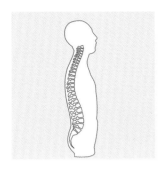

Lateral radiograph of lumbar spine

1 - Rib XII (floating rib)
2 - Body of vertebra
3 - Transverse (costal)
    process
4 - Spinous process
5 - Intervertebral foramen

6 - Intervertebral disc
7 - Inferior articular process
8 - Superior articular process
9 - Lumbosacral transition
10 - Sacral promontory

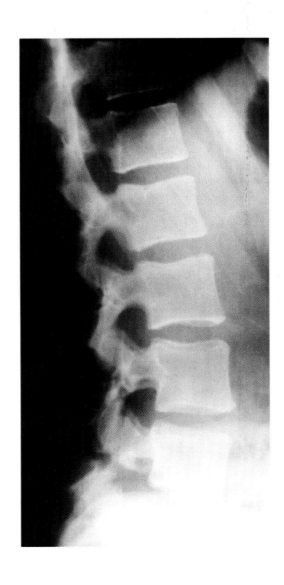

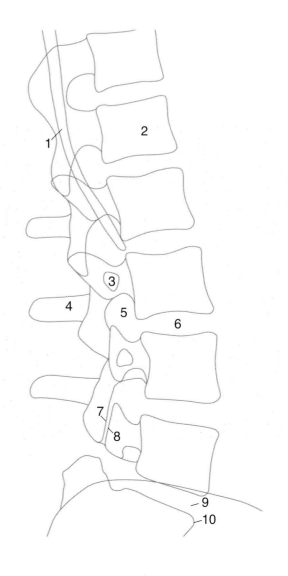

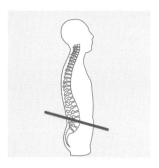

Axial CT of lumbar vertebra

1 - Body of vertebra
2 - Pedicle
3 - Transverse process (costal process)
4 - Vertebral foramen
5 - Superior articular process (zygapophyseal joint)
6 - Lamina
7 - Inferior articular process (zygapophyseal joint)
8 - Spinous process

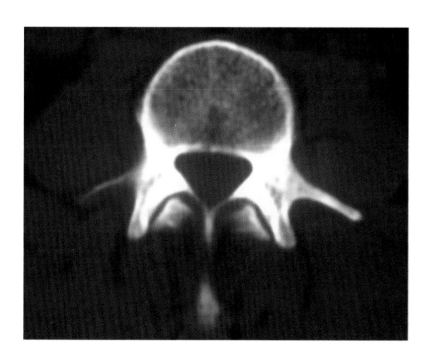

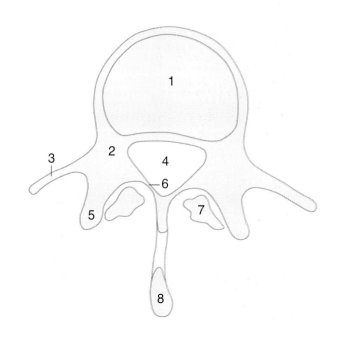

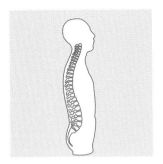

3D CT SSD reconstruction of lumbar vertebra, superior aspect

1 - Body of vertebra
2 - Transverse process (costal process)
3 - Pedicle
4 - Vertebral foramen
5 - Superior articular process of lower vertebra
6 - Inferior articular process of upper vertebra
7 - Lamina
8 - Spinous process
9 - Mamillary process

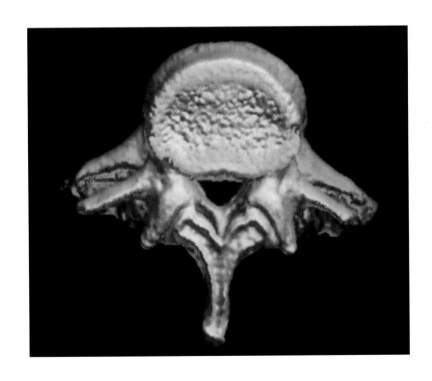

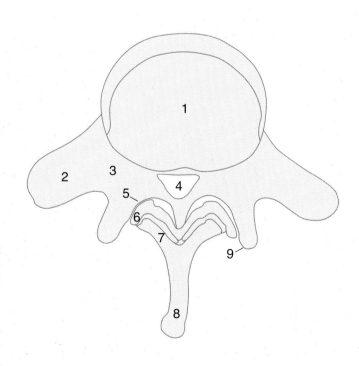

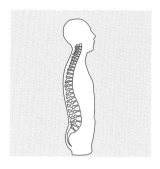

3D CT SSD reconstruction of lumbar vertebrae, posterosuperior aspect

1 - Body of vertebra
2 - Transverse process (costal process)
3 - Vertebral canal
4 - Superior articular process of lower vertebra
5 - Inferior articular process of upper vertebra
6 - Zygapophyseal joint
7 - Mamillary process
8 - Spinous process

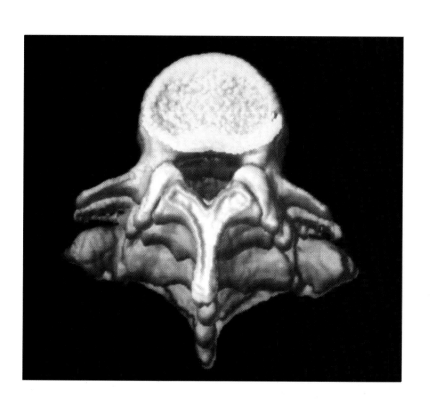

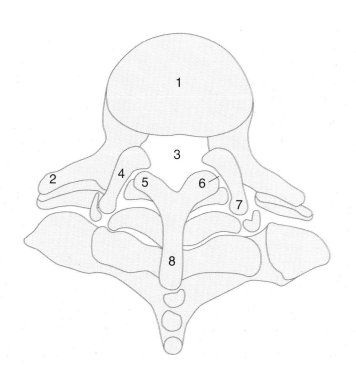

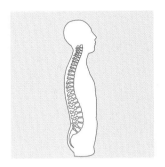

3D CT SSD reconstruction of lumbar vertebrae, lateral aspect

1 - Intervertebral foramen
2 - Spinous process
3 - Body of vertebra
4 - Intervertebral disc

5 - Superior articular process
6 - Transverse process
7 - Inferior articular process

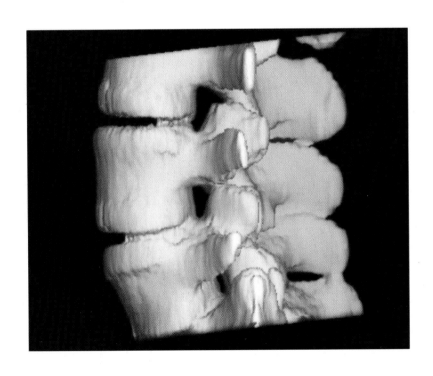

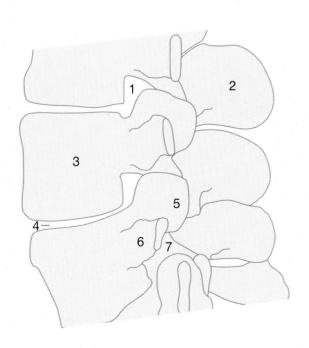

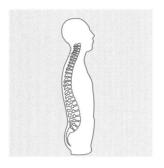

Parasagittal MR of lumbosacral spine

1 - Psoas major muscle
2 - Body of thoracic
    vertebra XI
3 - TXII/LI intervertebral
    foramen (for T12 root)
4 - Erector spinae muscle

5 - Pedicle
6 - Zygapophyseal joint
7 - L4 spinal nerve root in
    intervertebral foramen
8 - Sacrum

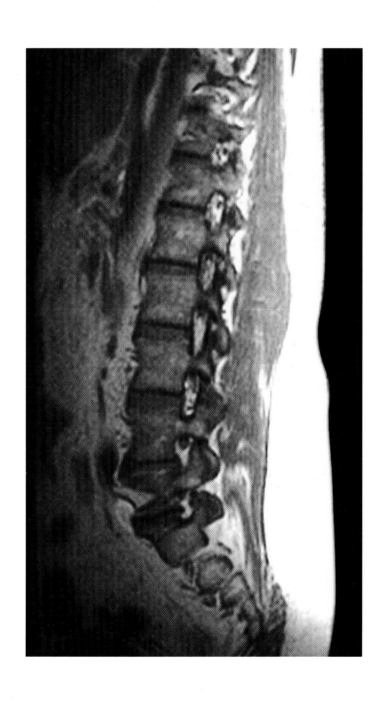

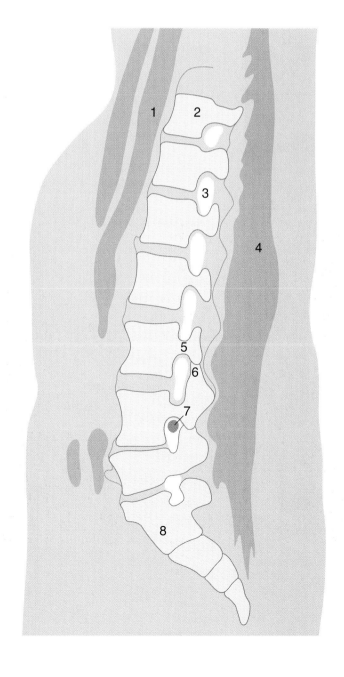

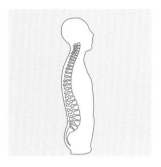

Sagittal MR of lumbosacral spine

1 - Body of thoracic vertebra X
2 - Spinous process
3 - Spinal cord
4 - Thecal sac (cerebrospinal fluid)
5 - Conus medullaris
6 - Intervertebral disc
7 - Filum terminale and cauda equina
8 - Anterior longitudinal ligament
9 - Interspinous ligament
10 - Basivertebral vein
11 - Posterior longitudinal ligament
12 - Lumbosacral junction
13 - Sacrum

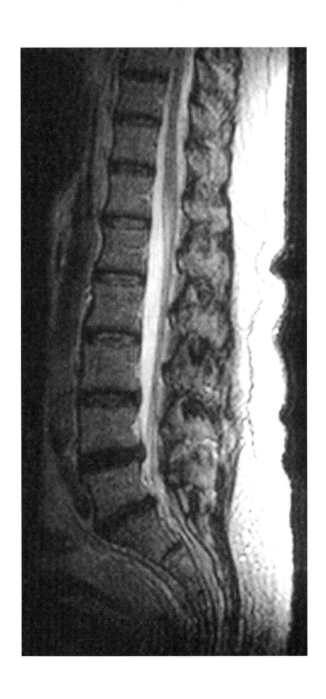

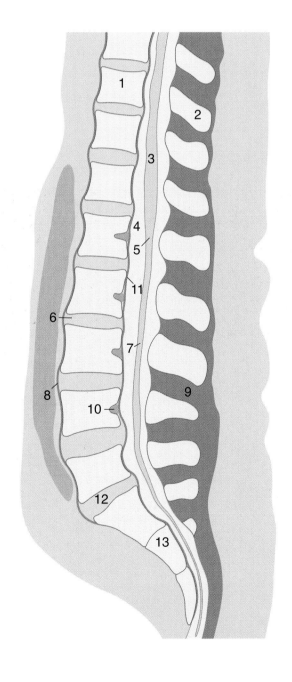

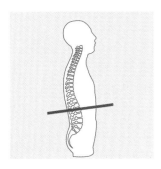

Axial MR of vertebral canal

1 - Aorta
2 - Body of lumbar vertebra I
3 - Cerebrospinal fluid in
  subarachnoid space
  (thecal sac)
4 - Spinal cord
5 - Pedicle
6 - Superior articular process
  of lumbar vertebra I

7 - Inferior articular process
  of thoracic vertebra XII
8 - Spinous process of
  thoracic vertebra XII
9 - Multifidus muscle
10 - Erector spinae muscle

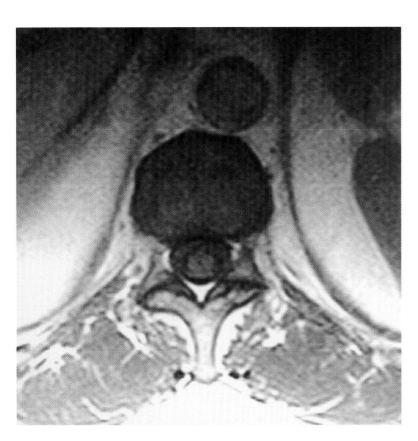

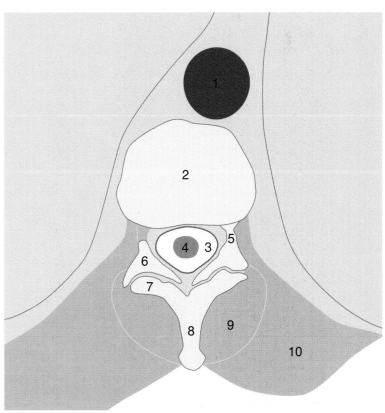

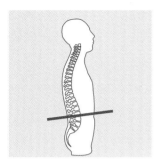

Axial MR of vertebral canal

1 - Aorta
2 - Right kidney
3 - Body of lumbar vertebra II
4 - Epidural fat
5 - Thecal sac and cauda equina
6 - Filum terminale
7 - Superior articular process of lumbar vertebra II
8 - Inferior articular process of lumbar vertebra I

9 - Ligamentum flavum
10 - Spinous process of lumbar vertebra I
11 - Multifidus muscle
12 - Erector spinae, longissimus thoracis muscle
13 - Erector spinae, iliocostalis lumborum muscle

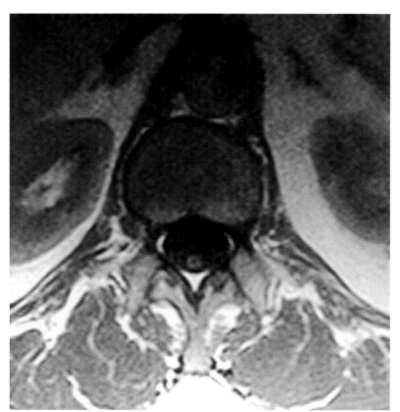

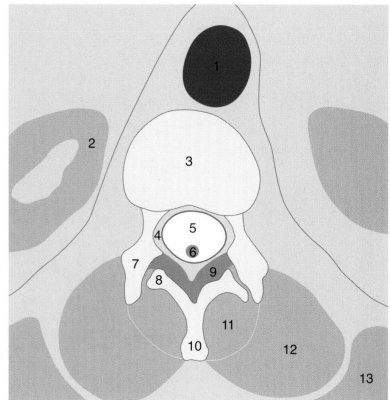

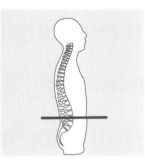

Axial MR of vertebral canal

1 - Inferior vena cava
2 - Aorta
3 - Psoas major muscle
4 - Body of lumbar vertebra III
5 - Thecal sac and cauda equina
6 - Intervertebral foramen
7 - Epidural fat

8 - Zygapophyseal joint
9 - Ligamentum flavum
10 - Multifidus muscle
11 - Spinous process of lumbar vertebra II
12 - Erector spinae muscle

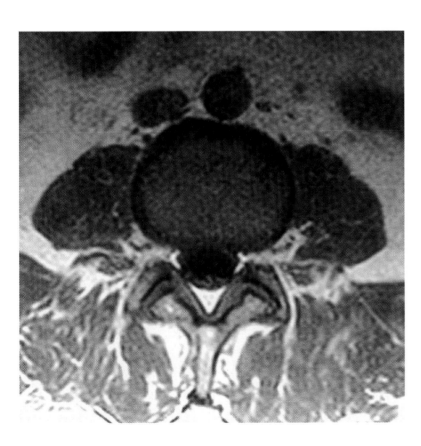

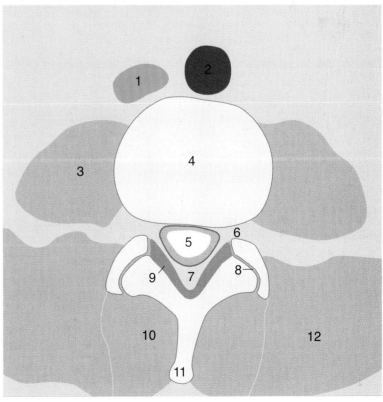

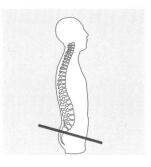

Axial MR of vertebral canal

1 - Sacro-iliac joint
2 - Lateral part of sacrum
3 - Body of sacrum
4 - Root sheath of sacral
    nerve I
5 - Root sheaths for sacral
    and coccygeal nerves

6 - Erector spinae muscle
7 - Median sacral crest
    (spinous tubercle)
8 - Attachment of
    interosseous sacro-iliac
    ligaments

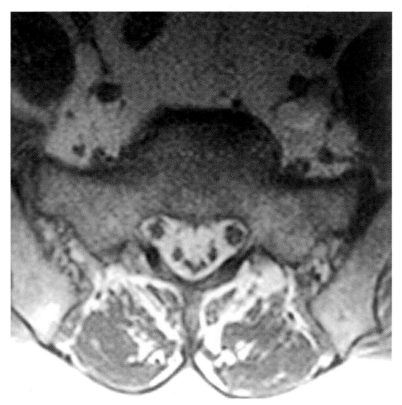

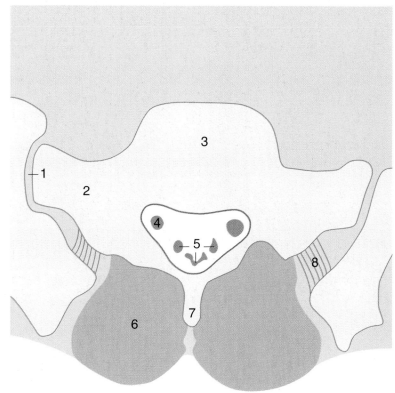

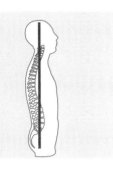

Coronal MR of thoracic spine

1 - Trapezius muscle
2 - Supraspinatus muscle
3 - Deltoid muscle
4 - Subscapularis muscle
5 - Infraspinatus muscle
6 - Teres minor muscle
7 - Spinal cord
8 - Body of vertebra

9 - Serratus anterior muscle
10 - Thecal sac
11 - Latissimus dorsi muscle
12 - Diaphragm
13 - Liver
14 - Right kidney
15 - Spleen
16 - Erector spinae muscle

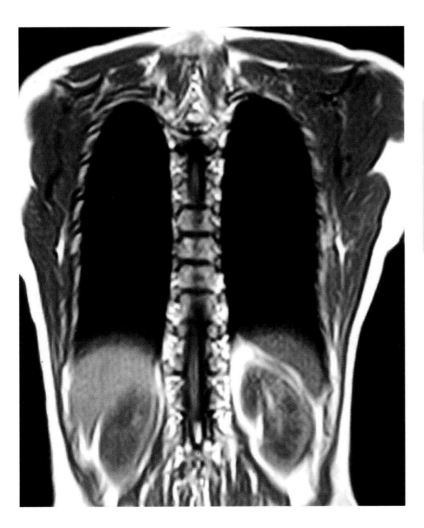

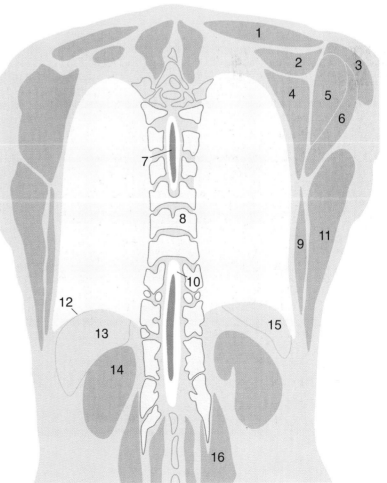

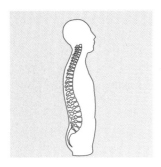

Myelogram of lumbosacral region, lateral view

1 - Spinal nerve roots in subarachnoid space
2 - Body of vertebra
3 - Lamina of vertebra
4 - Intervertebral disc indentation in anterior thecal margin

5 - Iliac crest
6 - Contrast medium in subarachnoid space

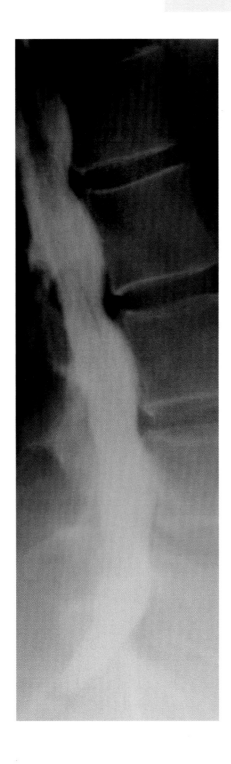

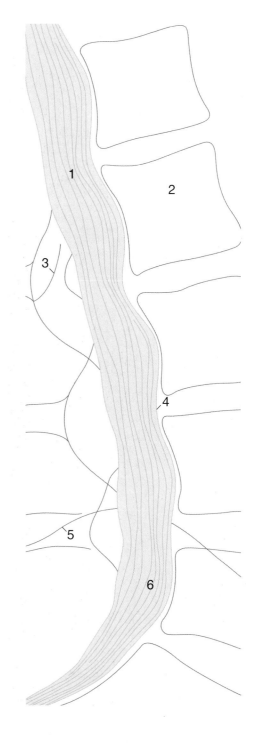

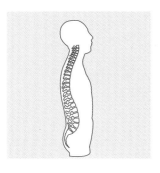

Myelogram of lumbosacral region, anteroposterior view

1 - Spinal nerve roots in subarachnoidal space

2 - Lateral extension of subarachnoid space around spinal nerve roots

3 - Terminal theca at sacral vertebra I

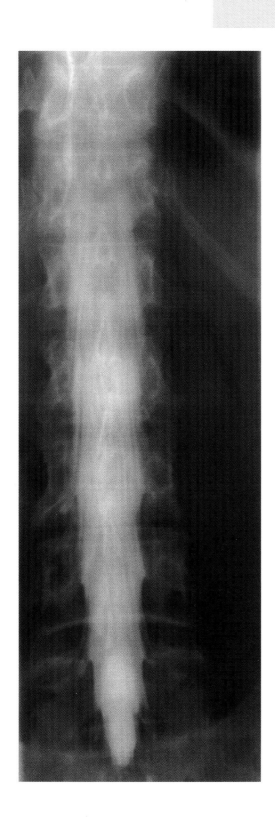

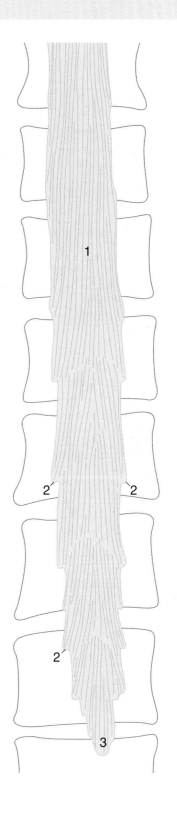

LIMBS

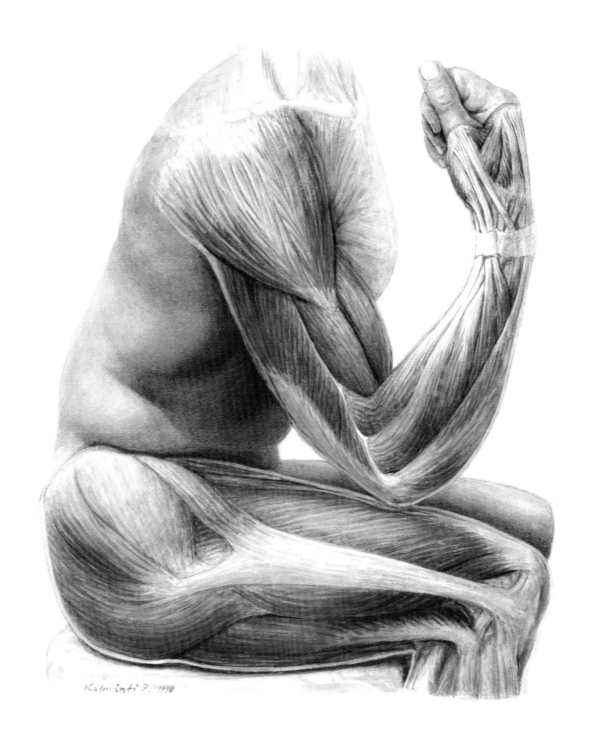

Kálmánfi J. 1998

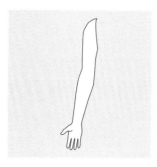

X-ray of shoulder, anteroposterior view

1 - Rib I
2 - Clavicle
3 - Acromion
4 - Acromioclavicular joint
5 - Coracoid process
6 - Scapula
7 - Glenoid fossa
8 - Greater tubercle of humerus

9 - Intertubercular groove
10 - Lesser tubercle of humerus
11 - Anatomical neck of humerus
12 - Surgical neck of humerus

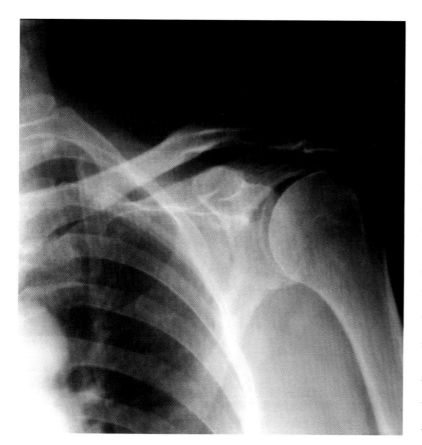

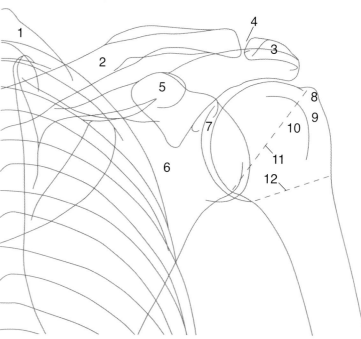

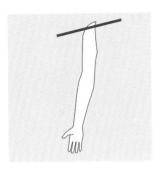

Axial MR of shoulder

1 - Clavicle
2 - Subclavius muscle
3 - Deltoid muscle
4 - Coracoid process
5 - Head of humerus
6 - Scapula

7 - Glenoid fossa of scapula
8 - Glenohumeral joint
9 - Supraspinatus muscle
10 - Spine of scapula
11 - Infraspinatus muscle

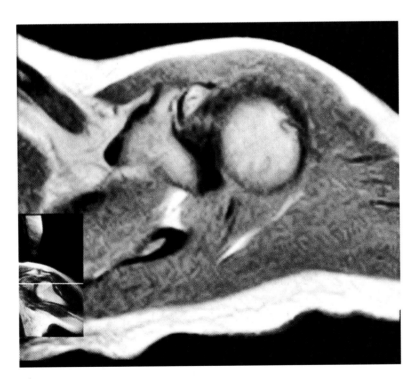

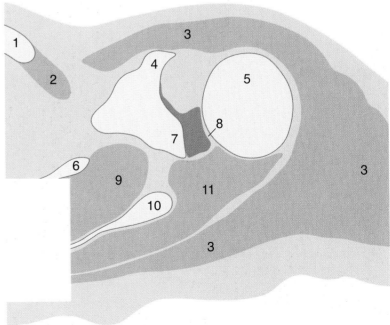

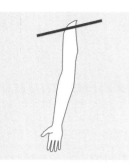

Axial MR of shoulder

1 - Pectoralis major and
    minor muscles
2 - Axillary fossa
3 - Deltoid muscle
4 - Serratus anterior muscle
5 - Coracoid process
6 - Tendon of subscapularis
    muscle

7 - Subscapularis muscle
8 - Glenoid fossa of scapula
9 - Head of humerus
10 - Infraspinatus muscle
11 - Posterior glenoid labrum

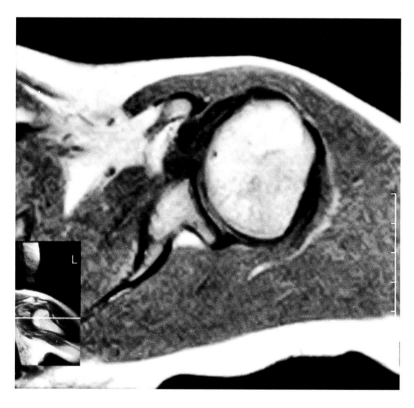

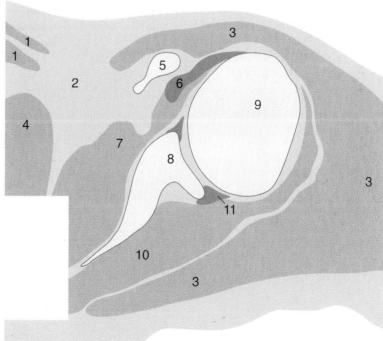

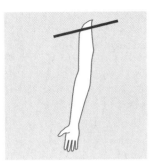

Axial MR of shoulder

1 - Pectoralis major muscle
2 - Axillary vein
3 - Deltoid muscle
4 - Axillary artery
    (surrounded by brachial
    plexus)
5 - Coracobrachialis muscle
6 - Short head of biceps
    brachii muscle
7 - Tendon of subscapularis
    muscle

8 - Head of humerus
9 - Serratus anterior muscle
10 - Axillary fossa (recess)
11 - Subscapularis muscle
12 - Glenohumeral joint
13 - Anterior glenoid labrum
14 - Posterior glenoid labrum
15 - Tendon of teres minor
     muscle
16 - Infraspinatus muscle
17 - Scapula

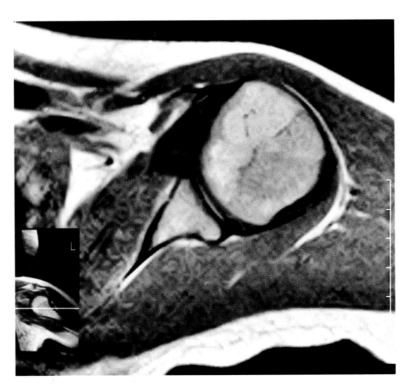

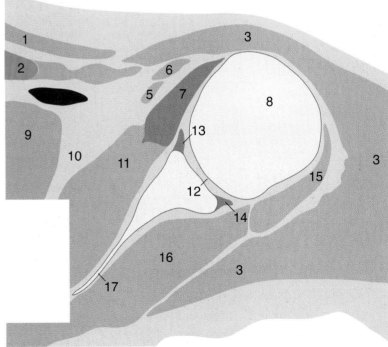

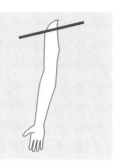

Axial MR of shoulder

1 - Pectoralis major muscle
2 - Pectoralis minor muscle
3 - Deltoid muscle
4 - Axillary vein
5 - Axillary artery (surrounded by brachial plexus)
6 - Coracobrachialis muscle
7 - Lesser tubercle (crest of lesser tubercle)
8 - Tendon of biceps brachii muscle
9 - Greater tubercle (crest of greater tubercle)
10 - Head of humerus
11 - Serratus anterior muscle
12 - Axillary fossa
13 - Subscapularis muscle
14 - Glenohumeral joint
15 - Infraspinatus muscle
16 - Teres minor muscle
17 - Scapula

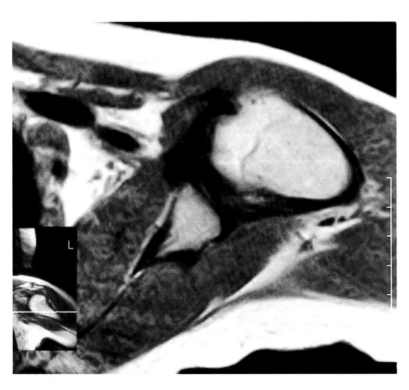

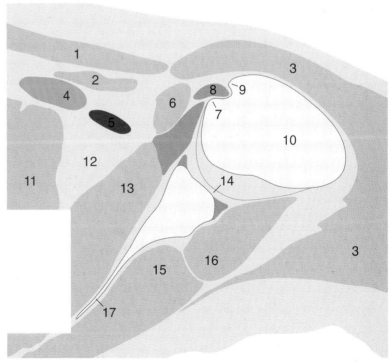

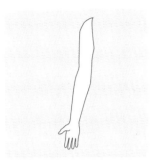

Axillary arteriogram, anteroposterior view

1 - Thorax (rib)
2 - Scapula
3 - Humerus, head
4 - Axillary artery
5 - Thoraco-acromial artery
   5a - Clavicular branch
   5b - Pectoral branch
   5c - Acromial branch
6 - Lateral thoracic artery
7 - Subscapular artery

8 - Anterior circumflex humeral artery
9 - Posterior circumflex humeral artery
10 - Circumflex scapular artery
11 - Thoracodorsal artery
12 - Deep brachial artery
13 - Brachial artery

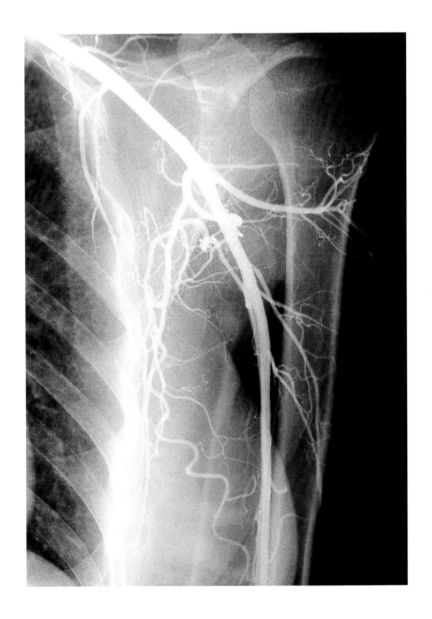

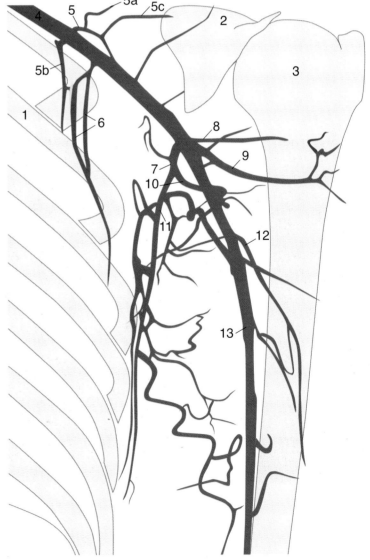

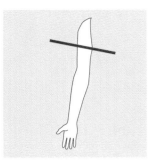

Axial CT of upper arm

1 - Biceps brachii muscle
2 - Brachialis muscle
3 - Humerus
4 - Deltoid muscle
5 - Brachial vessels and branches of the brachial plexus in the medial bicipital groove

6 - Medial head of triceps muscle
7 - Long head of triceps muscle
8 - Lateral head of triceps muscle

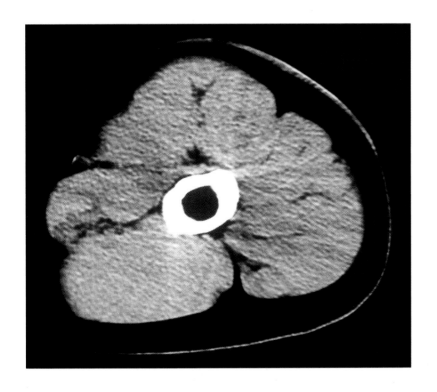

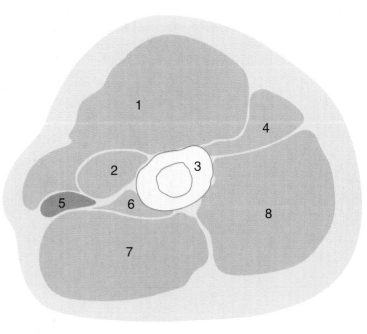

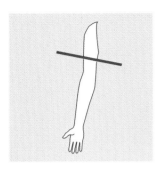

Axial CT of upper arm

1 - Biceps brachii muscle
2 - Brachial vessels and branches of the brachial plexus in the medial bicipital groove

3 - Brachialis muscle
4 - Humerus
5 - Brachioradialis muscle
6 - Triceps brachii muscle

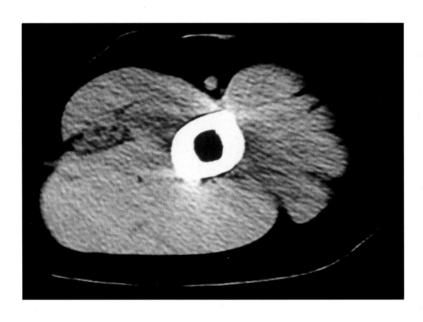

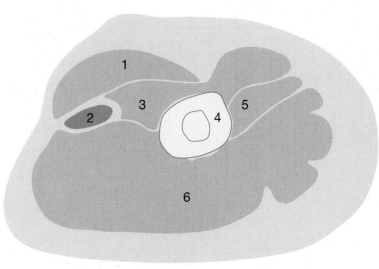

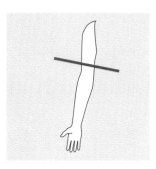

Axial CT of upper arm

1 - Biceps brachii muscle
2 - Cephalic vein
3 - Brachial artery, brachial
    vein and median nerve
4 - Basilic vein

5 - Brachialis muscle
6 - Brachioradialis muscle
7 - Humerus
8 - Triceps brachii muscle

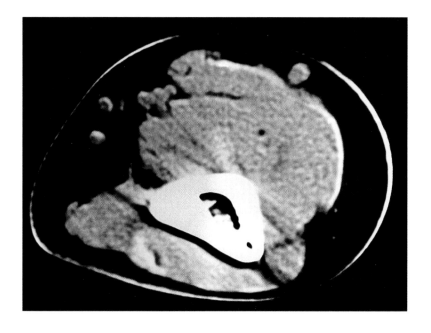

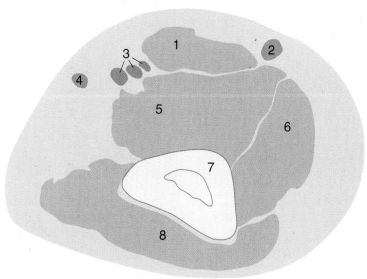

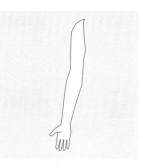

X-ray of elbow in slight pronation, anteroposterior view

1 - Lateral supracondylar crest
2 - Medial supracondylar crest
3 - Lateral epicondyle of humerus
4 - Medial epicondyle of humerus
5 - Capitulum of humerus
6 - Trochlea of humerus
7 - Olecranon
8 - Head of radius
9 - Coronoid process of ulna
10 - Neck of radius
11 - Tuberosity of radius
12 - Shaft of of radius
13 - Shaft of ulna

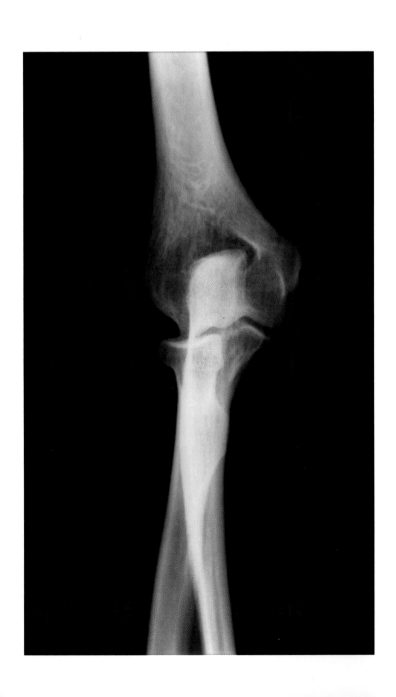

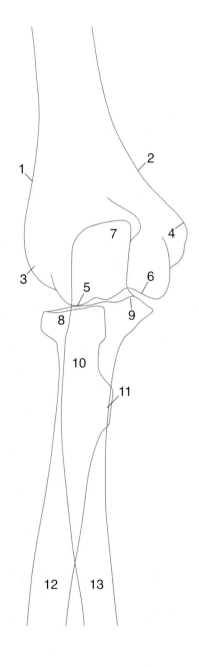

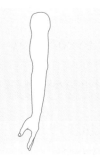

X-ray of elbow in supination, lateral view

1 - Humerus
2 - Olecranon fossa
3 - Trochlear notch
4 - Olecranon
5 - Coronoid process
6 - Head of radius
7 - Neck of radius
8 - Tuberosity of radius
9 - Shaft of radius
10 - Ulna

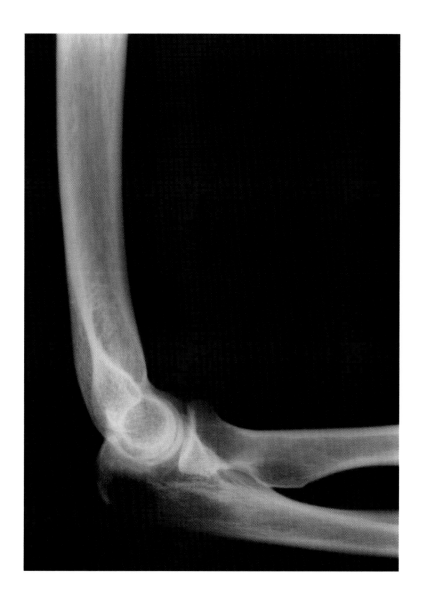

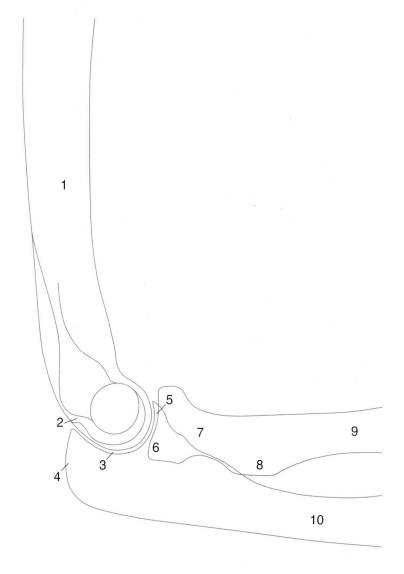

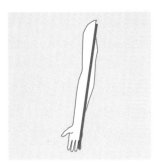

Sagittal MR of elbow, humero-ulnar joint

1 - Biceps brachii muscle
2 - Humerus
3 - Triceps brachii muscle, medial head
4 - Tendon of biceps brachii muscle
5 - Brachialis muscle
6 - Trochlea of humerus
7 - Olecranon fossa of humerus
8 - Olecranon of ulna
9 - Coronoid process of ulna
10 - Pronator teres and flexor carpi radialis muscles
11 - Flexors of forearm

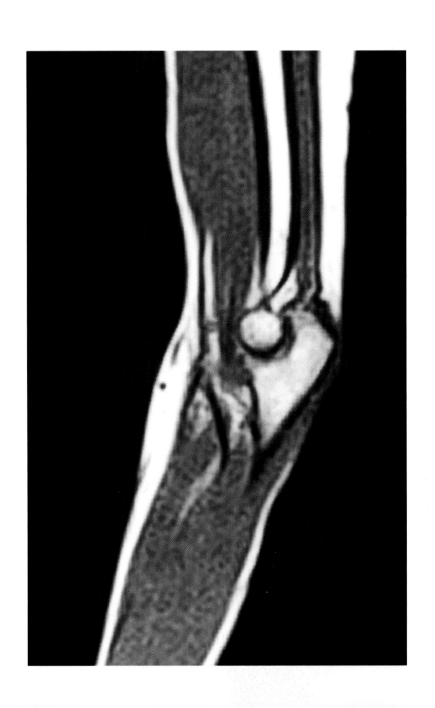

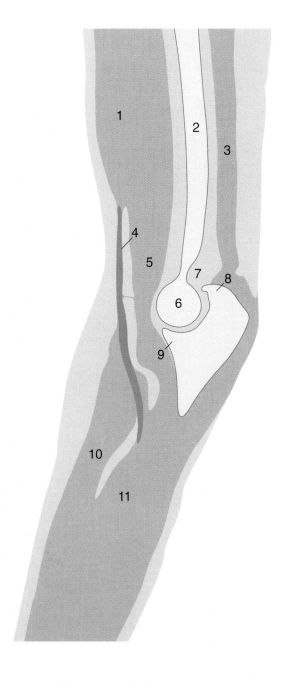

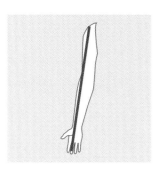

Sagittal MR of elbow, humeroradial joint

1 - Tendon of biceps brachii muscle
2 - Brachialis muscle
3 - Triceps brachii muscle, lateral head
4 - Capitulum of humerus
5 - Head of radius

6 - Brachioradialis muscle, and flexor carpi radialis longus and brevis muscles (radial extensors)
7 - Supinator muscle
8 - Extensors of forearm

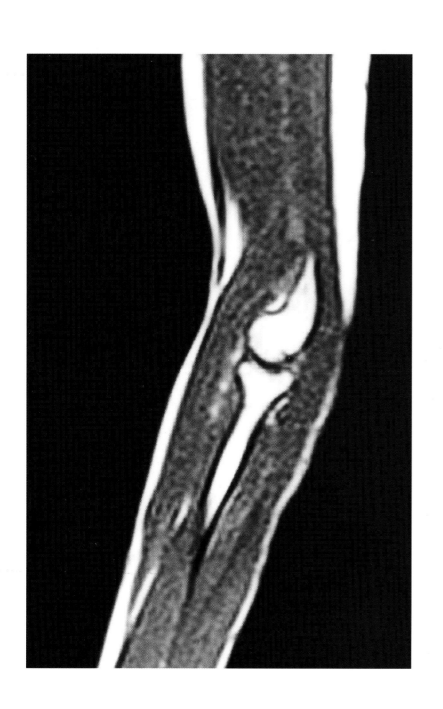

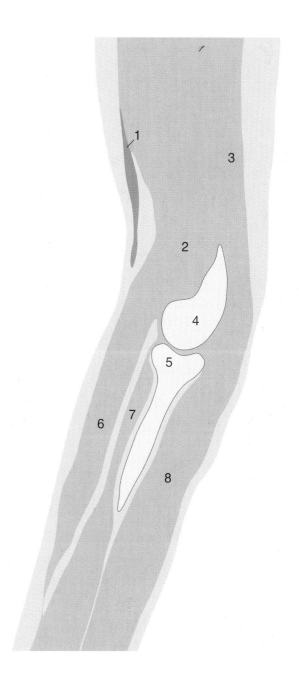

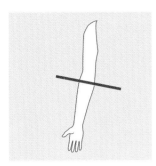

Axial CT of forearm

1 - Palmaris longus muscle
2 - Flexor carpi radialis muscle
3 - Pronator teres muscle
4 - Radial artery
5 - Brachioradialis muscle
6 - Extensor carpi radialis longus muscle
7 - Flexor digitorum superficialis muscle
8 - Ulnar artery
9 - Tendon of biceps brachii muscle
10 - Radius

11 - Supinator muscle
12 - Extensor carpi radialis brevis muscle
13 - Flexor carpi ulnaris muscle
14 - Flexor digitorum profundus muscle
15 - Ulna
16 - Extensor digitorum muscle
17 - Anconeus muscle
18 - Extensor carpi ulnaris muscle

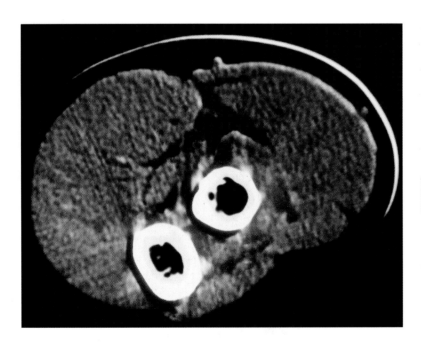

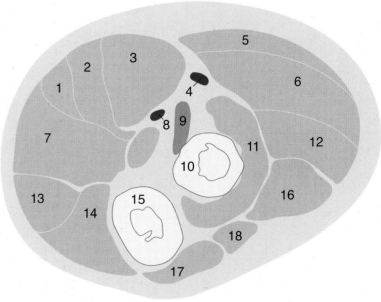

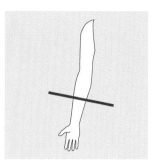

Axial CT of forearm

1 - Brachioradialis muscle
2 - Flexor carpi radialis muscle
3 - Pronator teres muscle
4 - Extensor carpi radialis longus and brevis muscles
5 - Flexor digitorum superficialis muscle
6 - Flexor digitorum profundus muscle

7 - Radius
8 - Flexor carpi ulnaris muscle
9 - Ulna
10 - Supinator muscle
11 - Extensor digitorum muscle
12 - Extensor carpi ulnaris muscle

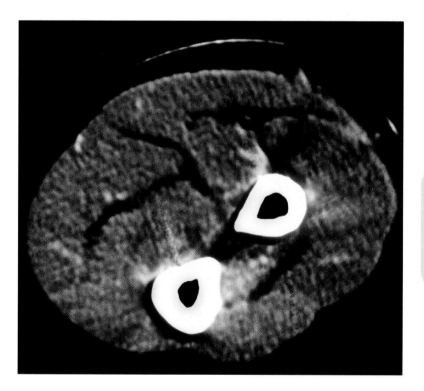

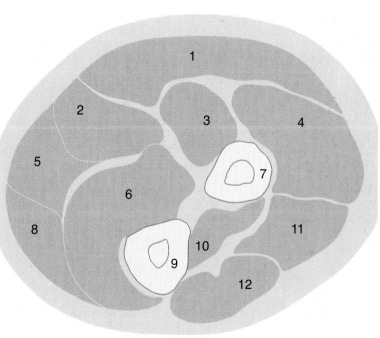

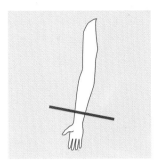

Axial CT of forearm

1 - Tendon of palmaris longus muscle
2 - Flexor digitorum superficialis muscle
3 - Radial artery
4 - Tendon of brachioradialis muscle
5 - Flexor digitorum profundus muscle
6 - Flexor pollicis longus muscle
7 - Radius
8 - Tendon of abductor pollicis longus muscle
9 - Flexor carpi ulnaris muscle
10 - Ulnar artery
11 - Pronator quadratus muscle
12 - Extensor pollicis longus and extensor indicis muscles
13 - Tendons of extensor carpi radialis longus and brevis muscles
14 - Extensor pollicis brevis muscle
15 - Ulna
16 - Extensor carpi ulnaris muscle
17 - Extensor digitorum and extensor digiti minimi muscles

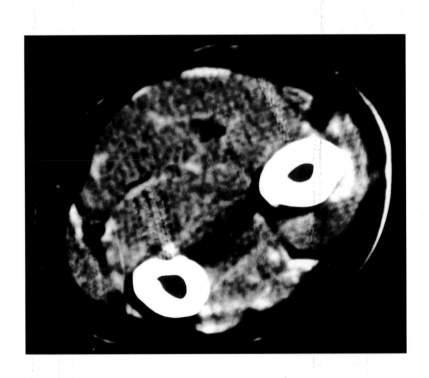

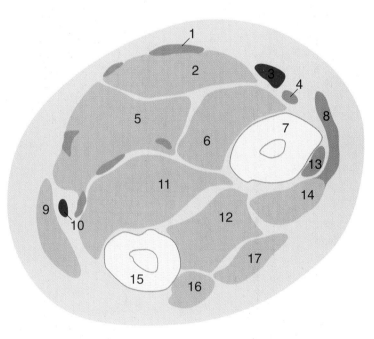

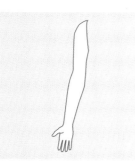

Brachial arteriogram, anteroposterior view

1 - Brachial artery
2 - Radial artery (weaker than normal, distal part blocked)
3 - Recurrent radial artery
4 - Recurrent ulnar artery
5 - Ulnar artery
6 - Common interosseous artery

7 - Posterior interosseous artery
8 - Anterior interosseous artery
9 - Recurrent interosseous artery
10 - Ulna
11 - Radius

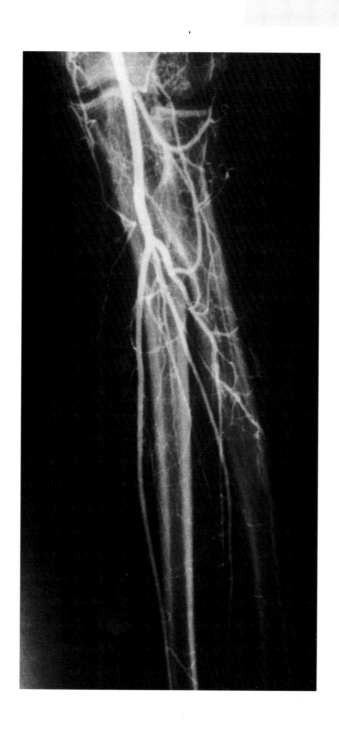

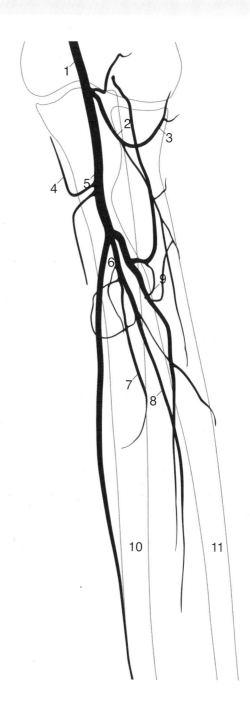

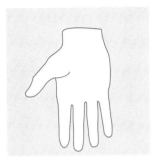

X-ray of hand, anteroposterior view

1 - Proximal phalanx of fifth finger
2 - Metacarpophalangeal joint
3 - Head of metacarpal III
4 - Sesamoid bone
5 - Shaft of metacarpal III
6 - Base of metacarpal III
7 - Hamulus (hook) of hamate
8 - Hamate
9 - Capitate
10 - Trapezoid
11 - Trapezium
12 - Pisiform
13 - Triquetral
14 - Lunate
15 - Scaphoid
16 - Styloid process of ulna
17 - Distal end (capitulum) of ulna
18 - Ulnar notch of radius
19 - Styloid process of radius

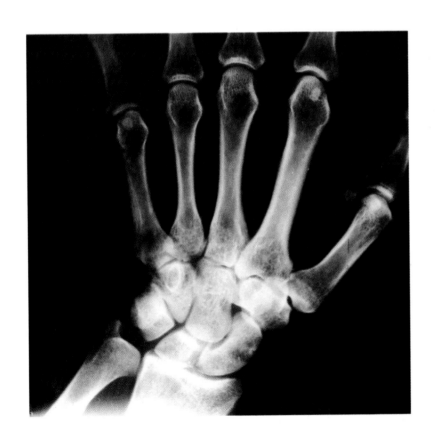

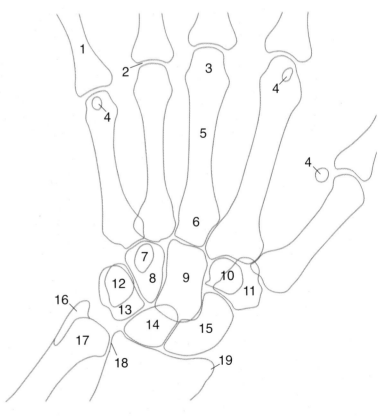

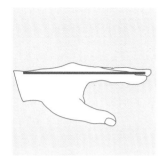

Coronal MR of wrist

1 - Proximal phalanx of fifth finger
2 - Tendon of flexor digitorum superficialis and profundus muscles
3 - Metacarpal V
4 - Dorsal and ventral interosseous muscles
5 - Adductor pollicis, transverse part
6 - First lumbrical muscle
7 - Adductor pollicis, oblique part
8 - Bases of metacarpals II-IV
9 - Metacarpal I
10 - Hamate
11 - Capitate
12 - Trapezoid
13 - Triquetral
14 - Lunate
15 - Scaphoid
16 - Articular disc of radiocarpal joint
17 - Ulna
18 - Styloid process of radius
19 - Tendon of brachioradialis muscle

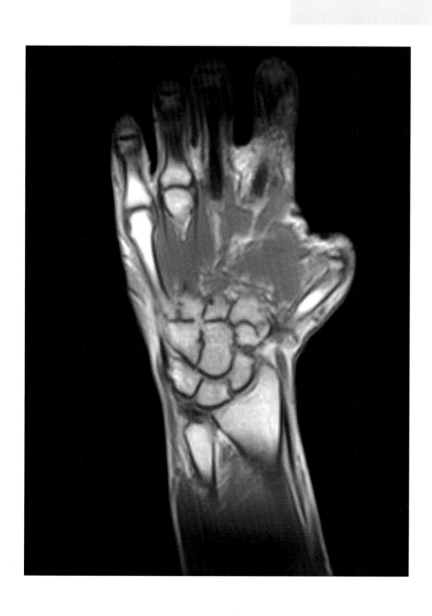

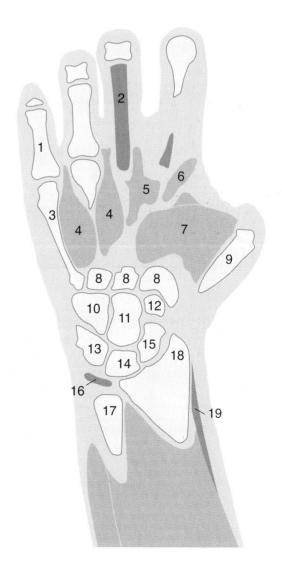

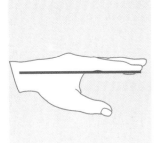

Coronal MR of wrist

1 - Abductor digiti minimi muscle

2 - Flexor digiti minimi brevis muscle

3 - Tendons of flexor digitorum superficialis and profundus muscles emerging from carpal tunnel

4 - Opponens pollicis muscle

5 - Pisiform

6 - Hamulus (hook) of hamate

7 - Trapezoid

8 - Trapezium

9 - Tendon of flexor pollicis longus muscle

10 - Metacarpal I

11 - Flexor carpi ulnaris muscle

12 - Ulna

13 - Abductor pollicis longus muscle

14 - Flexor digitorum superficialis and profundus muscles

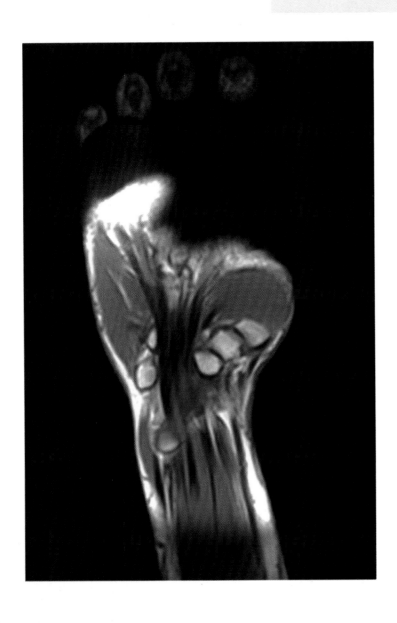

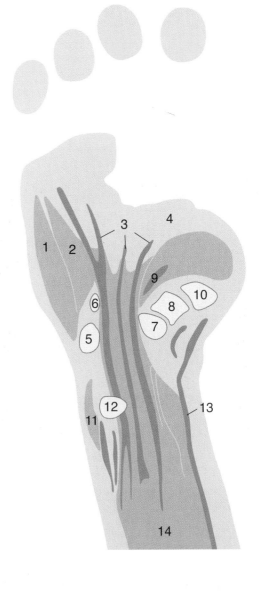

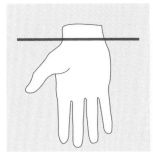

Axial MR of wrist

1 - Pisiform
2 - Ulnar vessels and nerve in Guyon's canal
3 - Flexor retinaculum
4 - Tendons of flexor digitorum superficialis and profundus muscles in carpal tunnel
5 - Tendon of palmaris longus muscle
6 - Tendon of flexor pollicis longus muscle
7 - Tendon of flexor carpi radialis muscle
8 - Tendons of abductor pollicis longus and extensor pollicis brevis muscles
9 - Triquetral
10 - Tendon of extensor carpi ulnaris muscle
11 - Capitate
12 - Tendons of extensor digitorum muscle
13 - Scaphoid
14 - Tendon of extensor carpi radialis brevis muscle
15 - Tendons of extensor pollicis longus and extensor carpi radialis longus muscles

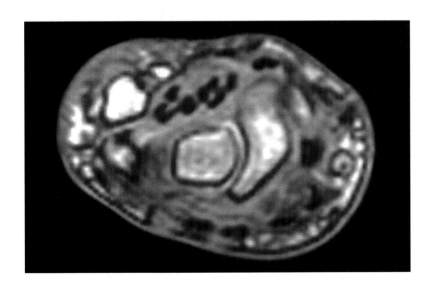

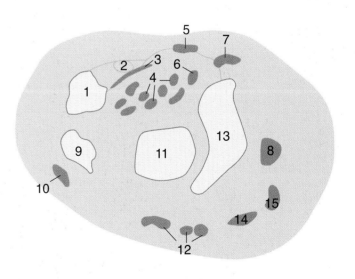

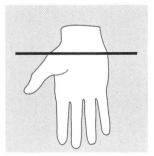

Axial MR of wrist

1 - Abductor digiti minimi muscle
2 - Palmar carpal ligament
3 - Ulnar artery and vein (together with the ulnar nerve) in Guyon's canal
4 - Flexor retinaculum
5 - Tendons of flexor digitorum superficialis and profundus muscles in carpal tunnel
6 - Median nerve
7 - Tendon of flexor pollicis longus muscle
8 - Tendon of flexor carpi radialis muscle
9 - Abductor pollicis brevis muscle
10 - Tendon of abductor pollicis longus muscle
11 - Tendon of extensor carpi ulnaris muscle
12 - Hamate
13 - Tendon of extensor digiti minimi muscle
14 - Dorsal venous plexus
15 - Tendons of extensor digitorum muscle
16 - Capitate
17 - Trapezoid
18 - Tendon of extensor carpi radialis brevis muscle
19 - Tendon of extensor carpi radialis longus muscle
20 - Trapezium
21 - Base of metacarpal I

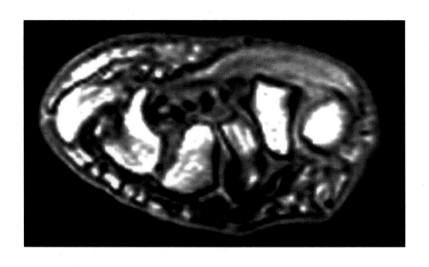

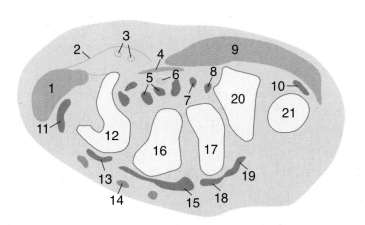

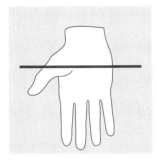

Axial MR of hand

1 - Abductor and flexor digiti
    minimi muscles
2 - Tendons of flexor
    digitorum superficialis
    muscle
3 - Tendons of flexor
    digitorum profundus
    muscle
4 - Flexor pollicis brevis
    muscle
5 - Tendon of flexor pollicis
    longus muscle
6 - Metacarpal V
7 - Adductor pollicis muscle
8 - Tendon of extensor digiti
    minimi muscle
9 - Tendons of extensor
    digitorum muscle
10 - Dorsal venous plexus
11 - Metacarpal I
12 - Dorsal and palmar
     interosseous muscles

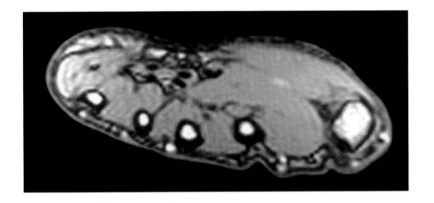
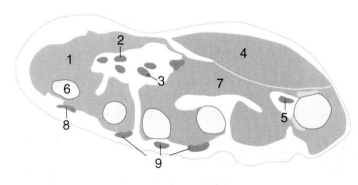
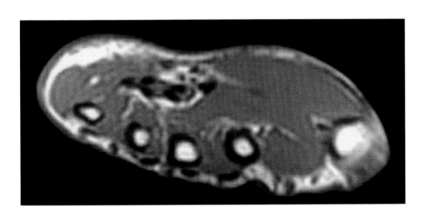
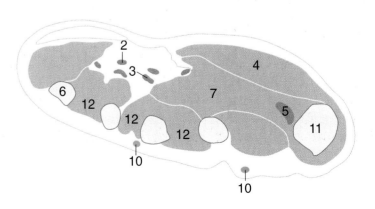

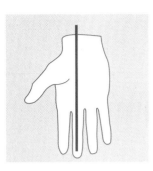

Sagittal MR of finger

1 - Distal phalanx

2 - Insertion of flexor digitorum profundus tendon on the base of distal phalanx

3 - Insertion of flexor digitorum superficialis tendon on the base of middle phalanx

4 - Flexor digitorum superficialis and profundus tendons

5 - Shaft of proximal phalanx

6 - Tendon of extensor digitorum muscle

7 - Head of metacarpal

8 - Shaft of metacarpal

9 - Palmar interosseous muscle

10 - Base of metacarpal

11 - Carpal bone

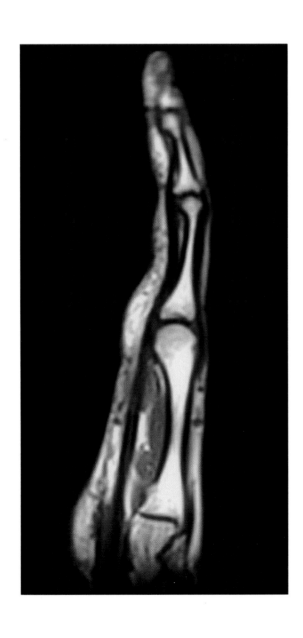

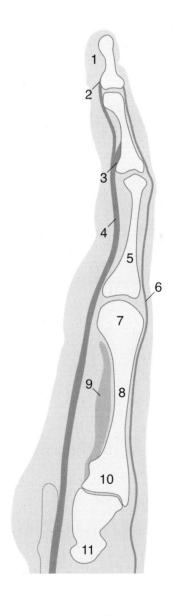

Arteriogram of forearm and wrist, anteroposterior view

1 - Radial artery
2 - Anterior interosseous artery (the posterior interosseous artery is not clearly visible)
3 - Ulnar artery
4 - Dorsal carpal branch of radial artery

5 - Deep palmar arch
6 - Superficial palmar branch of radial artery
7 - Princeps pollicis artery
8 - Superficial palmar arch (incomplete)
9 - Common palmar digital arteries

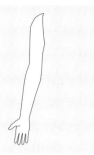

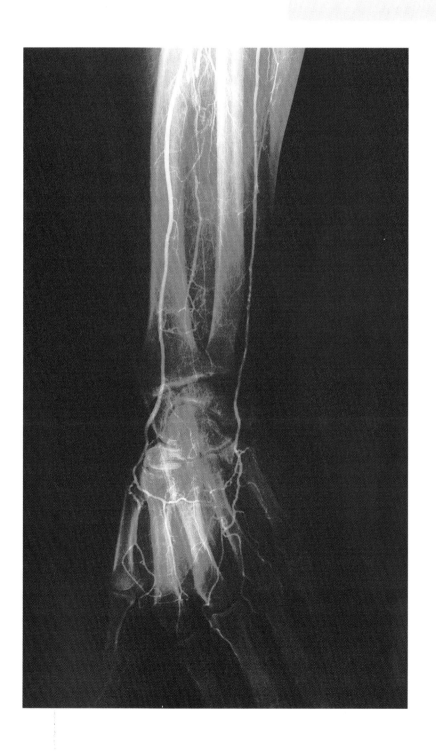

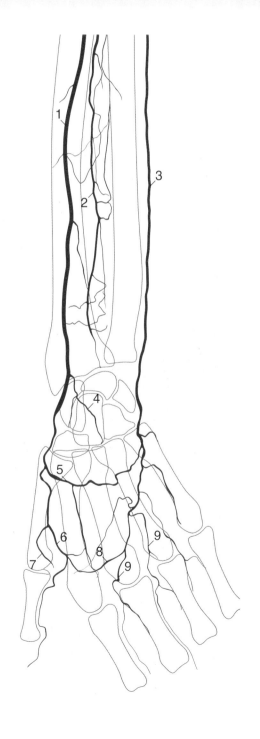

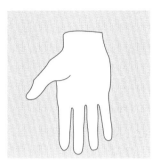

Arteriogram of hand

1 - Ulnar artery
2 - Radial artery
3 - Dorsal palmar branch
4 - Superficial palmar branch of radial artery
5 - Deep palmar arch
6 - Deep branch of ulnar artery
7 - Superficial palmar arch
8 - Princeps pollicis artery
9 - Common palmar digital arteries
10 - Palmar metacarpal artery
11 - Proper palmar digital arteries

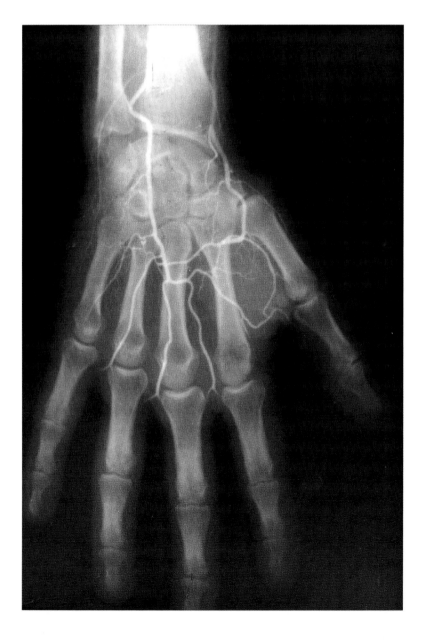

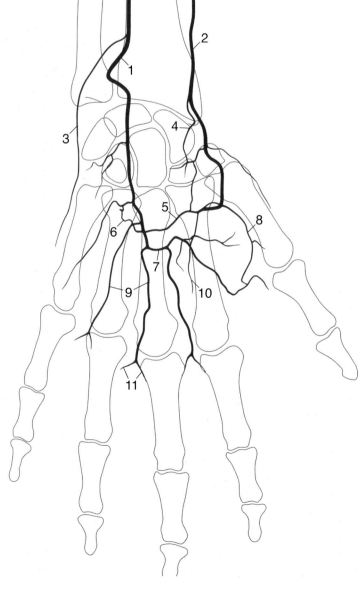

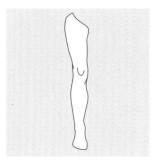

X-ray of hip, anteroposterior view

1 - Sacro-iliac joint
2 - Ilium
3 - Acetabulum
4 - Head of femur
5 - Neck of femur
6 - Greater trochanter
7 - Intertrochanteric crest
8 - Obturator foramen
9 - Ischial tuberosity
10 - Ramus of ischium
11 - Lesser trochanter
12 - Shaft of femur

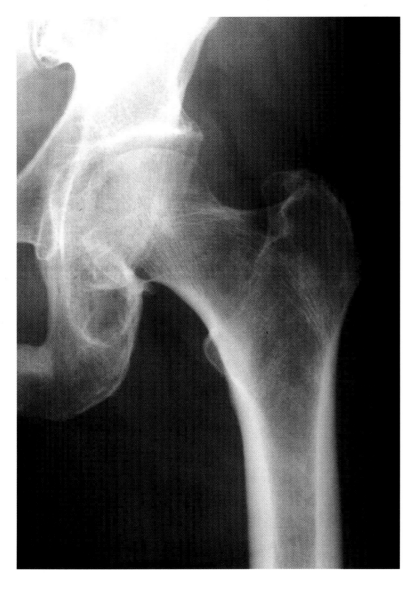

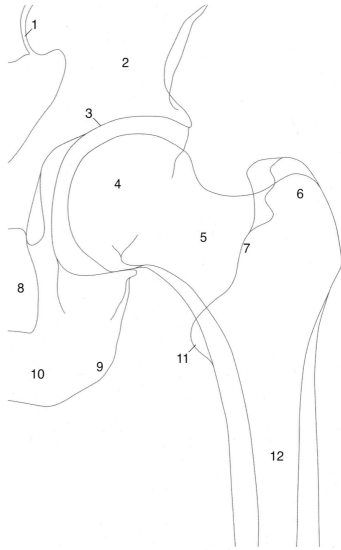

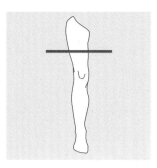

Axial MR of thigh

1 - Vastus lateralis muscle
2 - Rectus femoris muscle
3 - Vastus medialis muscle
4 - Sartorius muscle
5 - Vastus intermedius muscle
6 - Femoral vein
7 - Femoral artery
8 - Femur
9 - Adductor longus muscle
10 - Adductor magnus muscle
11 - Gracilis muscle
12 - Biceps femoris muscle (short head)
13 - Sciatic nerve
14 - Biceps femoris muscle (long head)
15 - Semitendinosus muscle
16 - Semimembranosus muscle

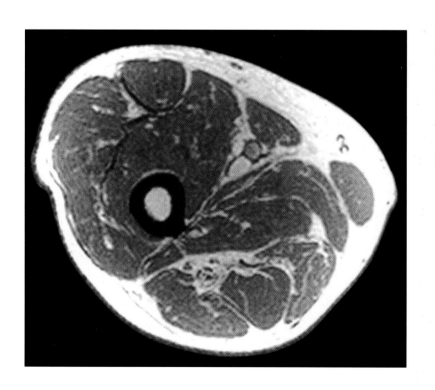

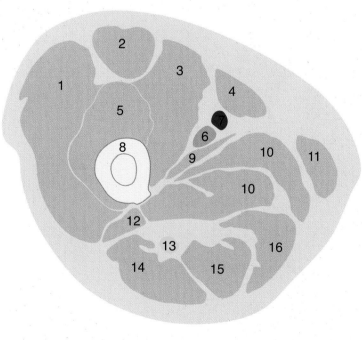

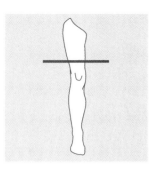

Axial MR of thigh

1 - Vastus lateralis muscle
2 - Rectus femoris muscle
3 - Vastus medialis muscle
4 - Sartorius muscle
5 - Vastus intermedius muscle
6 - Femur
7 - Femoral vein
8 - Femoral artery

9 - Adductor magnus muscle
10 - Biceps femoris (short head)
11 - Sciatic nerve
12 - Semimembranosus muscle
13 - Gracilis muscle
14 - Great saphenous vein
15 - Biceps femoris (long head)
16 - Semitendinosus muscle

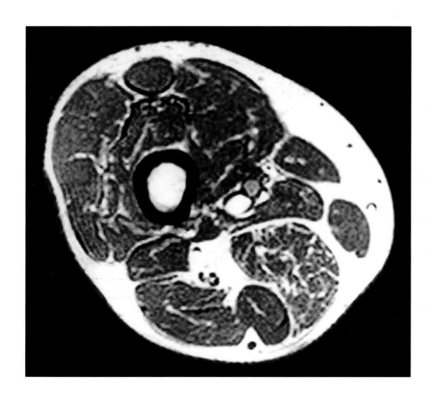

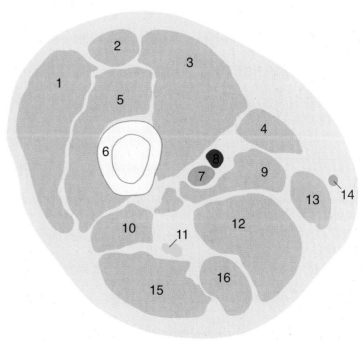

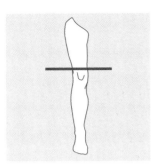

Axial MR of thigh

1 - Tendon of quadriceps
    femoris muscle
2 - Vastus lateralis muscle
3 - Femur
4 - Vastus medialis muscle
5 - Popliteal vein
6 - Popliteal artery
7 - Biceps femoris muscle
8 - Common peroneal
    (fibular) nerve

 9 - Tibial nerve
10 - Semimembranosus
     muscle
11 - Sartorius muscle
12 - Gracilis muscle
13 - Great saphenous vein
14 - Tendon of
     semitendinosus muscle

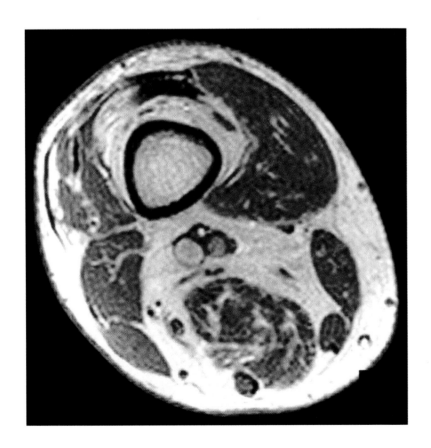

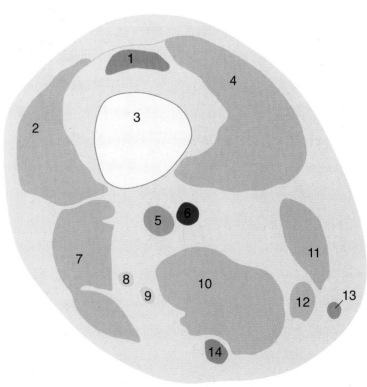

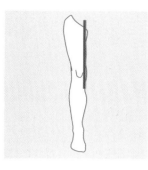

Sagittal MR of thigh

1 - Gluteus maximus muscle
2 - Obturator externus muscle
3 - Pectineus muscle
4 - Quadratus femoris muscle
5 - Adductor longus muscle
6 - Adductor magnus and brevis muscles
7 - Sartorius muscle
8 - Semitendinosus muscle
9 - Vastus medialis muscle
10 - Semimembranosus muscle
11 - Medial condyle of femur

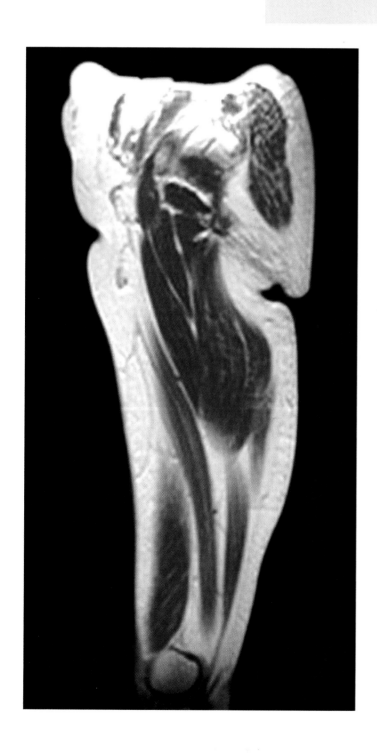

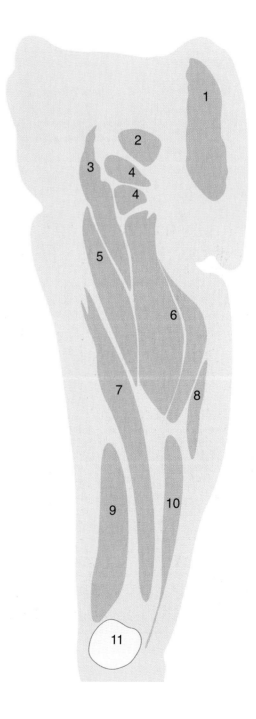

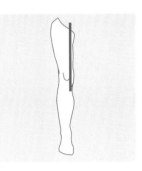

Sagittal MR of thigh

1 - Iliopsoas muscle
2 - Head of femur
3 - Quadratus femoris muscle
4 - Gluteus maximus muscle
5 - Sartorius muscle
6 - Vastus medialis muscle
7 - Adductor magnus muscle
8 - Semimembranosus muscle
9 - Semitendinosus muscle
10 - Tendon of adductor magnus muscle
11 - Medial condyle of femur
12 - Gastrocnemius muscle

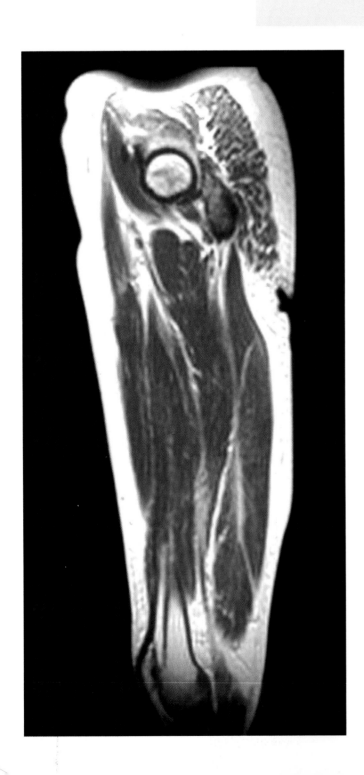

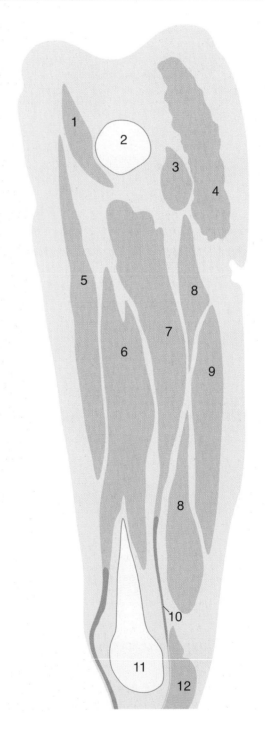

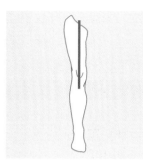

Sagittal MR of thigh

1 - Gluteus medius and
    minimus muscles
2 - Gluteus maximus muscle
3 - Sartorius muscle
4 - Femur

5 - Vastus medialis and
    intermedius muscle
6 - Rectus femoris muscle
7 - Adductor magnus muscle
8 - Biceps femoris muscle

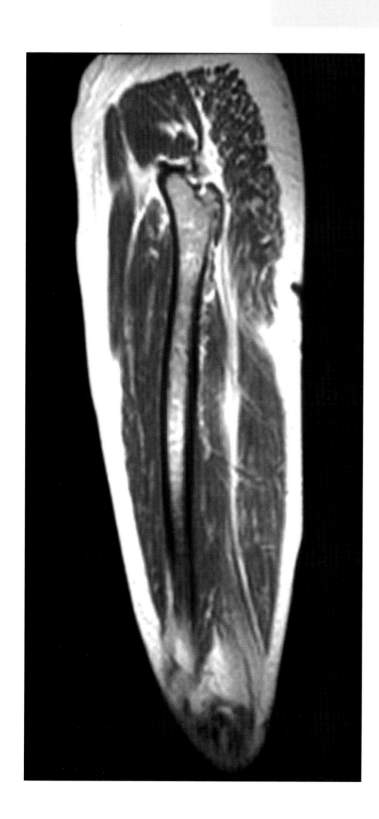

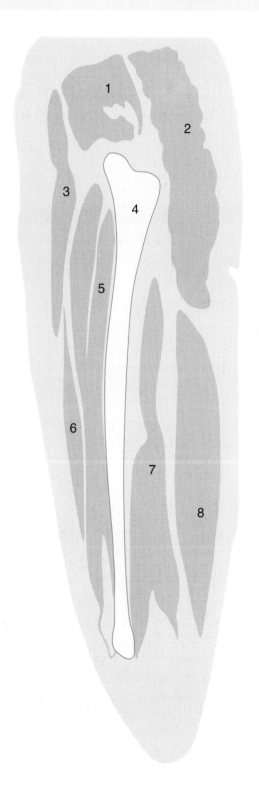

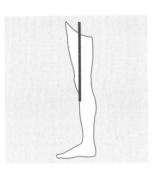

Coronal MR of thigh

1 - Gluteus medius muscle
2 - Gluteus minimus muscle
3 - Acetabulum
4 - Greater trochanter
5 - Head of femur
6 - Urinary bladder
7 - Obturator internus muscle
8 - Obturator externus muscle
9 - Iliopsoas muscle
10 - Adductor magnus and adductor brevis muscles
11 - Urogenital diaphragm
12 - Adductor longus muscle
13 - Gracilis muscle
14 - Vastus lateralis and vastus intermedius muscles
15 - Vastus medialis muscle
16 - Adductor canal and femoral vessels
17 - Sartorius muscle
18 - Lateral condyle of femur
19 - Medial condyle of femur

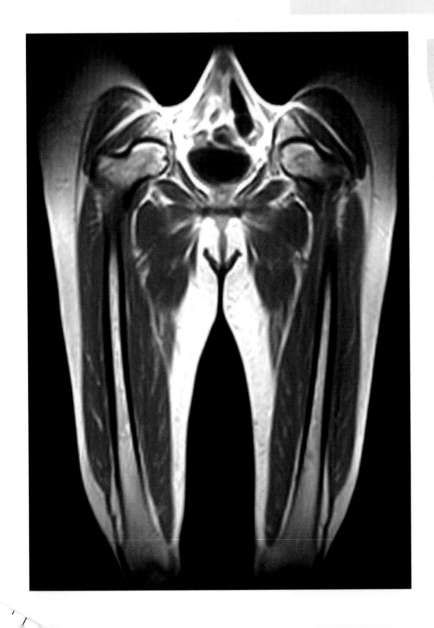

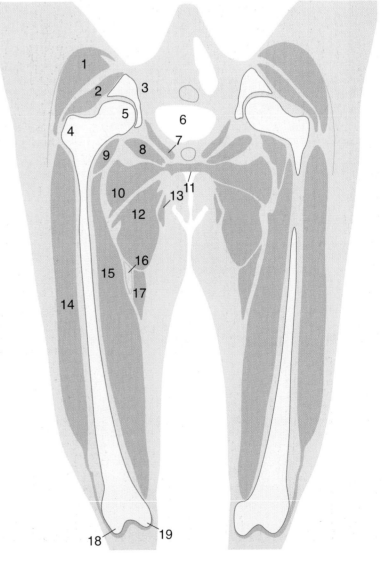

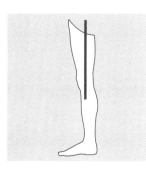

Coronal MR of thigh

1 - Gluteus medius muscle
2 - Gluteus minimus muscle
3 - Greater trochanter
4 - Obturator internus muscle
5 - Intertrochanteric crest
6 - Obturator externus muscle
7 - Vagina
8 - Adductor minimus muscle
9 - Adductor magnus muscle

10 - Adductor brevis muscle
11 - Gracilis muscle
12 - Vastus lateralis and vastus intermedius muscles
13 - Adductor longus muscle
14 - Adductor canal and femoral vessels
15 - Sartorius muscle
16 - Vastus medialis muscle

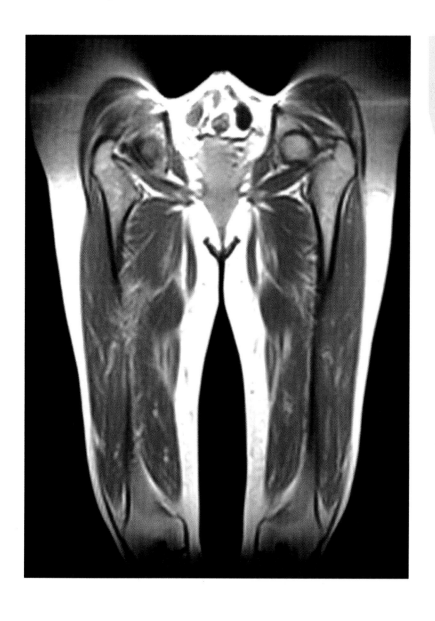

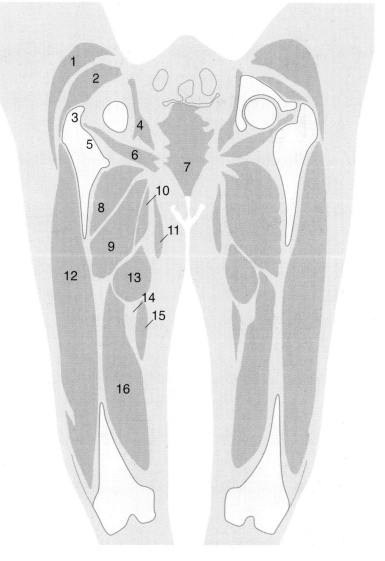

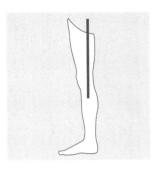

Coronal MR of thigh

1 - Gluteus maximus muscle
2 - Anal canal
3 - Levator ani muscle
4 - Ischio-anal fossa
5 - Biceps femoris muscle
6 - Semitendinosus muscle

7 - Adductor magnus muscle
8 - Gracilis muscle
9 - Semimembranosus
    muscle
10 - Popliteal fossa

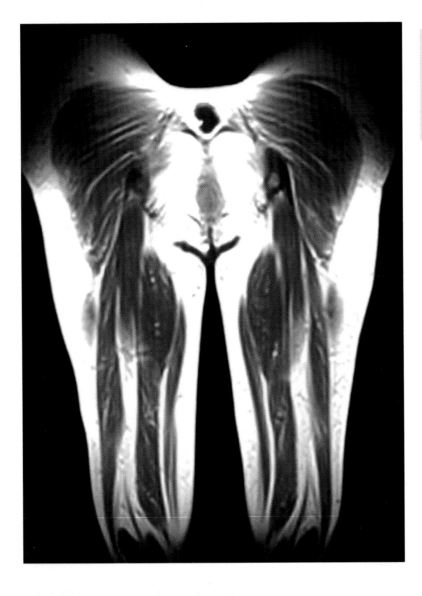

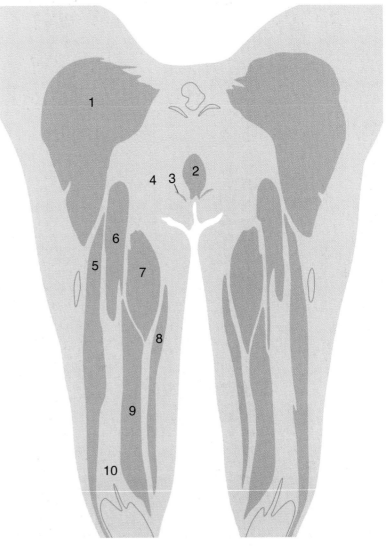

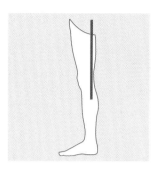

Coronal MR of thigh

1 - Gluteus maximus muscle
2 - Sacrum
3 - Anus
4 - Ischial tuberosity
5 - Adductor magnus muscle
6 - Biceps femoris muscle

7 - Semitendinosus muscle
8 - Gracilis muscle
9 - Semimembranosus muscle
10 - Popliteal fossa

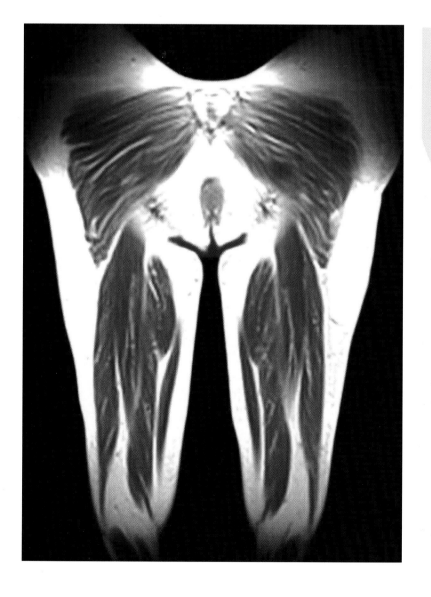

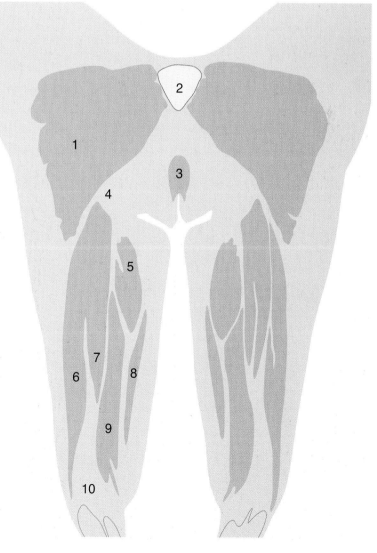

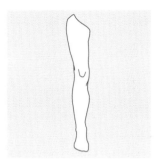

External iliac and femoral arteriogram, anteroposterior view

1 - External iliac artery
2 - Superficial circumflex iliac artery
3 - Femoral artery
4 - Lateral circumflex femoral artery
5 - Ascending branch
6 - Transverse branch
7 - Descending branch
8 - Deep femoral artery
9 - Medial circumflex femoral artery
10 - Ascending branch
11 - Descending branch
12 - Perforating arteries
13 - Superficial femoral artery

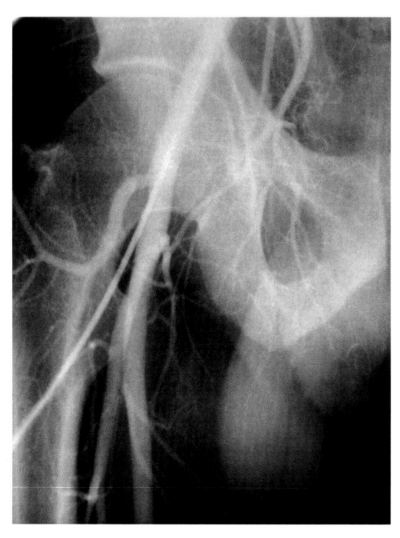

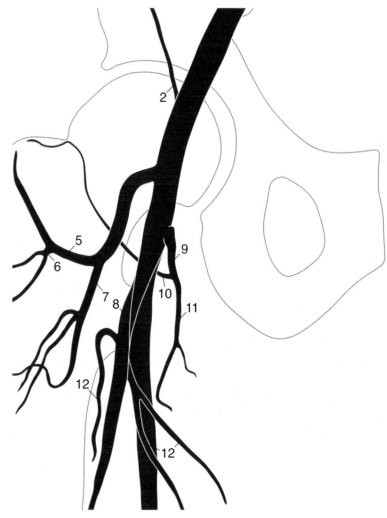

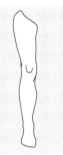

Inguinal and pelvic lymphangiography, front view

1 - External iliac lymph nodes and vessels
2 - Obturator foramen
3 - Pubic symphysis
4 - Pelvic brim
5 - Acetabulum
6 - Head of femur
7 - Greater trochanter
8 - Inguinal lymph nodes
9 - Inferior ramus of pubis
10 - Lesser trochanter
11 - Lymph vessels from the lower extremity

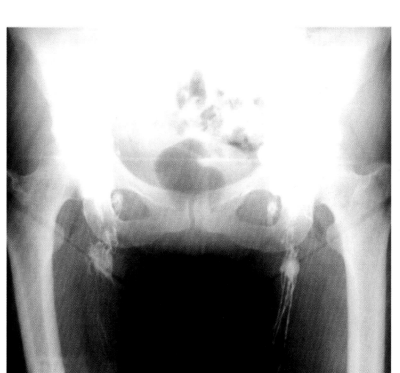

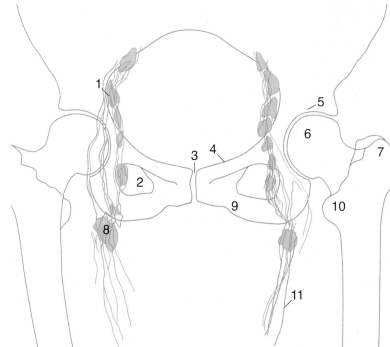

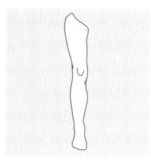

Femoral and popliteal arteriogram, anteroposterior view

1 - Perforating branches
of deep femoral artery
2 - Superficial femoral
artery
3 - Muscular branches
of superficial femoral
artery
4 - Femur

5 - Descending genicular
artery emerging from the
adductor canal
6 - Popliteal artery
7 - Superior lateral genicular
artery
8 - Superior medial genicular
artery

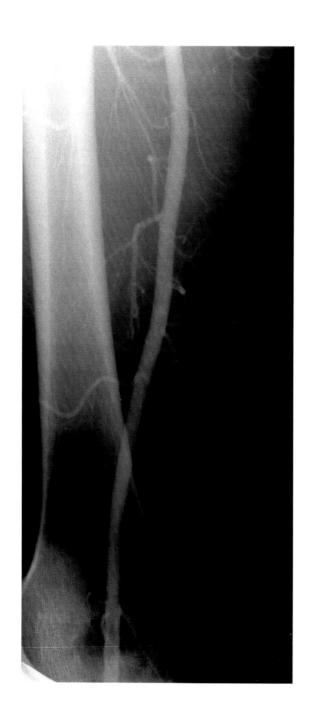

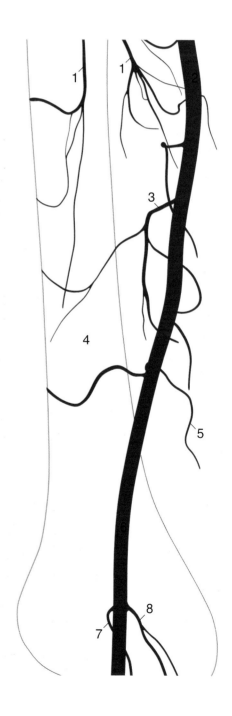

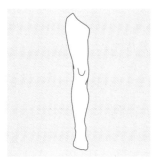

X-ray of knee of an adolescent, anteroposterior view

1 - Femur
2 - Patella
3 - Lateral epicondyle of femur
4 - Medial epicondyle of femur
5 - Lateral condyle of femur
6 - Intercondylar notch (fossa)
7 - Medial condyle of femur
8 - Lateral condyle of tibia
9 - Lateral intercondylar tubercle

10 - Medial intercondylar tubercle
11 - Superior articular facet of tibia (medial tibial plateau)
12 - Medial condyle of tibia
13 - Head of fibula
14 - Neck of fibula
15 - Tuberosity of tibia
16 - Epiphysial plate (growth cartilage)

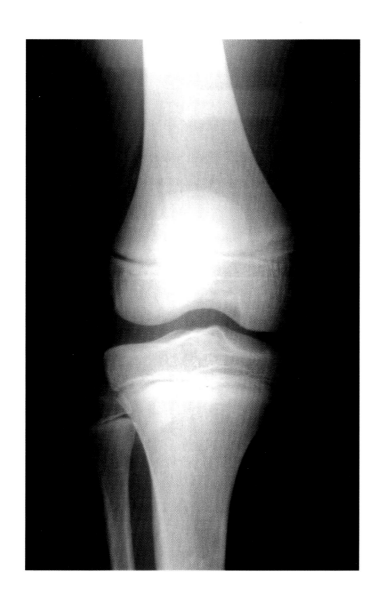

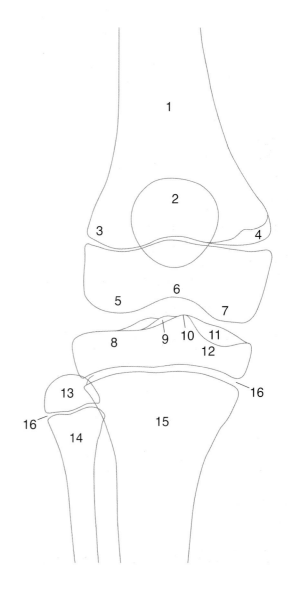

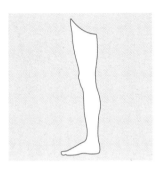

X-ray of knee of an adolescent, lateral view

1 - Femur
2 - Base (upper pole) of patella
3 - Articular facet of patella
4 - Apex (lower pole) of patella
5 - Epiphysial plate (growth cartilage)
6 - Medial condyle of femur
7 - Lateral condyle of femur
8 - Intercondylar eminence
9 - Proximal epiphysis of tibia
10 - Head of fibula
11 - Shaft of tibia
12 - Shaft of fibula

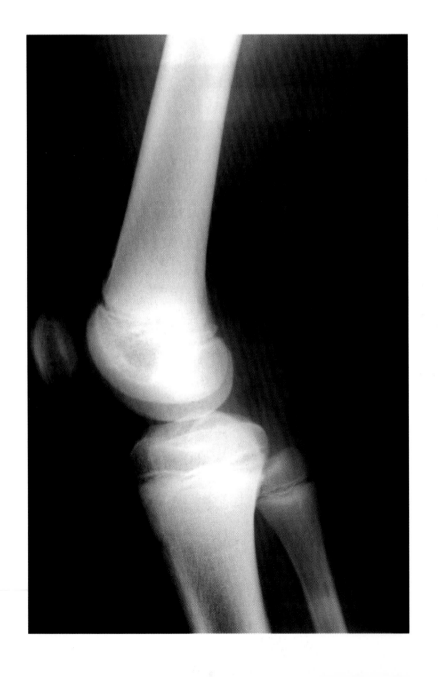

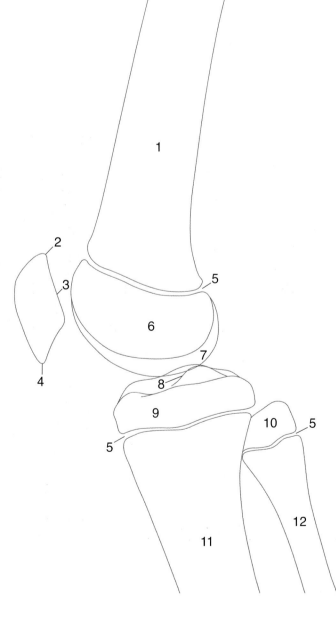

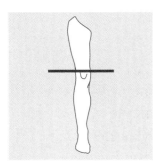

Axial MR of knee

1 - Tendon of quadriceps
    femoris muscle
2 - Lateral patellar
    retinaculum
3 - Medial patellar
    retinaculum
4 - Vastus lateralis muscle
5 - Femur
6 - Vastus medialis muscle
7 - Biceps femoris muscle
8 - Common peroneal
    (fibular) nerve

9 - Tibial nerve
10 - Popliteal vein
11 - Popliteal artery
12 - Semimembranosus
     muscle
13 - Tendon of
     semitendinosus muscle
14 - Gracilis muscle
15 - Sartorius muscle
16 - Great saphenous vein

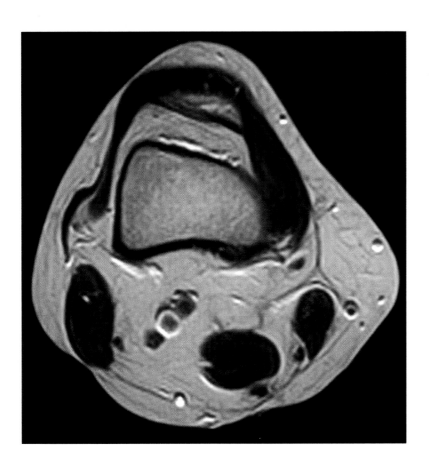

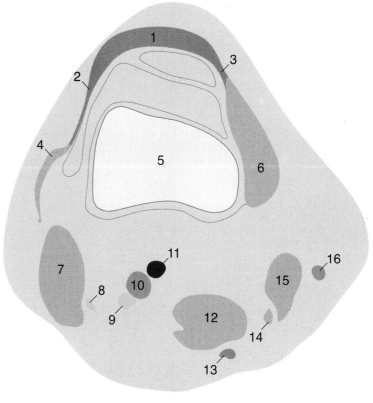

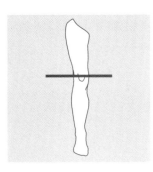

Axial MR of knee

1 - Patella
2 - Lateral patellar retinaculum
3 - Medial patellar retinaculum
4 - Vastus lateralis muscle
5 - Femur
6 - Vastus medialis muscle
7 - Biceps femoris muscle
8 - Lateral head of gastrocnemius muscle
9 - Popliteal artery
10 - Medial head of gastrocnemius muscle
11 - Common peroneal (fibular) nerve
12 - Popliteal vein
13 - Tibial nerve
14 - Semimembranosus muscle
15 - Tendon of semitendinosus muscle
16 - Gracilis muscle
17 - Sartorius muscle
18 - Great saphenous vein

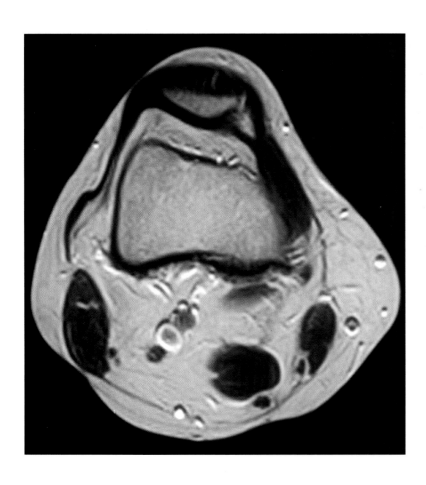

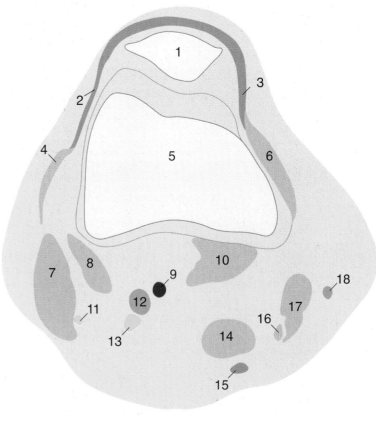

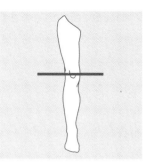

Axial MR of knee

1 - Patella
2 - Lateral patellar retinaculum
3 - Medial patellar retinaculum
4 - Biceps femoris muscle
5 - Lateral condyle of femur
6 - Medial condyle of femur
7 - Common peroneal (fibular) nerve
8 - Lateral head of gastrocnemius muscle
9 - Popliteal artery
10 - Popliteal vein
11 - Tibial nerve
12 - Medial head of gastrocnemius muscle
13 - Semimembranosus muscle
14 - Tendon of semitendinosus muscle
15 - Gracilis muscle
16 - Sartorius muscle
17 - Great saphenous vein
18 - Small saphenous vein

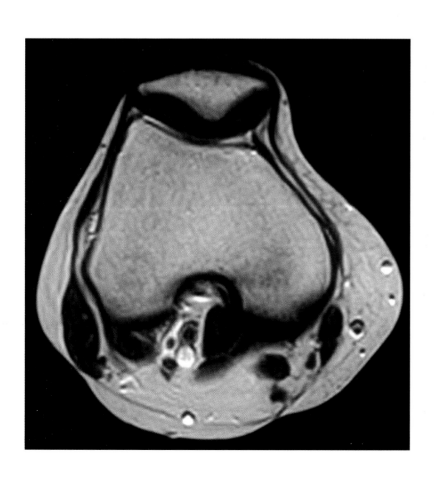

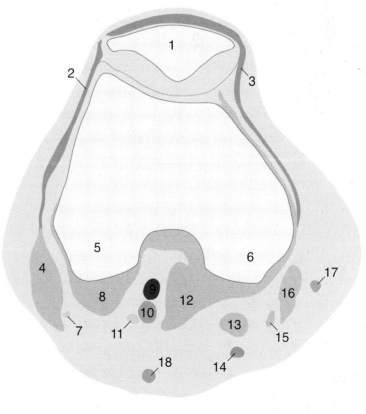

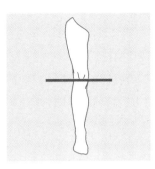

Axial MR of knee

1 - Patella
2 - Lateral patellar retinaculum
3 - Medial patellar retinaculum
4 - Lateral condyle of femur
5 - Intercondylar notch
6 - Medial condyle of femur
7 - Biceps femoris muscle
8 - Common peroneal (fibular) nerve
9 - Lateral head of gastrocnemius muscle and plantaris muscle

10 - Tibial nerve
11 - Popliteal vessels
12 - Medial head of gastrocnemius muscle
13 - Tendon of semitendinosus muscle
14 - Tendon of semimembranosus muscle
15 - Gracilis muscle
16 - Sartorius muscle
17 - Great saphenous vein
18 - Small saphenous vein

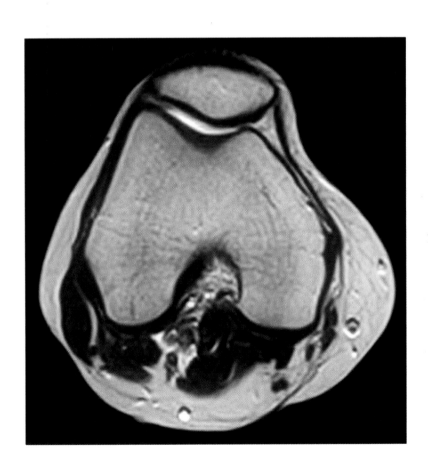

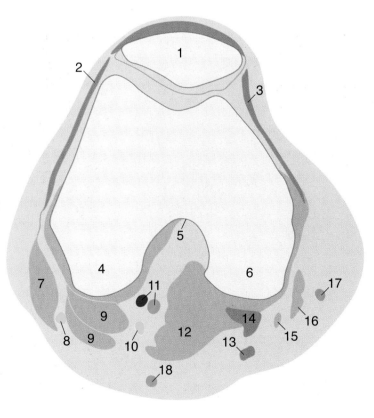

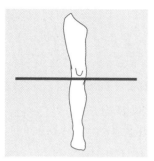

Axial MR of knee

1 - Patellar ligament
2 - Fat pad of knee joint
3 - Lateral condyle of femur
4 - Medial condyle of femur
5 - Anterior cruciate ligament
6 - Intercondylar fossa
7 - Biceps femoris muscle
8 - Lateral head of gastrocnemius muscle
9 - Popliteal vessels
10 - Small saphenous vein
11 - Medial head of gastrocnemius muscle
12 - Semitendinosus tendon
13 - Gracilis tendon
14 - Great saphenous vein
15 - Sartorius tendon
16 - Semimembranosus tendon

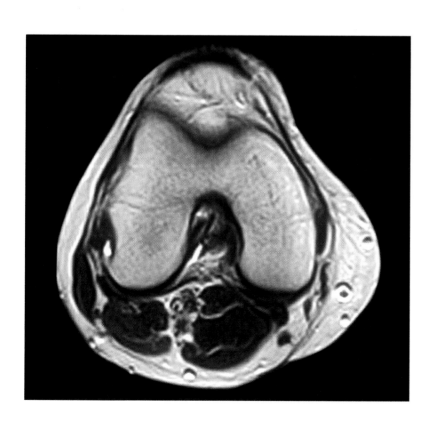

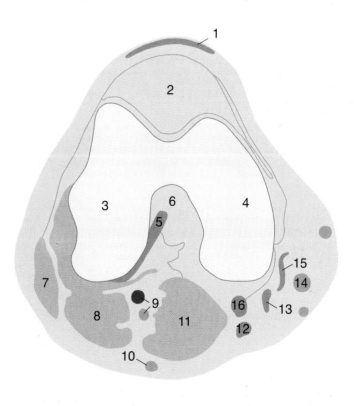

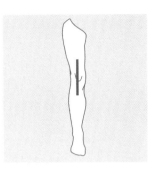

Sagittal MR of knee

1 - Tendon of quadriceps femoris muscle
2 - Suprapatellar bursa
3 - Lateral condyle of femur
4 - Biceps femoris muscle
5 - Patella
6 - Patellar ligament
7 - Anterior horn of lateral meniscus

8 - Posterior horn of lateral meniscus
9 - Tibia
10 - Gastrocnemius muscle (lateral head)
11 - Tibialis anterior muscle
12 - Head of fibula
13 - Soleus muscle

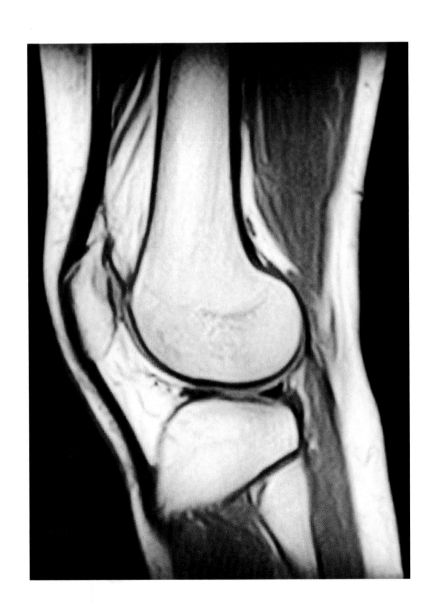

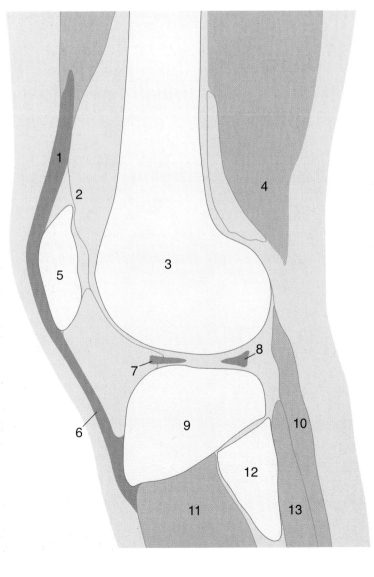

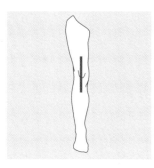

Sagittal MR of knee

1 - Quadriceps femoris muscle
2 - Suprapatellar bursa
3 - Biceps femoris muscle
4 - Patella
5 - Fat pad
6 - Lateral condyle of femur
7 - Anterior horn of lateral meniscus

8 - Tibia
9 - Posterior horn of lateral meniscus
10 - Tendon of popliteus muscle
11 - Plantaris muscle
12 - Head of fibula
13 - Tibialis anterior muscle
14 - Soleus muscle

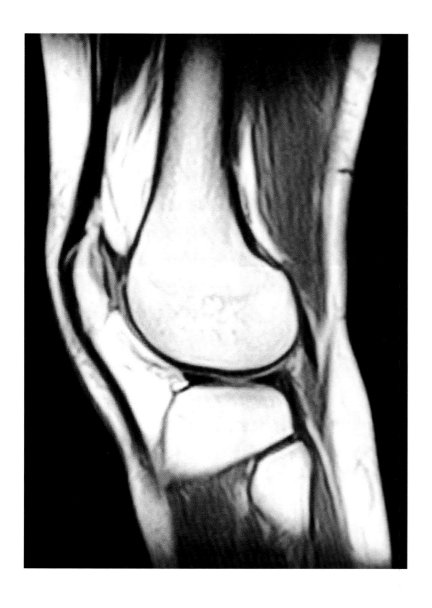

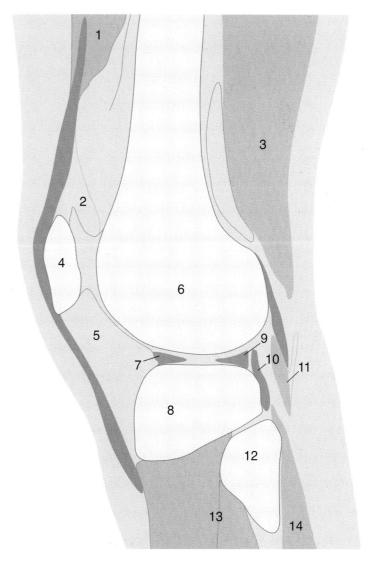

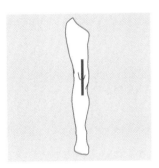

Sagittal MR of knee

1 - Quadriceps femoris
    muscle
2 - Femur
3 - Popliteal vessels
4 - Patella
5 - Fat pad
6 - Alar fold
7 - Anterior cruciate ligament

8 - Posterior cruciate ligament
9 - Fibrous capsule
10 - Patellar ligament
11 - Tibia
12 - Popliteus muscle
13 - Gastrocnemius muscle
     (medial head)

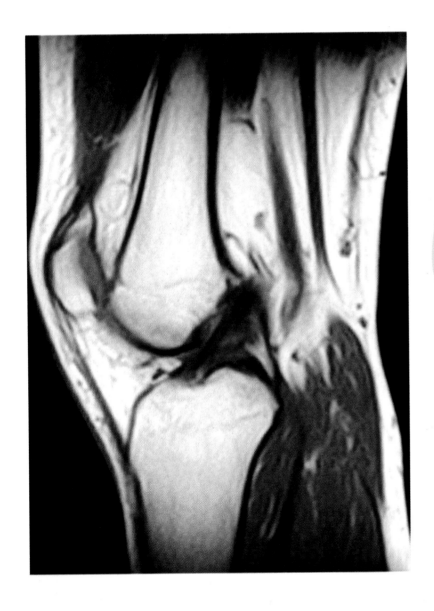

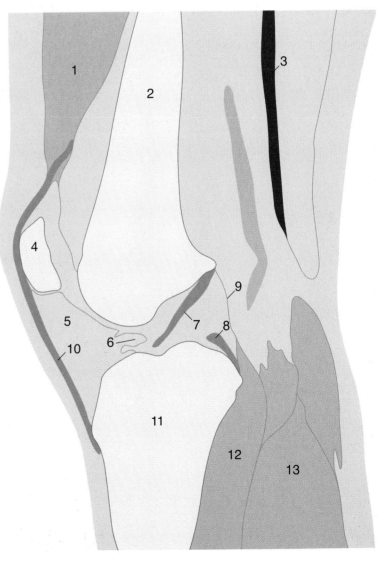

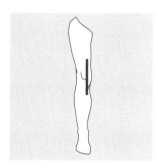

Sagittal MR of knee

1 - Quadriceps femoris
    muscle
2 - Femur
3 - Vastus medialis muscle
4 - Popliteal vessels
5 - Semimembranosus
    muscle
6 - Fat pad

7 - Posterior cruciate
    ligament
8 - Fibrous capsule
9 - Tibia
10 - Popliteus muscle
11 - Gastrocnemius muscle
    (medial head)

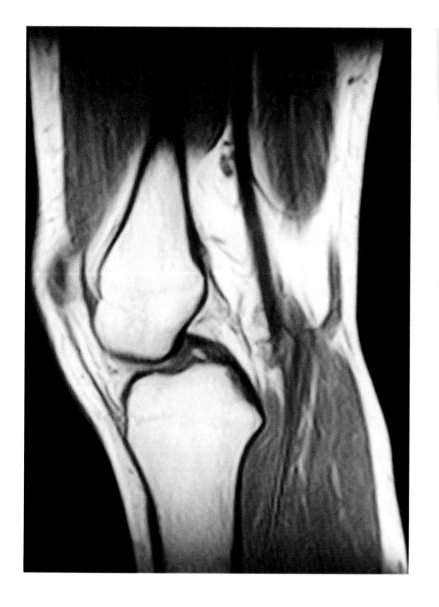

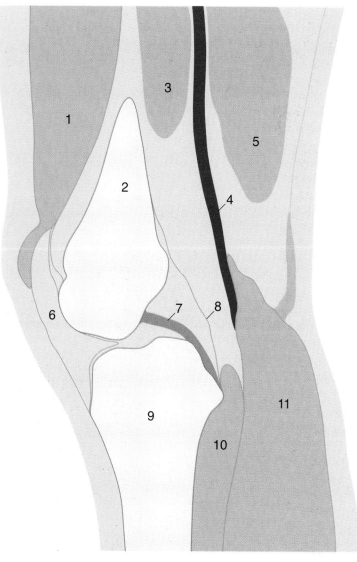

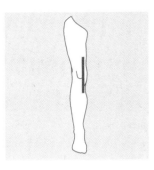

Sagittal MR of knee

1 - Vastus medialis muscle
2 - Semimembranosus muscle
3 - Medial patellar retinaculum
4 - Femur
5 - Gastrocnemius muscle (medial head)

6 - Anterior horn of medial meniscus
7 - Articular cartilage
8 - Posterior horn of medial meniscus
9 - Medial condyle of tibia
10 - Popliteus muscle
11 - Soleus muscle

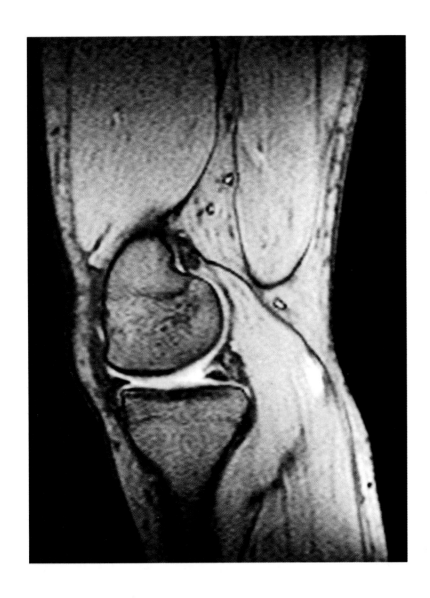

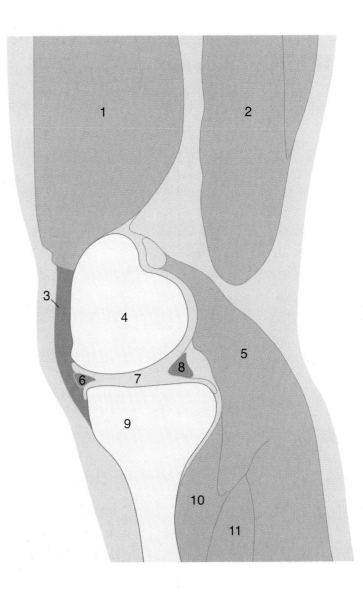

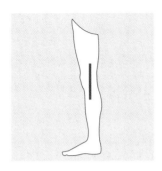

Coronal MR of knee

1 - Vastus medialis muscle
2 - Vastus lateralis muscle
3 - Iliotibial tract
4 - Medial collateral ligament
5 - Medial condyle of femur
6 - Lateral condyle of femur
7 - Medial meniscus
8 - Anterior horn of lateral meniscus
9 - Tibia
10 - Tibialis anterior muscle

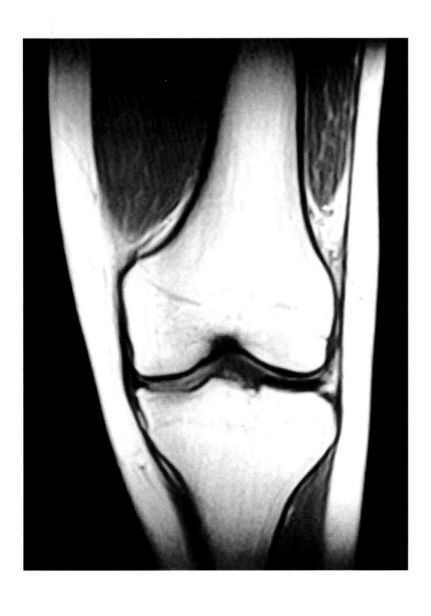

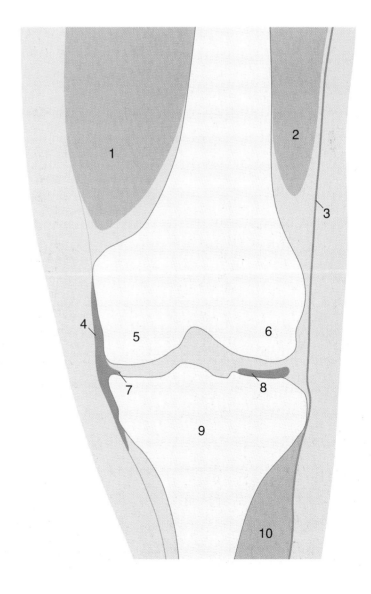

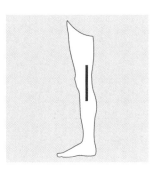

Coronal MR of knee

1 - Vastus medialis muscle
2 - Vastus lateralis muscle
3 - Medial collateral ligament
4 - Medial condyle of femur
5 - Posterior cruciate ligament

6 - Lateral condyle of femur
7 - Medial meniscus
8 - Anterior horn of lateral meniscus
9 - Tibia
10 - Tibialis anterior muscle

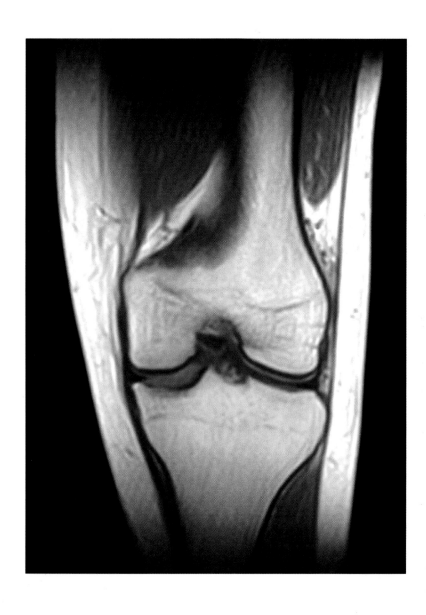

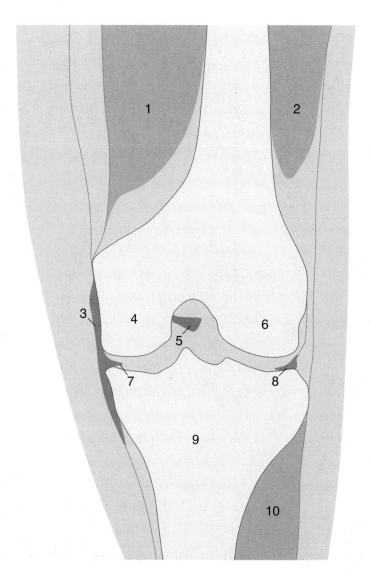

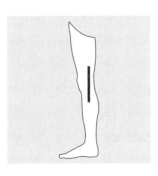

Coronal MR of knee

1 - Sartorius muscle	6 - Medial meniscus
2 - Popliteal fossa (fat)	7 - Intercondylar eminence
3 - Medial condyle of femur	8 - Lateral meniscus
4 - Anterior cruciate ligament	9 - Tibia
5 - Lateral condyle of femur	10 - Tibialis anterior muscle

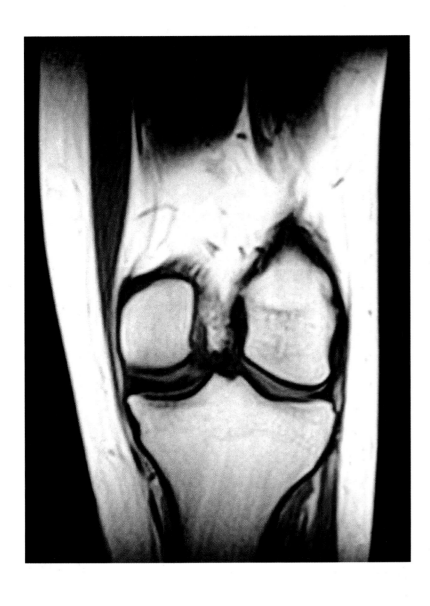
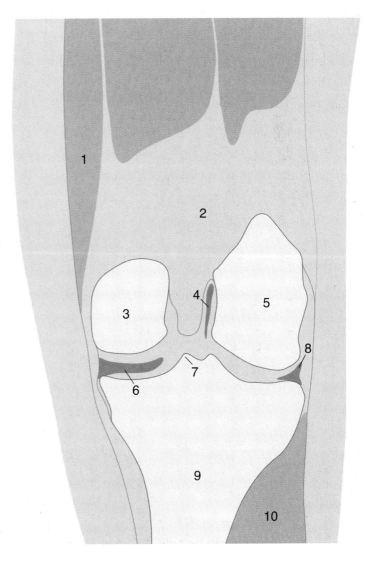

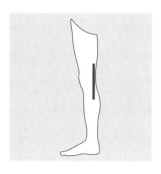

Coronal MR knee

1 - Sartorius muscle
2 - Popliteal fossa (fat)
3 - Biceps femoris muscle
4 - Medial condyle of femur
5 - Lateral condyle of femur
6 - Medial meniscus

7 - Anterior cruciate ligament
8 - Intercondylar eminence
9 - Lateral meniscus
10 - Tibia
11 - Tibialis anterior muscle

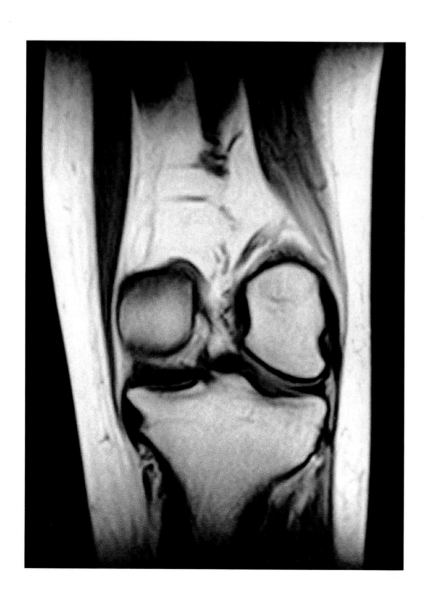

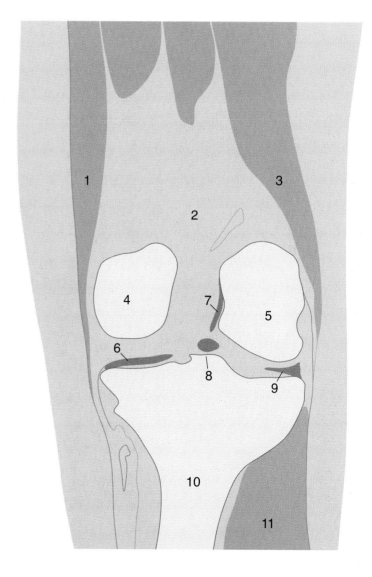

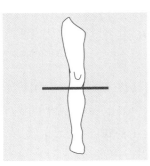

Axial MR of calf

1 - Tibia
2 - Tibialis anterior muscle
3 - Extensor digitorum longus muscle
4 - Tibialis posterior muscle
5 - Tendon of semitendinosus muscle
6 - Anterior intermuscular septum
7 - Soleus muscle (tibial head)
8 - Popliteus muscle

9 - Peroneus longus muscle
10 - Fibula
11 - Popliteal vessels
12 - Great saphenous vein
13 - Soleus muscle (fibular head)
14 - Gastrocnemius muscle, medial head
15 - Gastrocnemius muscle, lateral head

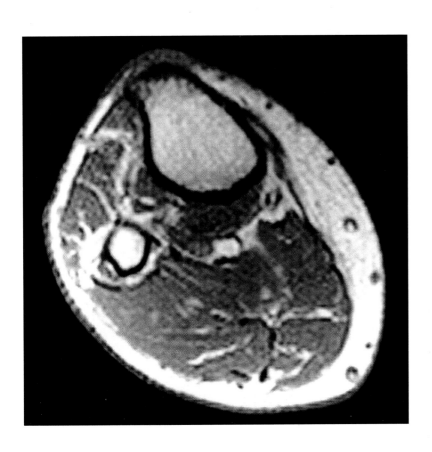

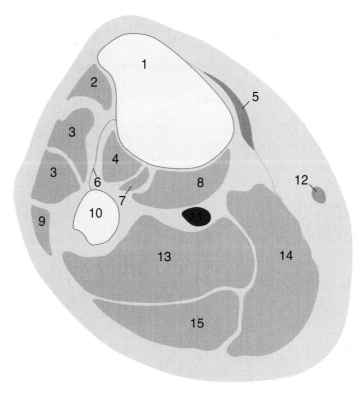

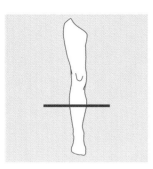

Axial CT of calf

1 - Tibia
2 - Tibialis anterior muscle
3 - Extensor hallucis longus muscle
4 - Tibialis posterior muscle
5 - Flexor digitorum longus muscle
6 - Great saphenous vein
7 - Extensor digitorum longus muscle

8 - Fibula
9 - Flexor hallucis longus muscle
10 - Peroneus brevis muscle
11 - Peroneus longus muscle
12 - Soleus muscle
13 - Gastrocnemius muscle, medial head
14 - Gastrocnemius muscle, lateral head

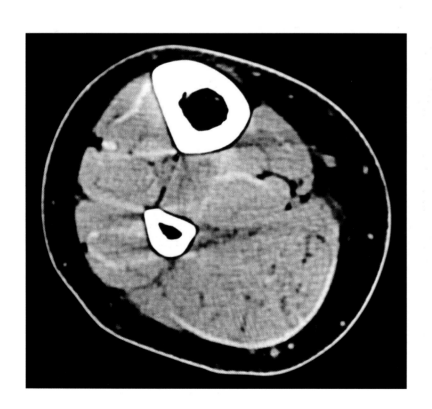

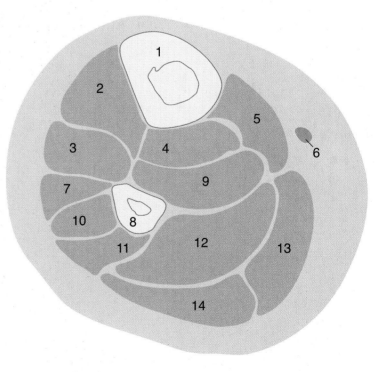

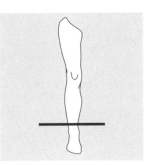

Axial CT of calf

1 - Extensors of ankle and digits
2 - Tibia
3 - Great saphenous vein
4 - Fibula
5 - Tibialis posterior muscle
6 - Flexor digitorum longus muscle
7 - Flexor hallucis longus muscle
8 - Peroneus brevis muscle
9 - Peroneus longus muscle
10 - Small saphenous vein
11 - Tendo calcaneus (Achilles' tendon)

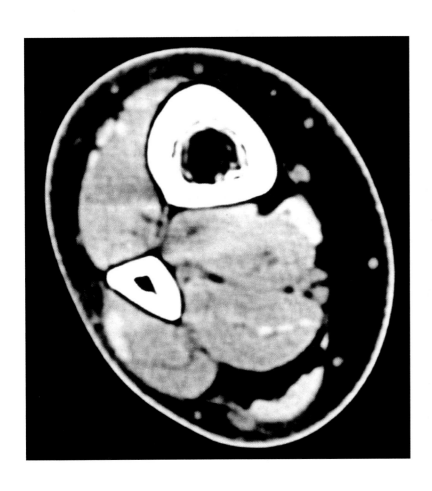

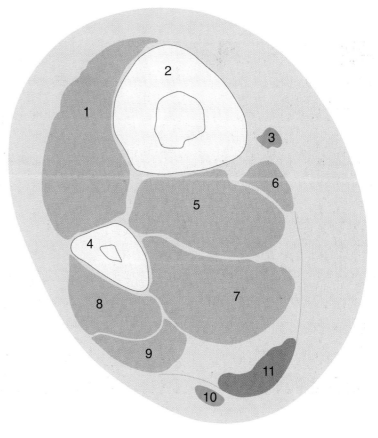

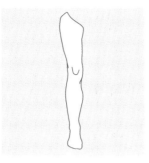

Arteriogram of leg, anteroposterior view

1 - Popliteal artery
2 - Inferior medial genicular artery
3 - Inferior lateral genicular artery
4 - Anterior tibial artery
5 - Fibular (peroneal) artery (less frequent variation of origin)

6 - Posterior tibial artery
7 - Muscular branches
8 - Fibula
9 - Tibia

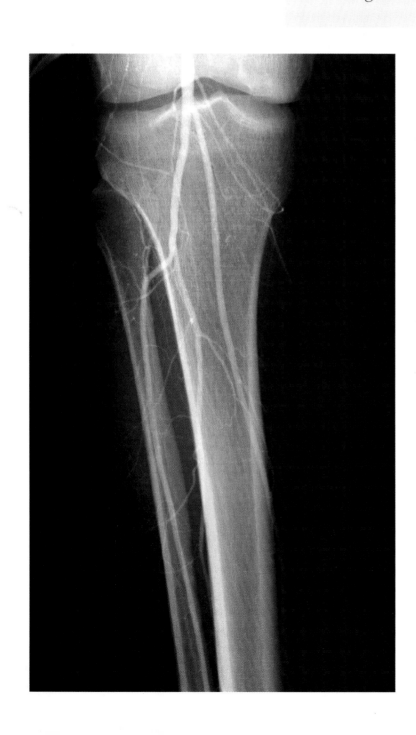

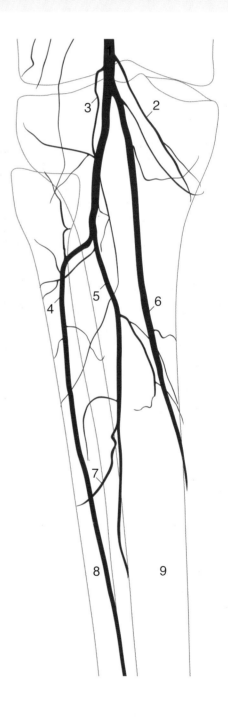

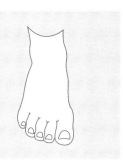

X-ray of ankle, anteroposterior view

1 - Fibula
2 - Tibia
3 - Tibiofibular syndesmosis
4 - Talocrural (tibiotalar) joint

5 - Lateral malleolus
6 - Trochlea of talus
7 - Medial malleolus

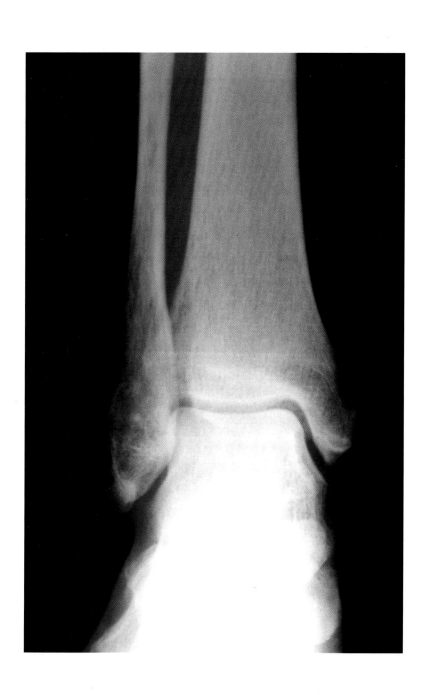

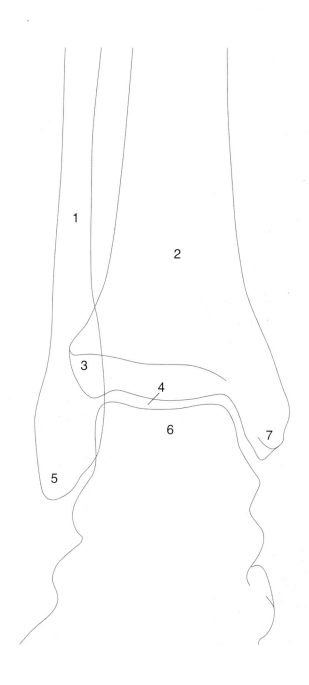

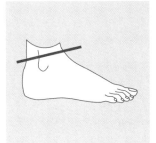

Axial MR of ankle

1 - Tendon of extensor digitorum longus muscle

2 - Tendon of extensor hallucis longus muscle

3 - Tendon of tibialis anterior muscle

4 - Extensor digitorum longus muscle

5 - Tibia

6 - Fibula

7 - Tendon of tibialis posterior muscle

8 - Tendon of flexor digitorum longus muscle

9 - Tendon of peroneus longus muscle

10 - Peroneus brevis muscle

11 - Flexor hallucis longus muscle

12 - Tendo calcaneus (Achilles' tendon)

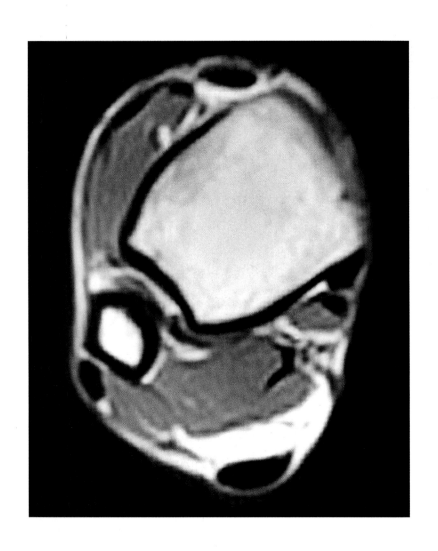

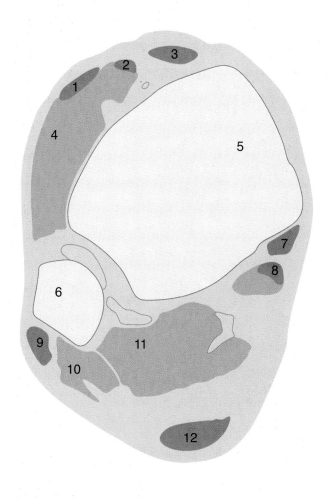

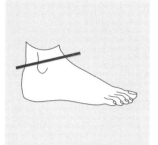

Axial MR of ankle

1 - Tendon of extensor digitorum longus muscle
2 - Extensor hallucis longus muscle and tendon
3 - Tendon of tibialis anterior muscle
4 - Extensor digitorum longus muscle
5 - Tibia
6 - Fibula
7 - Tendon of tibialis posterior muscle
8 - Tendon of flexor digitorum longus muscle
9 - Tendon of peroneus longus muscle
10 - Peroneus brevis muscle
11 - Flexor hallucis longus muscle
12 - Tendon of flexor hallucis longus muscle
13 - Posterior tibial artery and vein
14 - Small saphenous vein
15 - Tendo calcaneus (Achilles' tendon)

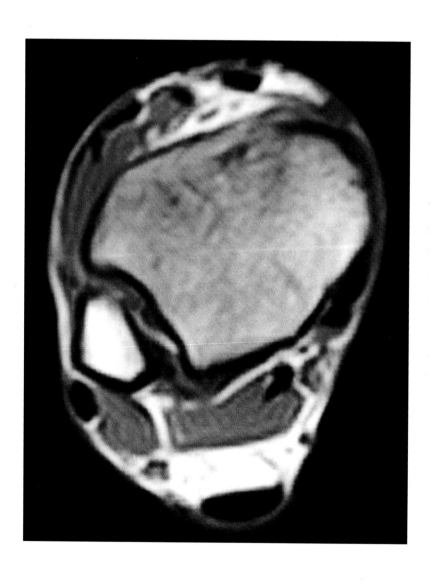

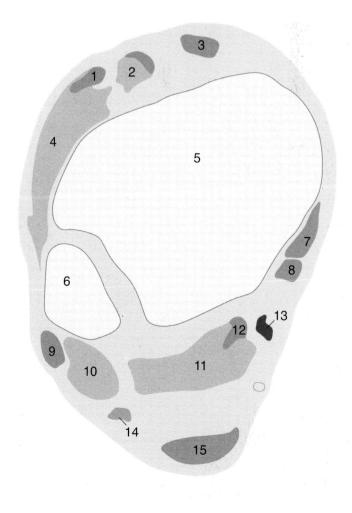

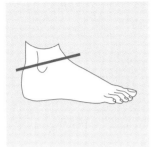

Axial MR of ankle

1 - Peroneus tertius tendon

2 - Tendon of extensor digitorum longus muscle

3 - Tendon of extensor hallucis longus muscle

4 - Tendon of tibialis anterior muscle

5 - Deltoid ligament and medial malleolus

6 - Trochlea of talus

7 - Lateral malleolus of fibula

8 - Tendons of tibialis posterior and flexor digitorum longus muscles

9 - Tendon of peroneus longus muscle

10 - Peroneus brevis muscle

11 - Flexor hallucis longus muscle and tendon

12 - Posterior tibial artery and vein

13 - Small saphenous vein

14 - Tendo calcaneus (Achilles' tendon)

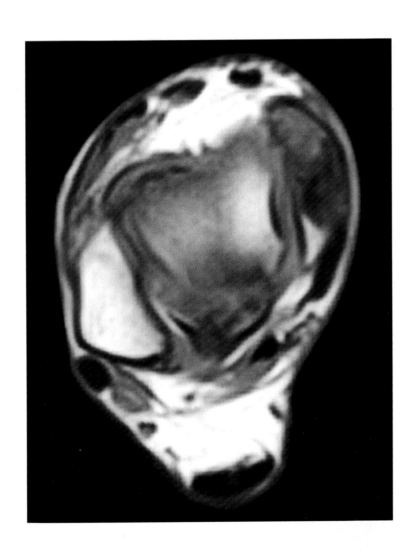

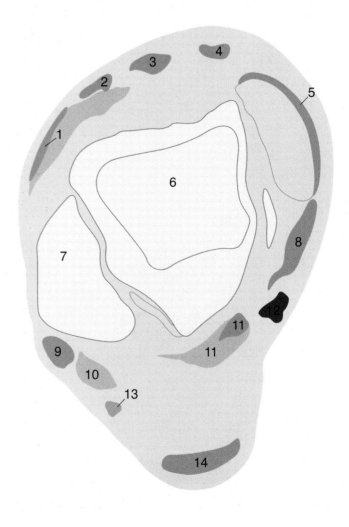

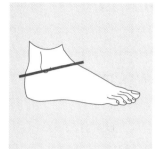

Axial MR of ankle

1 - Tendon of extensor digitorum longus muscle
2 - Tendon of extensor hallucis longus muscle
3 - Tendon of tibialis anterior muscle
4 - Extensor digitorum longus muscle
5 - Trochlea of talus
6 - Tendon of tibialis posterior muscle
7 - Tendon of flexor digitorum longus muscle
8 - Fibula, lateral malleolus
9 - Tendons of peroneus brevis and longus muscles
10 - Tendon of flexor hallucis longus muscle
11 - Posterior tibial artery and vein
12 - Small saphenous vein
13 - Tendo calcaneus (Achilles' tendon)

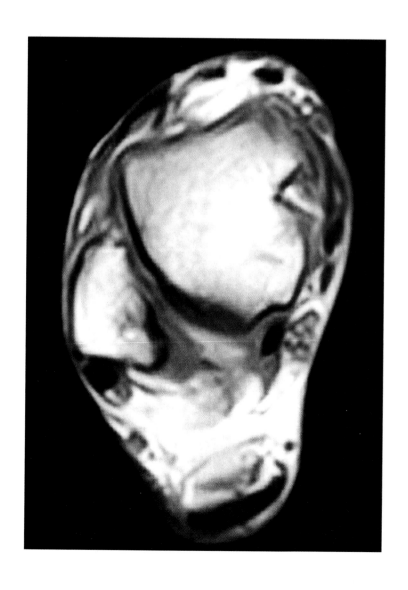

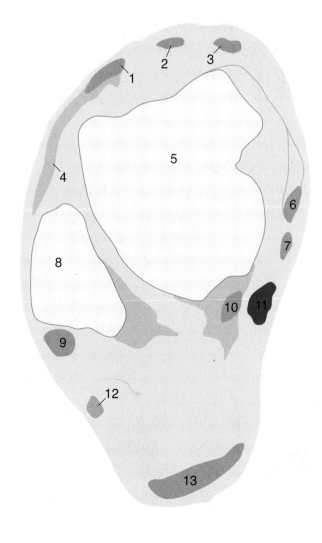

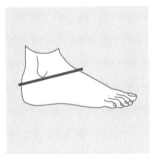

Axial MR of ankle

1 - Tendon of extensor
    digitorum longus muscle
2 - Tendon of extensor
    hallucis longus muscle
3 - Tendon of tibialis
    anterior muscle
4 - Fibular collateral ligament
    (talofibular part)
5 - Talus
6 - Tendon of tibialis
    posterior muscle
7 - Tendon of flexor
    digitorum longus muscle

8 - Lateral malleolus
9 - Calcaneus
10 - Tendon of flexor hallucis
     longus muscle
11 - Posterior tibial artery
     and vein
12 - Tendons of peroneus
     longus and brevis
     muscles
13 - Small saphenous vein
14 - Tendo calcaneus
     (Achilles' tendon)

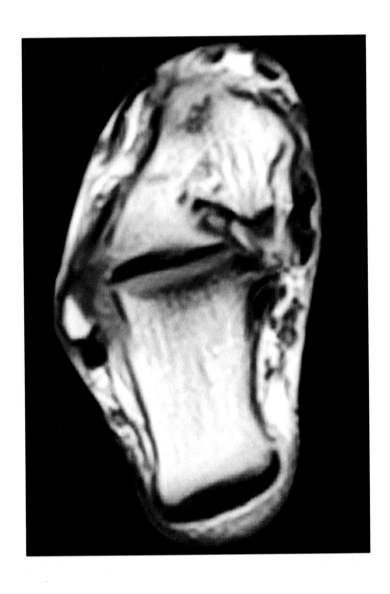

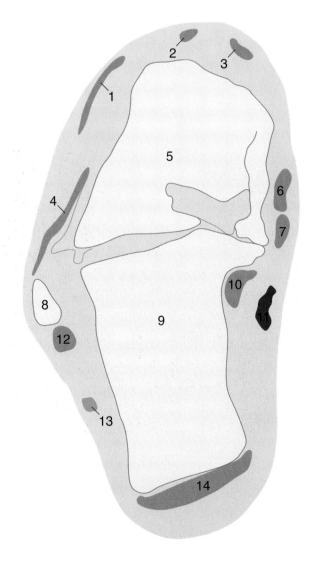

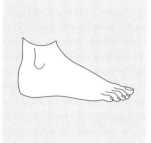

X-ray of foot, lateral view

1 - Tibia
2 - Talocrural (tibiotalar) joint
3 - Posterior process of talus
4 - Trochlea of talus (medial malleolar facet)
5 - Neck of talus
6 - Head of talus
7 - Talonavicular joint (constituent of talocalcaneonavicular joint)
8 - Subtalar (posterior talocalcanean) joint

9 - Sustentaculum tali
10 - Anterior talocalcanean joint (constituent of talocalcaneonavicular joint)
11 - Navicular
12 - Calcanean tuberosity
13 - Calcaneocuboid joint
14 - Cuboid
15 - Lateral cuneiform
16 - Medial cuneiform
17 - Metatarsal I
18 - Tuberosity of metatarsal V

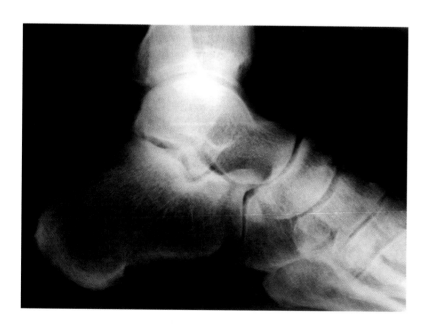

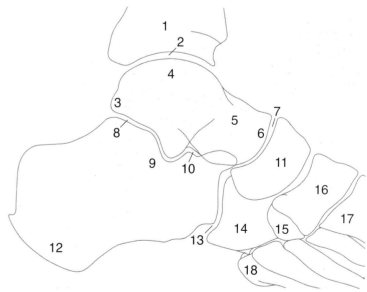

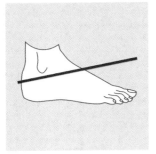

Axial MR of foot

1 - Tendon of peroneus tertius muscle and tendon of extensor digitorum longus muscle
2 - Tendon of extensor hallucis longus muscle
3 - Tendon of tibialis anterior muscle
4 - Great saphenous vein
5 - Head of talus
6 - Tendon of tibialis posterior muscle
7 - Lateral process of talus
8 - Talocalcanean (subtalar) joint
9 - Talocalcaneonavicular joint
10 - Tendon of flexor digitorum longus muscle
11 - Tendon of flexor hallucis longus muscle
12 - Tendon of peroneus brevis muscle
13 - Tendon of peroneus longus muscle
14 - Calcaneus
15 - Medial plantar neurovascular bundle
16 - Lateral plantar neurovascular bundle
17 - Quadratus plantae (flexor accessorius) muscle
18 - Small saphenous vein
19 - Tendo calcaneus (Achilles' tendon)

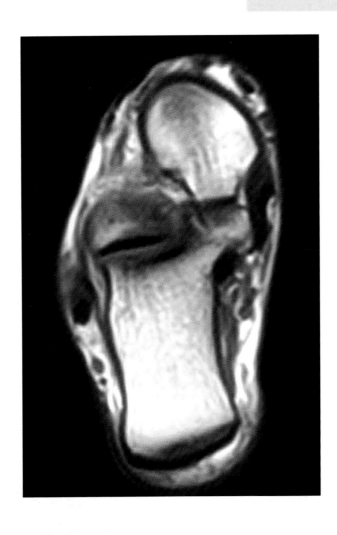

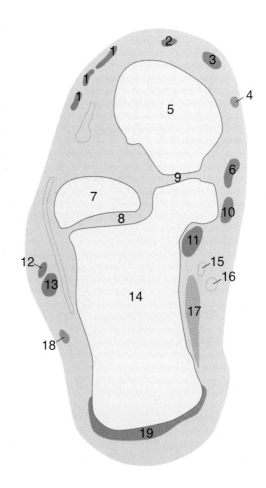

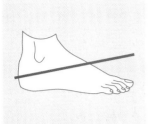

Axial MR of foot

1 - Extensor digitorum brevis and extensor hallucis brevis muscles
2 - Tendon of peroneus tertius muscle
3 - Tendon of extensor digitorum longus muscle
4 - Tendon of extensor hallucis longus muscle
5 - Tendon of tibialis anterior muscle
6 - Navicular
7 - Calcaneus
8 - Plantar calcaneonavicular ligament (spring ligament)
9 - Tendon of flexor hallucis longus muscle
10 - Tendon of flexor digitorum longus muscle
11 - Tendon of peroneus brevis muscle
12 - Tendon of peroneus longus muscle
13 - Quadratus plantae (flexor accessorius) muscle
14 - Abductor hallucis muscle

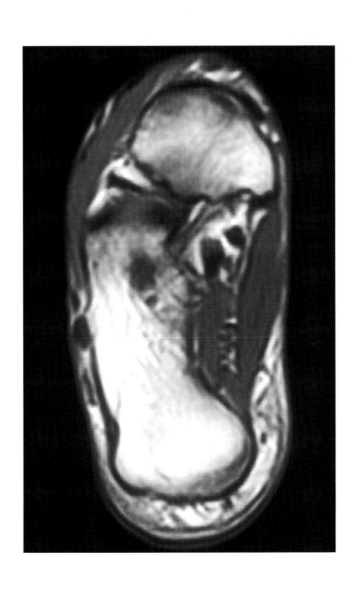

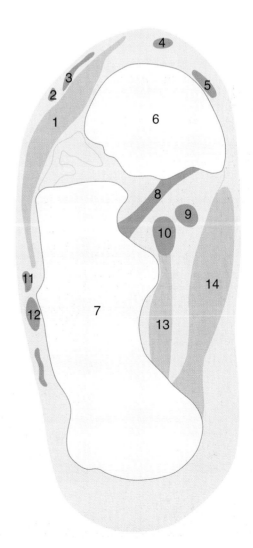

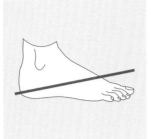

Axial MR of foot

1 - Tendon of extensor digitorum longus muscle
2 - Extensor digitorum brevis and extensor hallucis brevis muscles
3 - Tendon of extensor hallucis longus muscle
4 - Tendon of tibialis anterior muscle
5 - Navicular
6 - Cuboid
7 - Calcaneocuboid joint
8 - Tendon of flexor hallucis longus muscle
9 - Tendon of flexor digitorum longus muscle
10 - Abductor hallucis muscle
11 - Tendon of peroneus brevis muscle
12 - Tendon of peroneus longus muscle
13 - Calcaneus
14 - Adductor hallucis muscle
15 - Calcanean tuberosity

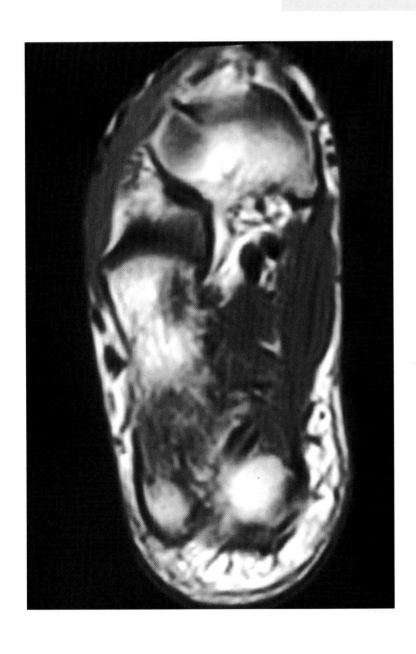

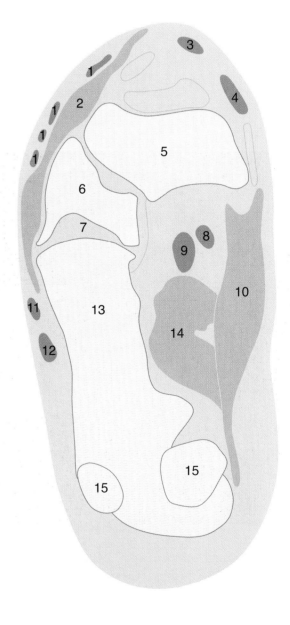

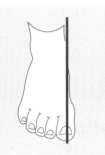

Sagittal MR of foot

1 - Medial malleolus
2 - Tendon of tibialis posterior muscle
3 - Tendon of flexor digitorum longus muscle
4 - Tuberosity of navicular
5 - Tendon of tibialis anterior muscle

6 - Medial cuneiform
7 - Metatarsal I
8 - Abductor hallucis muscle
9 - Posterior tibial vessels
10 - Tendon of flexor hallucis longus muscle

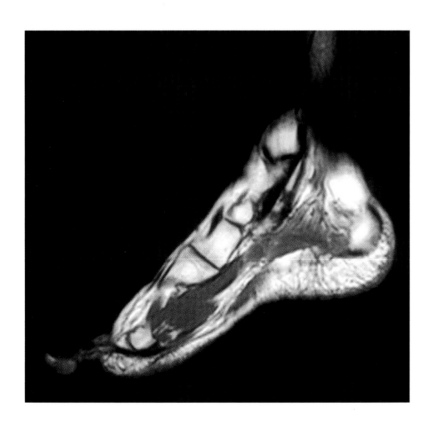

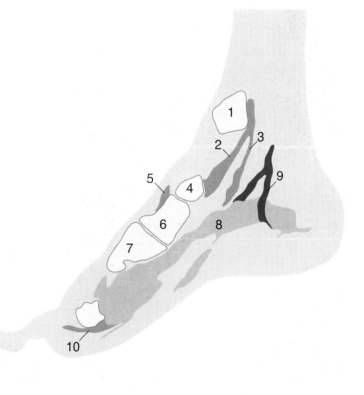

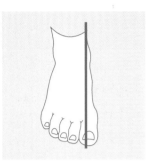

Sagittal MR of foot

1 - Tendon of tibialis anterior muscle
2 - Tibia
3 - Tendon of tibialis posterior muscle
4 - Tendon of flexor digitorum longus muscle
5 - Tendon of flexor hallucis longus muscle
6 - Tendon of tibialis anterior muscle
7 - Navicular
8 - Sustentaculum tali
9 - Calcaneus
10 - Tendo calcaneus (Achilles' tendon)
11 - Medial cuneiform
12 - Tendon of flexor digitorum longus muscle
13 - Metatarsal I
14 - Interosseous muscles
15 - Flexor digitorum brevis muscle
16 - Proximal phalanx
17 - Middle phalanx
18 - Distal phalanx

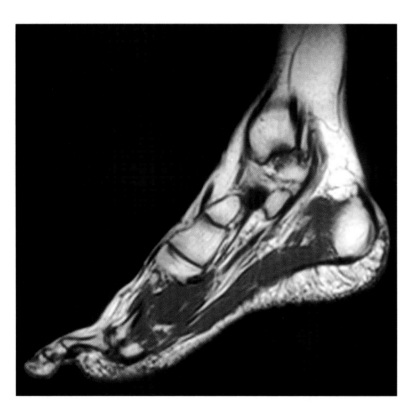

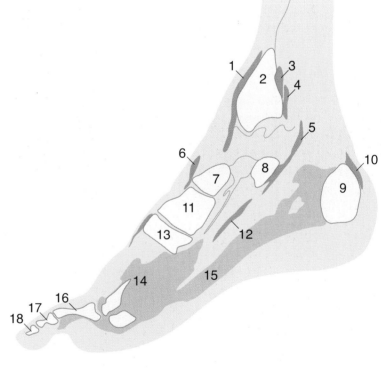

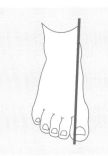

Sagittal MR of foot

1 - Tibia
2 - Tendon of tibialis anterior muscle
3 - Head of talus
4 - Trochlea of talus
5 - Interosseous talocalcanean ligament
6 - Calcaneus
7 - Navicular

8 - Sustentaculum tali
9 - Medial cuneiform
10 - Tendon of flexor digitorum longus muscle
11 - Flexor digitorum brevis muscle
12 - Calcanean tuberosity
13 - Plantar aponeurosis

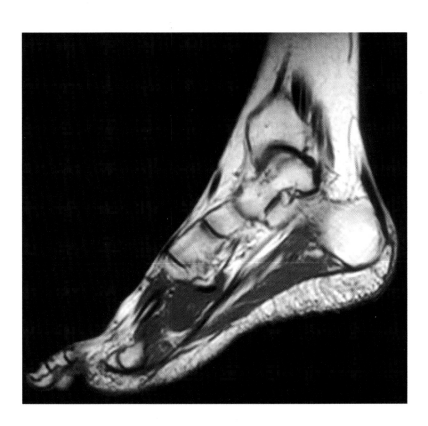

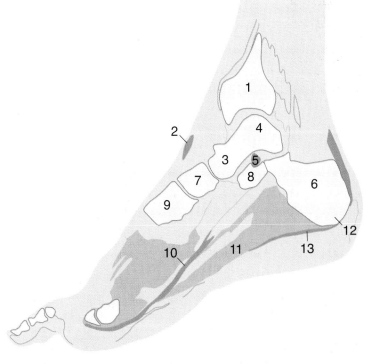

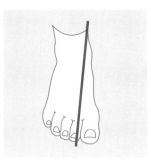

Sagittal MR of foot

1 - Tendon of extensor digitorum longus muscle
2 - Tibia
3 - Flexor hallucis longus muscle
4 - Triceps surae muscle
5 - Tendo calcaneus (Achilles' tendon)
6 - Tendon of tibialis anterior muscle
7 - Talus
8 - Interosseous talocalcanean ligament
9 - Tendon of extensor hallucis longus muscle
10 - Navicular
11 - Calcaneus
12 - Medial and intermediate cuneiforms
13 - Metatarsal II
14 - Interosseous muscles
15 - Abductor digiti minimi muscle

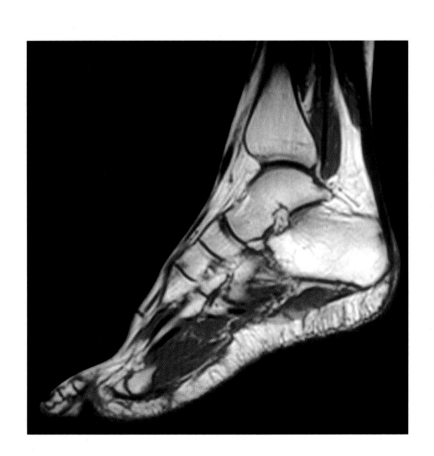
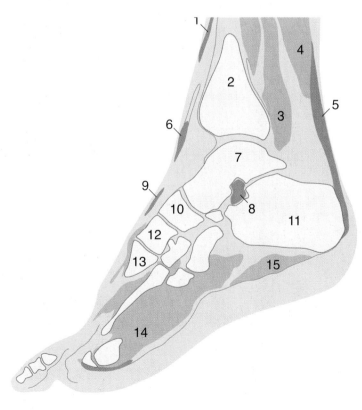

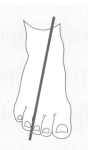

Sagittal MR of foot

1 - Tendon of extensor hallucis longus muscle
2 - Tibia
3 - Flexor hallucis longus muscle
4 - Tendon of extensor digitorum longus muscle
5 - Talus
6 - Interosseous talocalcanean ligament
7 - Calcaneus
8 - Navicular
9 - Extensor digitorum brevis muscle
10 - Intermediate cuneiform
11 - Lateral cuneiform
12 - Cuboid
13 - Long plantar ligament
14 - Metatarsal IV
15 - Abductor digiti minimi muscle
16 - Head of metatarsal V

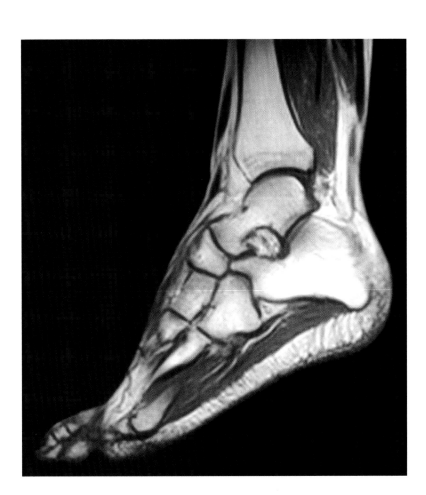

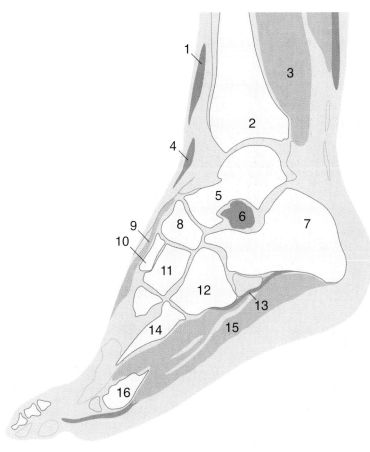

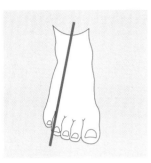

Sagittal MR of foot

1 - Tendon of extensor
hallucis longus
muscle
2 - Tibia
3 - Flexor hallucis
longus muscle
4 - Extensor digitorum
longus muscle
5 - Talus
6 - Navicular

7 - Interosseous
talocalcanean ligament
8 - Calcaneus
9 - Lateral cuneiform
10 - Cuboid
11 - Long plantar ligament
12 - Metatarsal IV
13 - Abductor digiti
minimi muscle
14 - Metatarsal V

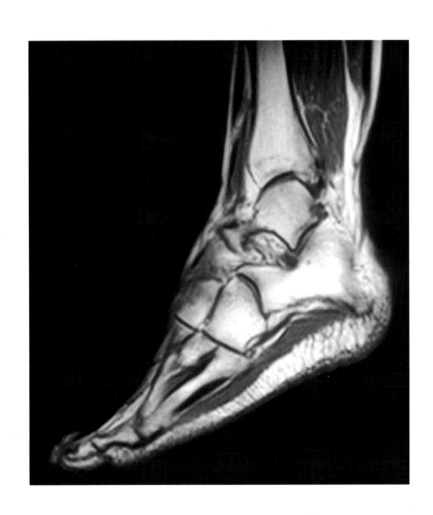

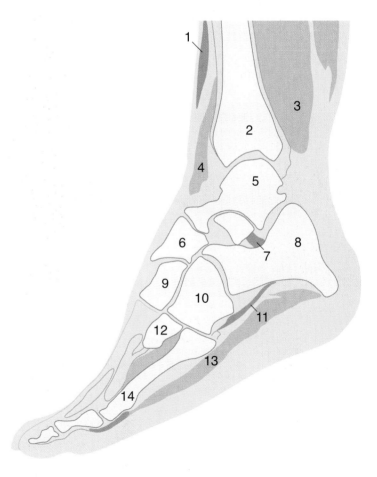

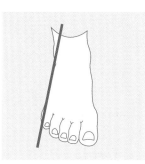

Sagittal MR of foot

1 - Extensor digitorum longus muscle
2 - Tibia
3 - Peroneus brevis and longus muscles
4 - Lateral malleolus of fibula
5 - Talus

6 - Tendon of peroneus brevis muscle
7 - Tendon of peroneus longus muscle
8 - Extensor digitorum brevis muscle
9 - Cuboid

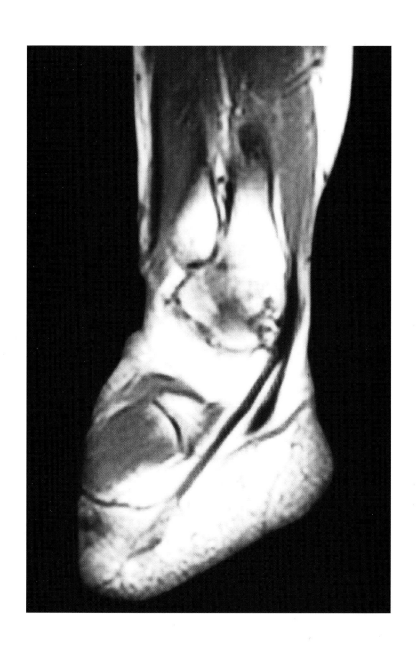

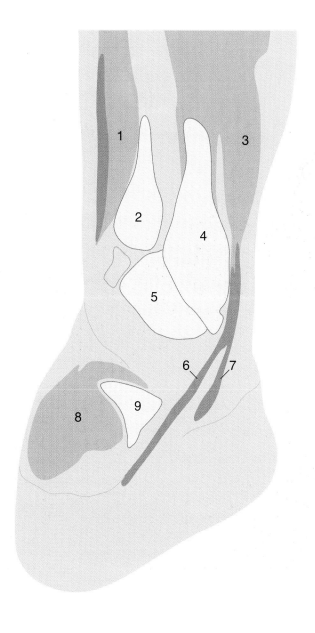

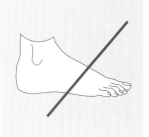

Coronal MR of foot

1 - Tendon of extensor hallucis longus muscle
2 - Metatarsal I
3 - Tendons of extensor digitorum longus muscle
4 - Plantar interosseous muscles
5 - Abductor hallucis and flexor hallucis brevis muscles (thenar eminence)
6 - Tendons of flexor digitorum longus muscle
7 - Shaft of metatarsal V
8 - Abductor digiti minimi muscle (hypothenar eminence)
9 - Plantar aponeurosis

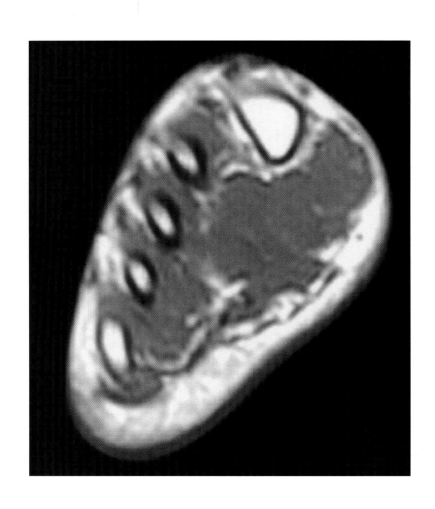

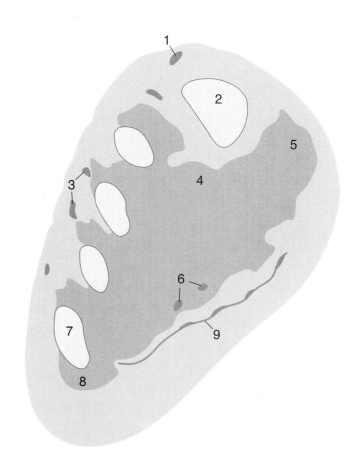

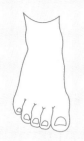

Arteriogram of foot

1 - Anterior tibial artery
2 - Posterior tibial artery
3 - Dorsalis pedis artery
4 - Calcanean branch of
   posterior tibial artery

5 - Medial plantar artery
6 - Lateral plantar artery
7 - Arcuate artery
8 - Dorsal metatarsal
   arteries

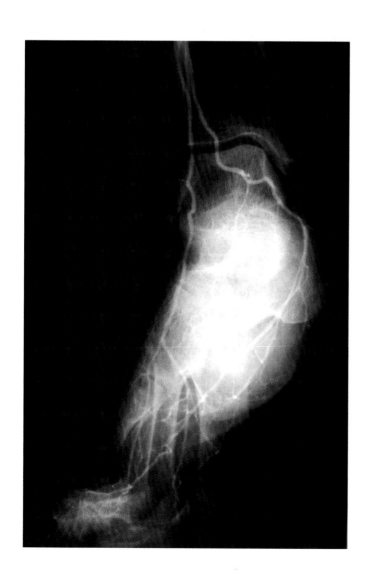

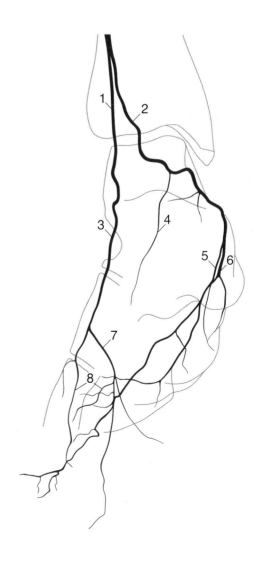

Subject Index